Synopsis of
Gynecologic Oncology

CLINICAL MONOGRAPHS IN OBSTETRICS AND GYNECOLOGY

E. J. QUILLIGAN, M.D., Editor
Chairman, Department of Obstetrics and Gynecology
University of Southern California School of Medicine
Los Angeles, California

Philip J. DiSaia, M.D., C. Paul Morrow, M.D., and Duane E. Townsend, M.D.,
Synopsis of Gynecologic Oncology

SYNOPSIS OF GYNECOLOGIC ONCOLOGY

PHILIP J. DISAIA, M.D.

C. PAUL MORROW, M.D.

DUANE E. TOWNSEND, M.D.

Los Angeles County/University of Southern California Medical Center
Women's Hospital
Department of Obstetrics and Gynecology
Section of Gynecologic Oncology
Los Angeles, California

This book was supported in part
by the generosity
of the
The Robert E. and May R. Wright Foundation
The University of Southern California School of Medicine

A WILEY BIOMEDICAL-HEALTH PUBLICATION

JOHN WILEY & SONS, New York · London · Sydney · Toronto

Library of Congress Cataloging in Publication Data:

DiSaia, Philip J   1937-
    Synopsis of gynecologic oncology.
    (Clinical monographs in obstertrics and gynecology) (A Wiley-biomedical health publication)
Includes bibliographies and index.
    1. Generative organs, Female--Cancer. I. Morrow, C. Paul, joint author. II. Townsend, Duane E., joint author.   III. Title.   IV. Series.
[DNLM: 1. Gynecologic neoplasms. WP145 D611s]
RC280. G5D48   616.9'94'65   74-34307
ISBN 0-471-21590-2

Printed in the United States of America
10 9 8 7 6

To

Jean, Linda, Barbara, Janis, Patti, Lydia, and Eleanor,
who labored in the completion of this work

Umit Tamer
whose artwork is used throughout this book

Series Preface

Just as a child has growth spurts, so do medicine and its specialties. For the past two decades the explosion of knowledge in obstetrics and gynecology has been truly astounding. These advances, the products of dedicated scientists and physicians, have enabled many patients to receive a quality of medical care unparalleled in United States history.

Unfortunately, the high level of medical care is not always available to every individual in the country. Among the reasons for the lack of availability are economics, uneven physician distribution, some would say a shortage of physicians, and ignorance. It is ignorance that should remain a totally unacceptable cause of inferior patient care. Changes in the examination procedure for specialty and subspecialty boards and the institution of recertification examinations would help to ensure adequate knowledge, though this insurance may be short-lived or minimal. Fundamentally, it is the physician himself who must see to his education.

I hope that this series of monographs on the current aspects of obstetrics and gynecology will assist the physicians who, despite heavy workloads, by rigid self-discipline maintain high standards of professional knowledge.

E. J. QUILLIGAN, M.D.

Los Angeles, California

Acknowledgments

This book began as a series of lectures to our students, residents, and fellows. Inevitably a written version of these lectures was assembled and distributed to our pupils for detailed study and review. In response to encouragement by students and colleagues and to an apparent absence of a similar publication, the working manual has been written to produce a comprehensive, clinically oriented review of pelvic cancer in women.

This product reflects not only the efforts of the authors but also the support and instruction of many others. Noteworthy among these are Edward J. Quilligan, M.D., Professor and Chairman of Department of Obstetrics and Gynecology, University of Southern California Medical School; Felix N. Rutledge, M.D., Gynecologist-in-Chief, The University of Texas, M. D. Anderson Hospital and Tumor Institute; Gilbert H. Fletcher, M.D., Head of Department of Radiotherapy, The University of Texas, M. D. Anderson Hospital and Tumor Institute; Daniel G. Morton, M.D., Professor and Chairman Emeritus, University of California at Los Angeles; Julian P. Smith, M.D., Associate Professor of Gynecology, The University of Texas, M. D. Anderson Hospital and Tumor Institute; John M. Morris, M.D., Ely Professor of Gynecology, Department of Obstetrics and Gynecology, Yale University School of Medicine; Charles J. Smith, M.D., Chairman of Department of Obstetrics and Gynecology, Mercy Hospital Medical Center; and James P. Nolan, M.D., Director of the Southern California Cancer Center in Los Angeles. To these great men we dedicate this book with gratitude.

PHILIP J. DISAIA, M.D.
C. PAUL MORROW, M.D.
DUANE E. TOWNSEND, M.D.

Los Angeles, California
October 1974

Contents

*Synopsis of
Gynecologic Oncology*

CHAPTER ONE

Staging and Classification

1-1   CLASSIFICATION AND STAGING OF
MALIGNANT TUMORS IN THE FEMALE PELVIS

The classification and staging of tumors in the female pelvis are considered not only by the Cancer Committee of the International Federation of Gynecology and Obstetrics (FIGO), but also by the International Union Against Cancer (UICC), especially its TNM Committee, by the Cancer Unit of the World Health Organization (WHO), by the Reference Centers of WHO for histopathological classification of ovarian tumors as well as of tumors in the uterus and the vagina, by the American Joint Committee, and finally by the International Congress of Radiology, especially its ICPR Committee. For several years opinions differed concerning the classification and staging of malignant tumors in the female pelvis. The Cancer Committee of FIGO has aimed at adjusting these opinions. It has been possible to reach international agreement on several main issues which are considered to be of great importance for research.

The TNM classification makes it possible to describe in detail the anatomical extent of the disease. If, however, used as the only method of classification, it will divide a series of treated cases into so many small groups that a statistical evaluation of the material is not possible. The Cancer Committee of FIGO stresses the importance of staging, and experience has shown that from a statistical, as well as from a prognostic point of view, it is advisable to group every type of malignant tumor into four stages.

Although the UICC adheres to the TNM classification, we wish to point out that there is, in principle, no important difference between the classification and staging adopted by the UICC and the one adopted by FIGO as far as carcinoma of the cervix uteri, carcinoma of the corpus uteri, and carcinoma of the vagina are concerned. The FIGO clinical

Reprinted from *Acta Obstet. Gynecol. Scand.* 50:1, 1971, and *Annual Report on Gynecological Cancer*, FIGO, Vol. 15, Sweden, 1973.

stage-grouping of carcinoma of the uterus and carcinoma of the vagina had already existed for many years when the proposals by the UICC were presented. Experience has shown that institutions in all countries of the world are using the FIGO clinical stage-grouping. The collaboration between the UICC and the Cancer Committee of FIGO is very important, and it is of value that the so-called TNM classifications of carcinoma of the uterus and carcinoma of the vagina follow the same lines as the clinical stage-grouping adopted by FIGO. In this respect, however, we have to remember that the stage-grouping is based exclusively on clinical examination.

1-2   GENERAL RULES (FIGO, JANUARY 1971) FOR CLINICAL CLASSIFICATION AND STAGING

Carcinoma of the Uterus and Vagina

Every case of carcinoma of the uterus and vagina should be classified and staged prior to definitive therapy.

Opinions differ as to which findings should serve as a basis for clinical classification and staging of carcinoma of the uterus and vagina. In order to obtain a correct and uniform classification and staging, the Cancer Committee considers it important that such examinations be used exclusively which can be carried out at any hospital by the physicians and surgeons. The following examinations fulfill this requirement: palpation, inspection, colposcopy, hysteroscopy, fractional curettage, roentgen examination of the lungs and skeleton, and, finally, intravenous urography. Some clinicians prefer to supplement their examination with lymphography, arteriography, venography, hysterography, laparoscopy, and so on. The Cancer Committee does not recommend these last mentioned examinations as a basis for staging. They may sometimes give information of importance, but it is evident that none of them is used as a routine. Furthermore, opinions differ among roentgenologists about the interpretation of findings observed by, for instance, lymphography, venography, or hysterography.

Carcinoma of the Cervix

Cases should be classified as carcinoma of the cervix if the primary growth is in the cervix. All histological types must be included.

The clinical staging of carcinoma of the cervix is based on palpation, inspection, colposcopy, endocervical curettage, roentgen examination of lungs and skeleton, and urography.

A conization or amputation of the cervix should be regarded as a clinical examination, and an invasive carcinoma of the cervix diagnosed in this way should be reported as invasive carcinoma.

In the past, cases of invasive carcinoma which were diagnosed only at the histological examination of the removed uterus were to be excluded from therapeutic statistics on invasive carcinoma. As the number of such cases is increasing, the Cancer Committee has seriously reconsidered this problem, and the Committee recommends that cases in which a microscopic focus is found in the removed uterus should be included among the Stage I cases.

The presence of a hydronephrosis or nonfunctioning kidney due to stenosis of the ureter by the cancer permits the allotment of a case to Stage III even if, according to the other findings, the case should be allotted to an earlier stage.

Subgrouping of Stage I

It is well known that opinions differ among pathologists concerning the criteria for early invasion of abnormal epithelium. The introduction of colposcopy and cytology into the clinical examination has increased the number of early carcinomas. The number of such cases at an institution will partly depend on the pathologist and his criteria for considering a case as invasive. Cases of early invasive carcinoma sometimes are treated in a different way than are cases of obviously invasive carcinoma. Therefore the Cancer Committee some years ago recommended a subdivision of the Stage I cases into Stage Ia—cases which cannot be diagnosed by clinical examination, and Stage Ib—all other cases of Stage I.

Stage Ia (microinvasive carcinoma) represents those cases of epithelial abnormalities in which histological evidence of early stromal invasion is unambiguous. The diagnosis is based on microscopical examination of tissue removed by biopsy, conisation, or portio amputation or of the removed uterus. Cases of early stromal invasion should thus be allotted to Stage Ia. The remainder of Stage I cases should be allotted to Stage Ib. As a rule these cases can be diagnosed by routine clinical examination.

Occult cancer is an evidently invasive cancer which cannot be diagnosed by routine clinical examination. They are as a rule diagnosed on a cone or on the amputated portio. They should be included in Stage Ib and should be marked "Stage Ib, occ".

Stage I cases can thus be indicated in the following ways:

Stage Ia   Carcinoma in situ with early stromal invasion diagnosed on tissue removed by biopsy, conisation, or portio amputation or on the removed uterus.

Stage Ib   Clinically invasive carcinoma confined to the cervix.

Stage Ib, occ Histologic invasive carcinoma of the cervix which could not be detected at routine clinical examination but which was diagnosed on a large biopsy, a cone or the amputated portio.

As a rule it is impossible clinically to estimate whether a cancer of the cervix has extended to the corpus or not. Extension to the corpus should therefore be disregarded.

Subgrouping of Stage II

Some years ago the Cancer Committee recommended a subgrouping of the Stage II cases into Stage IIa—no parametrial involvement, and Stage IIb—obvious parametrial involvement. This subgrouping has been widely used but was not officially approved by the General Assembly until its meeting in April 1970 in New York. The clinical staging is of importance not only to compare therapeutic results, but also to give information of value when planning therapy. Irrespective of the method of therapy applied, the treatment is different if the parametrium is obviously involved or not, and therefore the Cancer Committee recommends the following subgrouping:

Stage IIa The carcinoma involves the vagina but not the lower third. No obvious extension to the parametrium.

Stage IIb The carcinoma involves the vagina but not the lower third. Obvious extension to the parametrium, but not onto the pelvic wall.

Subgrouping of Stage III

For the same reasons as above, the Cancer Committee recommends a subgrouping of the Stage III cases along the same lines as for Stage II, that is:

Stage IIIa   The carcinoma involves the lower third of the vagina but has not extended onto the pelvic wall.

Stage IIIb   The carcinoma has extended onto the pelvic wall.

A patient with a growth to the pelvic wall by a short and indurated, but not nodular, parametrium should be allotted to Stage IIb. It is impossible at clinical examination to decide whether a smooth and indurated parametrium is truly cancerous or only inflammatory. Therefore, the case should be placed in Stage III only if the parametrium is nodular out on the pelvic wall or the growth itself extends out on the pelvic wall.

The presence of hydronephrosis or non-functioning kidney due to stenosis of the ureter by cancer permits a case to be allotted to Stage III even if according to the other findings the case should be allotted Stage I or Stage II.

Stage IV

The presence of a bullous edema as such should not permit a case to be allotted to Stage IV. Ridges and furrows into the bladder wall should be interpreted as signs of submucous involvement of the bladder if they remain fixed to the growth at palposcopy (i.e. examination from the vagina or the rectum during cystoscopy). A cytological finding of malignant cells in washings from the urinary bladder requires further examination and a biopsy from the wall of the bladder.

Definitions of the Different Clinical Stages in Carcinoma of the Cervix Uteri to Be Used From January 1, 1971

Preinvasive carcinoma
Stage 0   Carcinoma *in situ*, intraepithelial carcinoma. Cases of Stage 0 should not be included in any therapeutic statistics.

Invasive Carcinoma
Stage I   Carcinoma strictly confined to the cervix (extension to the corpus should be disregarded).
Stage Ia   Microinvasive carcinoma (early stromal invasion).
Stage Ib   All other cases of Stage I. Occult cancer should be marked "occ".
Stage II   The carcinoma extends beyond the cervix but has not extended onto the pelvic wall. The carcinoma involves the vagina, but not the lower third.
Stage IIa   No obvious parametrial involvement.
Stage IIb   Obvious parametrial involvement.
Stage III   The carcinoma has extended onto the pelvic wall. On rectal examination there is no cancer-free space between the tumor and the pelvic wall. The tumor involves the lower third of the vagina.
            All cases with a hydro-nephrosis or non-functioning kidney.

Stage IIIa No extension onto the pelvic wall.

Stage IIIb Extension onto the pelvic wall and/or hydro-nephrosis or non-functioning kidney.

Stage IV The carcinoma has extended beyond the true pelvis or has clinically involved the mucosa of the bladder or rectum. A bullous edema as such does not permit allotment of a case to Stage IV.

Stage IVa Spread of the growth to adjacent organs.

Stage IVb Spread to distant organs.

Carcinoma of the Corpus

A case should be classified as carcinoma of the corpus uteri when the primary site of the growth is in the corpus. Cases of mixed mesenchymal tumors and so-called carcinosarcoma should be excluded.

Stage 0 Carcinoma *in situ*. Histological findings suspicious of malignancy.
Cases of Stage 0 should not be included in any therapeutic statistics.

Stage I The carcinoma is confined to the corpus.

The great majority of cases of carcinoma of the corpus will be allotted to Stage I. The factors which decide the prognosis in carcinoma of the corpus Stage I are (1) the age and the general condition of the patient, (2) the size of the uterine cavity, and (3) the histological pattern.

Several years ago the Annual Report on the Results of Treatment in Carcinoma of the Uterus recommended a subdivision of the Stage I cases with regard to operability. Patients of old age and patients suffering from extragenital disease were considered as poor operative risks. Experience has obviously shown that no absolute criteria can be given for "poor operative risk." Such a judgment depends on the ability and skill of the surgeon. The Cancer Committee of FIGO considers a subdivision with regard to operability of limited value. We will not deny, however, that, especially in presentations of therapeutic results in carcinoma of the corpus, it is of value to know the number of patients suffering from serious extragenital disease, as for instance nephrocardiovascular disabilities, and the number of patients of 70 or 80 years of age, respectively.

Studies of large series of endometrial carcinoma limited to the corpus have shown that the prognosis to some extent is related to the size of the uterus. However, enlargement of the uterus may be caused by fibroids, adenomyosis, and so on. Therefore the size of the uterus cannot serve as a basis for subgrouping Stage I cases. The length of the uterine cavity, however, measured with a sound from the external os, may give information of value for therapy. The Cancer Committee recommends a subdivision of the Stage I cases with regard to the length of the sound. Cases with a sound of 8 cm or less should be allotted to Stage Ia, and cases with a sound of more than 8 cm to Stage Ib.

The histopathology as such should not serve as a basis for clinical stage-grouping. Experience, however, has demonstrated that highly differentiated adenocarcinomas, frequently with papillary structures, as well as differentiated carcinomas with partly solid areas, have a tendency to grow exophytically in the uterine cavity, while predominantly solid and entirely undifferentiated anaplastic tumors frequently tend to deeply invade the myometrium at an early stage of development. Thus, these last mentioned tumors are more malignant, and experience has shown that they have a worse prognosis than the differentiated ones. A subdivision of the Stage I cases with regard to the histological structures will facilitate the interpretation of a series of carcinomas of the corpus Stage I. Therefore, the Cancer Committee recommends *a subdivision of the Stage I cases into:*

G1   Highly differentiated adenomatous carcinomas.
G2   Differentiated adenomatous carcinomas with partly solid areas.
G3   Predominantly solid or entirely undifferentiated carcinomas.

Stage II   The carcinoma has involved the corpus and the cervix.
As far as prognosis and therapy are concerned, it is important to know whether the cancer has extended to the cervix. The extension of the carcinoma to the endocervix is confirmed by fractional curettage or hysteroscopy. The scraping of the cervix should be the first step of the curettage, and the specimens from the cervix should be examined separately. Occasionally it may be difficult to decide whether the endocervix is involved by the cancer or not. In such cases the simultaneous presence of normal cervical glands and cancer in the same piece will give the final diagnosis. In questionable cases the histological examination of the curettage should decide whether the origin of the cancer is in the corpus or in the cervix. If a clear decision cannot be made, an adenocarcinoma should be allotted to carcinoma of the corpus and an epidermal carcinoma to carcinoma of the cervix.

Stage III and Stage IV   Extension of the carcinoma outside the uterus should refer a case to Stage III or Stage IV. The presence of metastases in the vagina permits, as such, allotment of a case to Stage III.

Every gynecologist and pathologist knows that there are cases in which it is clinically as well as histologically impossible to decide whether the cancer primarily is a cancer of the corpus uteri or a cancer of the ovary. Previously such cases were diagnosed as carcinoma uteri et ovarii, but this is not adequate. As a rule it is possible from the history of the patient and from the clinical examination to decide which tumor is likely to be the primary one. In rare cases this may, however, be impossible. Such rare cases should be included in the statistics on carcinoma of the corpus as well as in the statistics on ovarian cancer. They should be reported separately.

Definitions of the Different Clinical Stages of Carcinoma
of the Corpus Uteri to Be Used From January 1, 1971

Stage 0   Carcinoma *in situ*. Histological finding suspicious of malignancy.
                Cases of Stage 0 should not be included in any therapeutic statistics.
Stage I   The carcinoma is confined to the corpus.
Stage Ia   The length of the uterine cavity is 8 cm or less.
Stage Ib   The length of the uterine cavity is more than 8 cm.

The Stage I cases should be subgrouped with regard to the histological type of the adenocarcinoma as follows:

G1   Highly differentiated adenomatous carcinomas.
G2   Differentiated adenomatous carcinomas with partly solid areas.
G3   Predominantly solid or entirely undifferentiated carcinomas.

Stage II   The carcinoma has involved the corpus and the cervis.
Stage III   The carcinoma has extended outside the uterus but not outside the true pelvis.
Stage IV   The carcinoma has extended outside the true pelvis or has obviously involved the mucosa of the bladder or rectum. A bullous edema as such does not permit allotment of a case to Stage IV.

Carcinoma of the Vagina

Cases should be classified as carcinoma of the vagina when the primary site of the growth is in the vagina. Tumors presenting in the vagina as secondary growths from either genital or extragenital sites should be excluded from registration.

A growth that has extended to the portio and reached the area of the external os should always be allotted to carcinoma of the cervix.

A growth that has extended to the vulva should be classified as a carcinoma of the vulva.

A growth that is limited to the urethra should be classified as a carcinoma of the urethra.

*Definitions of the Different Clinical Stages in Carcinoma of the
Vagina to be Used from January 1, 1962*

Preinvasive carcinoma
Stage 0   Carcinoma *in situ*, intraepithelial carcinoma.

Invasive carcinoma
Stage I   The carcinoma is limited to the vaginal wall.
Stage II   The carcinoma has involved the subvaginal tissue but has not extended onto the pelvic wall.
Stage III   The carcinoma has extended onto the pelvic wall.
Stage IV   The carcinoma has extended beyond the true pelvis or has involved the mucosa of the bladder or rectum. A bullous edema as such does not permit allotment of a case to Stage IV.

Carcinoma of the Vulva

Cases should be classified as carcinoma of the vulva when the primary site of the growth is in the vulva. Tumors present in the vulva as secondary growths from either a genital or extragenital site should be excluded from registration, as should cases of malignant melanoma (see also "Carcinoma of the Vagina").

Many attempts have been made to classify and stage carcinoma of the vulva (Simon, 1932; Taussig, 1940; Berven, 1961; Cosbie, 1951), but none of the proposals has been internationally accepted.

Carcinoma of the vulva tends to give metastases primarily to the inguinal nodes. Only exceptionally the primary site of metastases from a carcinoma of the vulva is in the deep pelvic lymph nodes. Therefore the TNM classification is well suited for this tumor. In 1967 the TNM Committee of the UICC proposed a classification for carcinoma of the vulva. The Cancer Committee of FIGO has expressed some criticism of the UICC proposal.

The Cancer Committee of FIGO wishes to express its sincere thanks to Mr. Stanley Way, Newcastle; Dr. Howard Ulfelder, Boston; Dr. Malcolm Stening, Sydney; and Dr. Folke Edsmyr, Stockholm; for their detailed investigation of the series of carcinoma of the vulva. It is important to point out that, in principle, the four colleagues came to the same conclusions. At the congress in Sydney the Cancer Committee discussed some minor differences in the recommendations presented by the above mentioned colleagues.

At the Radiumhemmet, a series of 721 cases of primary invasive epidermoid cancer of the vulva treated by primary surgery has been investigated by Edsmyr and Kottmeier. In April 1971 the General Assembly of FIGO approved a TNM classification and a stage-grouping of carcinoma of the vulva proposed by the Cancer Committee. The FIGO classification differs to some extent from the UICC proposal.

TNM Classification and Clinical Staging of Carcinoma of the Vulva
Adopted in 1970, to be used from January 1, 1971

T   Primary tumor
T1   Tumor confined to the vulva—2 cm or less in larger diameter.
T2   Tumor confined to the vulva—more than 2 cm in diameter.
T3   Tumor of any size with adjacent spread to the urethra and/or vagina and/or perineum and/or anus.
T4   Tumor of any size infiltrating the bladder mucosa and/or the rectum mucosa or both, including the upper part of the urethra mucosa, and/or fixed to the bone.

N   Regional lymph nodes
NO   No nodes palpable.
N1   Nodes palpable in either groin, not enlarged, mobile (not clinically suspicious of neoplasm).
N2   Nodes palpable in either groin or both groins, enlarged, firm and mobile (clinically suspicious of neoplasm).
N3   Fixed or ulcerated nodes.

M   Distant metastases
M0   No clinical metastases.
M1a   Palpable deep pelvic lymph nodes.
M1b   Other distant metastases.

Clinical Stage Groups

Stage I	T1 N0 M0	Stage IV	T1 N3 M0
	T1 N1 M0		T2 N3 M0
			T3 N3 M0
Stage II	T2 N0 M0		T4 N3 M0
	T2 N1 M0		T4 N0 M0
			T4 N1 M0
Stage III	T3N0 M0		T4 N2 M0
	T3 N1 M0		
	T3 N2 M0		All other conditions
	T1 N2 M0		containing Mla orMlb.
	T2 N2 M0		

If cytology or histology of lymph nodes reveals malignant cells, the symbol + (plus) should be added to N. If such examinations do not reveal malignant cells, the symbol - (minus) should be added to N.

Carcinoma of the Urethra

Cases should be classified as carcinoma of the urethra when it is evident that the primary site of the growth is in the urethra.

It is important to separate cases of carcinoma at the external urethral os from cases originating deeper in the urethra. In 1969 the TNM Committee of the UICC proposed a TNM classification of carcinoma of the urethra in women. For the present, the Cancer Committee of FIGO has not proposed a stage-grouping for carcinoma of the urethra.

Carcinoma of the Ovary

Ovarian carcinoma is a common malignant tumor. It cannot be regarded as an entity. Therapeutic statistics on ovarian cancer are of limited value if attention is not paid to the histological type of the growth. Experience has shown that there is no clear correlation between clinical and histological malignancy in ovarian tumors. This holds valid for various types of neoplasms, but especially for epithelial tumors, granulosa cell tumors, and virilizing tumors.

The Cancer Unit of WHO has set up a special Reference Center for histopathological classification of various ovarian tumors. The Cancer Committee of FIGO is pleased to have a close collaboration with this Reference Center.

In 1961 the Cancer Committee of FIGO proposed a histopathological classification of the common primary epithelial ovarian tumors. This proposal has been slightly modified. The Reference Center of WHO has not yet presented its final recommendations, but it is important to know that, in principle, the Reference Center and FIGO are working along the same lines.

Histopathological Classification of Ovarian Tumors

Cases of germ cell tumors, hormone-producing neoplasia, and metastatic carcinomas should be excluded from therapeutic statistics on ovarian epithelial tumors.

Histological Classification of the Common Primary Epithelial
Tumors of the Ovary to be Used from January 1, 1971.

I. Serous Cystomas
    a. Serous benign cystadenomas
    b. Serous cystadenomas with proliferating activity of the epithelial cells and nuclear abnormalities but with no infiltrative destructive growth (low potential malignancy)
    c. Serous cystadenocarcinomas

II. Mucinous Cystomas
    a. Mucinous benign cystadenomas
    b. Mucinous cystadenomas with proliferating activity of the epithelial cells and nuclear abnormalities but with no infiltrative destructive growth (low potential malignancy)
    c. Mucinous cystadenocarcinomas

III. Endometrioid Tumors (similar to adenocarcinomas in the endometrium)
    a. Endometrioid tumors
    b. Endometrioid tumors with proliferating activity of the epithelial cells and nuclear abnormalities but with no infiltrative destructive growth (low potential malignancy)
    c. Endometrioid adenocarcinomas

IV. Mesonephric Tumors
    a. Benign mesonephric tumors
    b. Mesonephric tumors with proliferating activity of the epithelial cells and nuclear abnormalities but with no infiltrative destructive growth (low potential malignancy)
    c. Mesonephric cystadenocarcinomas

Concomitant carcinoma, unclassified carcinoma (tumors which cannot be allotted to one of the groups I, II, III, or IV)

It has been proposed that cases which according to the above classification are tumors of low potential malignancy, that is, Ib, IIB, IIIb, and IVb, should be called borderline cases. The Cancer Committee of FIGO cannot accept this term, especially as histologically unquestionably benign tumors of papillary nature may give rise to implantation of metastases which spontaneously disappear after removal of the primary growth. Such tumors should not be included among cases of Ib, IIb, IIIb, or IVb. The Cancer Committee is aware of the fact that ovarian neoplasms alotted to the group "low potential malignancy" may be of different biological behavior. At present there is, however, no method to subdivide these cases.

For ovarian tumors it is desirable to have a clinical stage-grouping like those in the other malignant tumors in the female pelvis. Sometimes it is impossible to come to a final diagnosis by inspection or palpation or by any of the other methods recommended for clinical staging of carcinoma of the uterus and vagina. Therefore, the Cancer Committee of FIGO has recommended that this clinical staging of ovarian cancer should be based on clinical examination as well as on findings at laparotomy. In some cases of malignant tumor in the pelvis or abdomen, the condition of the patient does not permit explorative laparotomy, and thus they cannot be clinically staged in detail. For the presentation of therapeutic results it is necessary, however, to receive information concerning the number of such patients who are thought to have an ovarian malignant tumor. They should be reported in the group "Special Category." In 1964 the General Assembly of FIGO approved a stage-grouping of ovarian carcinoma based on findings at clinical examination and laparotomy. In 1966 the TNM Committee of th UICC proposed a TNM classification of ovarian cancer. This classification is not based, however, on studies of a large consecutive series of cases. It was under trial in the years 1967-1971.

Since 1964 the Cancer Committee of FIGO has investigated several series of ovarian cancer. The therapy and prognosis in ovarian carcinoma are to a great extent dependent on the anatomical extent of the growth and on the penetration of the ovarian capsule by the tumor. Opinions still differ whether the presence of ascites as such will have an influence on the final outcome. On the basis of the studies carried out, the Cancer Committee in 1970 recommended a definitive stage-grouping of ovarian cancer as follows:

Stage-Grouping for Primary Carcinoma of the Ovary

Based on findings at clinical examination and surgical exploration. The final histology (and cytology when required) after surgery is to be considered in the staging.

Stage I   Growth limited to the ovaries
Stage Ia   Growth limited to *one* ovary; no ascites
             (i)   No tumor on the external surface; capsule intact
             (ii) Tumor present on the external surface or/and capsule ruptured
Stage Ib   Growth limited to *both* ovaries; no ascites
             (i)   No tumor on the external surface; capsule intact
             (ii) Tumor present on the external surface or/and capsule(s) ruptured
Stage Ic   Tumor either Stage Ia or Stage Ib, but with ascites* present or positive peri-
             toneal washings
Stage II   Growth involving one or both ovaries with pelvic extension.
Stage IIa   Extension and/or metastases to the uterus and/or tubes.
Stage IIb   Extension to other pelvic tissues.
Stage IIc   Tumor either Stage IIa or Stage IIb, but with ascites* present or positive peri-
             toneal washings
Stage III   Growth involving one or both ovaries with intraperitoneal metastases outside
             the pelvis and/or positive retroperitoneal nodes. Tumor limited to the true
             pelvis with histologically proven malignant extension to small bowel or
             omentum.

---

*Ascites is peritoneal effusion which in the opinion of the surgeon is pathological or/and clearly exceeds normal amounts.

Stage IV   Growth involving one or both ovaries with distant metastases. If pleural effu-
             sion is present there must be positive cytology to allot a case to Stage IV.
             Parenchymal liver metastases equals Stage IV.

Special category. Unexplored cases which are thought to be ovarian carcinoma.

The foregoing rules on the classification and staging of malignant tumors in the female
pelvis were accepted by the General Assembly of FIGO in New York on April 12, 1970.
(Modified October 1974-Information contributed by Dr. Howard Ulfelder.)

CHAPTER TWO

Cancer
of the Cervix

2-1 PREINVASIVE CARCINOMA OF THE CERVIX

Within the past two decades, there has been a great deal of new information regarding the nature, diagnosis, and treatment of precancerous lesions of the uterine cervix. These studies have advanced the understanding of this disease, permitting a more sophisticated approach to its management. Such lesions are generally called dysplasia and, later, carcinoma *in situ* (Fig. 2-1). For the convenience of this review, these surface squamous epithelial lesions will be collectively termed cervical intraepithelial neoplasia (CIN). When necessary, the specific lesions will be mentioned for clarification. Although similar adenomatous lesions can rarely occur in the endocervical glands (Fig. 2-2), our discussion is directed to the squamous epithelium on the portio of the cervix.

Etiology

The etiologic agent or agents responsible for the genesis of CIN as well as of invasive cervical carcinoma are unknown. However, it has been conclusively demonstrated that for a woman to develop a squamous cell cancer of the uterine cervix, sexual intercourse must take place. On the other hand, adenocarcinoma of the cervix, which accounts for approximately 5% of cervical neoplasms, can arise in virgins. Herpes virus Type II is suspect as an etiologic agent for cervical neoplasms. Studies regarding herpes virus are inconclusive and in some cases contradictory. Investigators from Australia have suggested that sperm may even be an inciting agent. In any event, it can be stated that cervical neoplasia is a venereal disease, that is, a disease transmitted by sexual intercourse.

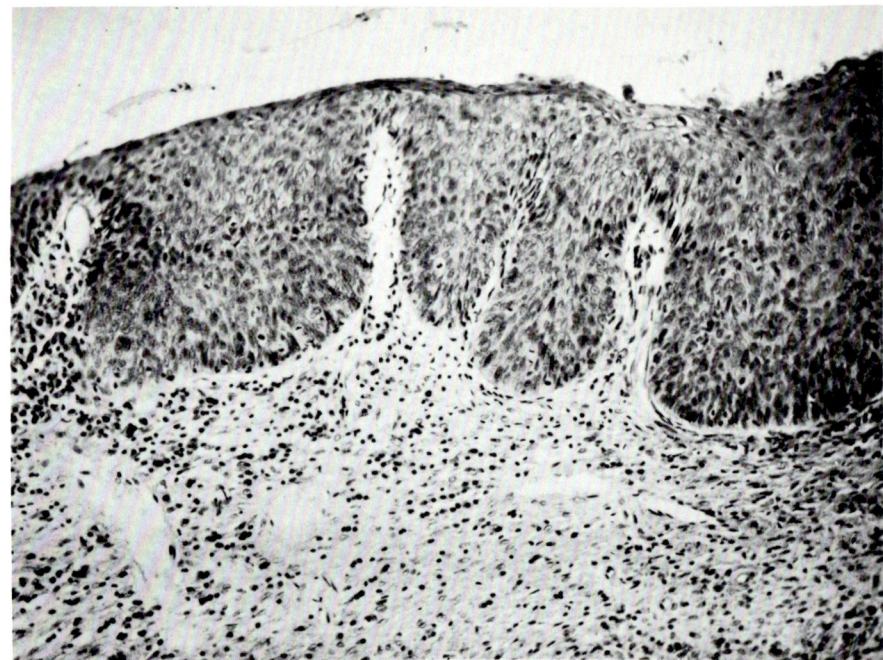

Fig. 2-1 Photomicrograph (150X) of carcinoma-*in-situ* of the cervix. Note complete loss of cellular polarity; all layers are pleomorphic.

Developmental Concepts

Prospective studies strongly suggest that cervical neoplasia is a spectrum of disease beginning as an early superficial lesion called dysplasia, which, if all conditions are favorable, will gradually progress to invasive carcinoma. Unfortunately, histopathologic studies of CIN cannot predict which lesion has a truly invasive potential. Although in the past some investigators tended to disregard the early forms of CIN (mild and moderate dysplasia), it is now the consensus that 10-15% of these will progress to invasive cancer if not treated.

The length of time necessary for the advanced forms of CIN (i.e., severe dysplasia and carcinoma *in situ*) to progress to invasive squamous cell carcinoma varies from 3 to 20 years. Studies by Kottmeier (Koss 1969) suggest that the most advanced forms of CIN will eventually progress to invasive cancer in 75% of the cases.

Because of our inability to predict which CIN has a true malignant potential, the treatment for these lesions has been haphazard and often quite radical.

Detection of CIN

The best detection technique for CIN is cytology. The generally accepted false-negative rate for the Papanicolaou test is between 10 and 20%. Poor sampling accounts for the greatest number of these errors. The best method for cervical sampling is an os aspiration coupled with an exocervical scrape. The vaginal pool technique that has been in vogue for

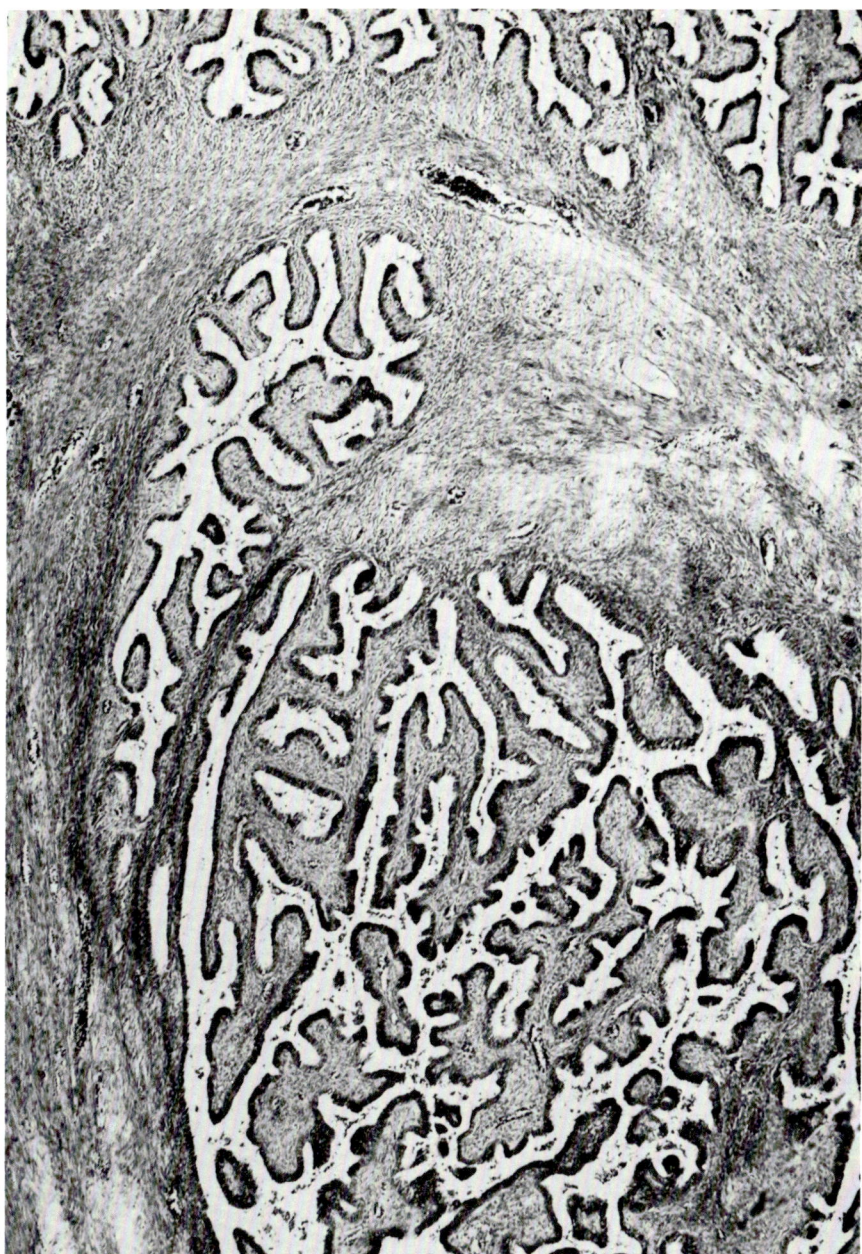

Fig. 2-2 Carcinoma *in situ* of the endocervix, discovered post-hysterectomy in an asymptomatic patient.

so many years has a false-negative rate of 40% and should no longer be employed. Self irrigation techniques are being promoted, but they have a false-negative rate of at least 20%. The self-irrigation method is applicable only in areas that lack adequate personnel to carry out proper cancer detection examinations.

Evaluation of CIN

Cytology may be the best method to detect CIN, but it is inadequate in the evaluation of this disease. Random cervical biopsy, invariably followed by conization of the cervix, has been the time honored means to evaluate the patient with an abnormal Pap test, that is, Class III or worse (dysplasia or worse). However, as the younger population is being screened by cytology, it is becoming evident that CIN begins in the late teens and early twenties. When conization is employed in these young individuals, the hazards and expenses of surgery and hospitalization are significant.

Colposcopy, a technique developed almost 50 years ago in Europe, is gaining recognition as the ideal means for evaluating a patient with an abnormal Pap test. Although cytology is highly accurate in predicting the probable nature of the CIN, it cannot determine its extent or location. On the other hand, coloposcopy, an office technique, can easily determine the location and extent of 90% of CIN lesions, eliminating the need for *diagnostic* conization in these cases.

Colposcopy emphasizes the transformation zone. In simplest terms, the transformation zone is the portion of the uterine cervix that at one time was covered by *columnar epithelium* which, through a process of *metaplasia*, has been *transformed* into *squamous epithelium*. Contrary to many beliefs, the exocervix is frequently covered by columnar epithelium, particularly in the teenage years. However, as a woman begins to menstruate there occur changes in the hormone balance as well as the vaginal pH which in turn promote a change from columnar to squamous epithelium.

Columnar epithelium on the exocervix appears red to the naked eye. The redness is due to the fact that only a single cell layer is covering the highly vascular cervical stroma. It is not surprising, therefore, that in the past physicians who saw this red area on the cervix thought that it represented an area of infection or erosion; hence, the terms *cervicitis* or *erosion* are often used to describe the "red" cervix. Colposcopically, columnar epithelium has a classic grapelike appearance and is easily discernible.

Columnar epithelium exists on the exocervix in well over half the female population during the adolescent and teenage years. At puberty, the metaplastic process accelerates, probably because of the hormonal changes and acidification of the vagina. It is postulated that during the active phases of metaplasia CIN begins. Metaplasia occurs throughout a woman's life but has been shown to be particulary dynamic during the teenage years. If an individual is sexually active during the periods of highly active metaplasia, there is a greater chance for CIN to develop.

Cervical intraepithelial neoplasia develops within the transformation zone invariably at the squamocolumnar junction. It probably begins as a small focal area that increases in size. The lesions stay superficial for many, many years, but some will eventually develop into invasive carcinoma. Since the lesions can be easily located by colposcopy, they can be biopsied and evaluated. In over 90% of women with a Pap test suggestive of CIN, colposcopy coupled with directed biopsy can easily exclude the presence of invasive carcinoma without the need for hospitalization or the expenses and hazards of conization. The physician can then offer the patient a variety of treatment techniques.

The colposcopic examination is similar to a regular gynecologic examination except that one introduces magnification of from 10 to 20 times and thus can more adequately evaluate the cervix. A cleansing solution, usually 3% acetic acid, is employed just before the colposcopic examination to dissolve mucus. The acetic acid also accentuates the colposcopic findings. The standard colposcopic examination is as follows:

1. Repeat cytology.
2. Carry out gross examination.
   a. Clean the cervix with acetic acid.
   b. Perform colposcopy.
3. Stain cervix with Lugol's solution (Schiller test).
4. Perform endocervical curettage if limits of lesion are not seen (not performed in pregnant patients).
5. Take colposcopically directed punch biopsies of suspicious lesions.

The entire examination procedure takes 5-10 minutes. Colposcopy itself requires 2 or 3 minutes during the examination process.

Depending on the result of the biopsies, one can triage the patient into one of various categories, thereby providing several treatment plans (Fig. 2-3). Generally, one can divide patients into two major categories, based on ability or inability to see the limits of the lesion.

Management

Entire Limits of Lesion Seen

If the entire limits of the lesion and the squamocolumnar junction are visible, it is only necessary to take one to three biopsies of the most colposcopically abnormal appearing area. Endocervical curettage (ECC) is not necessary in these patients, since there will not be disease beyond the upper extension of the lesion. Nevertheless, ECC has been

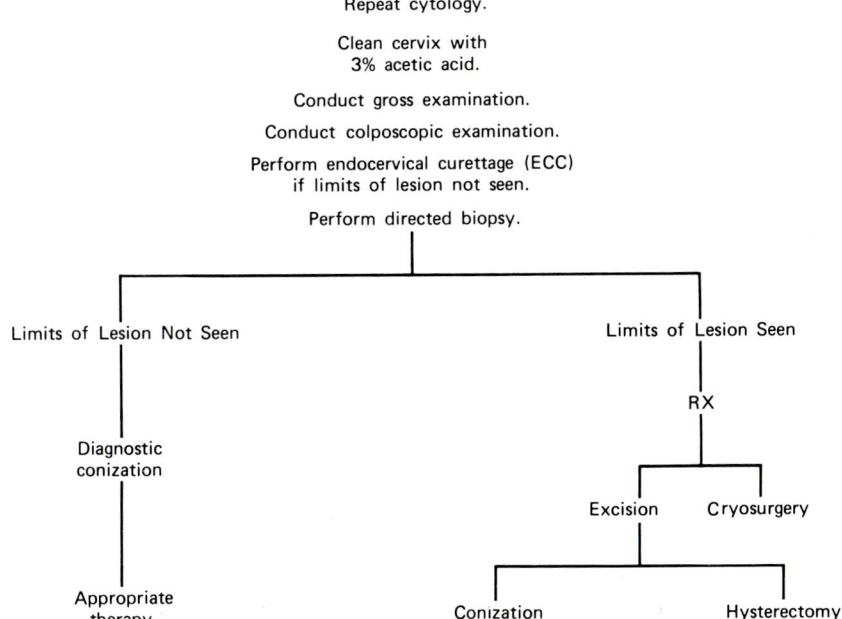

Fig. 2-3 Management of the abnormal Pap test.

performed almost routinely in our program for several reasons. First, it permits an expedient grouping of patients into two major categories based on the presence or absence of neoplastic disease in the endocervical curettings. Second, the multifocal concept of cervical neoplasia is an unproved entity and needs to be substantiated or refuted. Third, early asymptomatic cytologically negative adenocarcinoma may be revealed by routine ECC. Fourth, patients with a negative ECC have rarely (i.e., 1:500) been found to have invasive cancer.

After the patients are evaluated and informed of their disease status several treatment techniques can be used. Outpatient methods include excision biopsy, cryosurgery, and hot cautery. Excision biopsy is used when lesions are 1 cm or less in size. Once the lesion is totally removed, patients are seen every 3 months for 1 year and then every 6 months thereafter. Larger lesions are treated by cryosurgery.

Surgical treatment is performed in a minority of patients when CIN is colposcopically visible. Therapeutic conization is used for individuals who refuse outpatient therapy or are considered poor follow-up risks.

Hysterectomy is restricted to patients who desire sterilization by this means or have some other gynecologic problem such as pelvic relaxation, uterine myoma, chronic salpingitis, or adenomyosis. A simple vaginal or abdominal hysterectomy is sufficient. Only when neoplastic disease extends onto the vagina (<5% of the time) is a vaginal cuff necessary.

Entire Limits of Lesion Not Seen

In about 10% of patients with an abnormal Pap test the lesion will extend well into the endocervical canal or will be present solely within the canal. In these patients a firm and vigorous ECC should be carried out since invasive cancer may be diagnosed by canal sampling. Patients in whom there is evidence only of CIN must undergo diagnostic conization. Depending on the results of the conization, further treatment may be necessary.

If frankly invasive cancer is found, radical surgery or irradiation is undertaken. When microinvasive cancer is present, a simple hysterectomy is sufficient. (See page 40)

If only CIN is present and the conization has cleared the lesion, treatment has been completed. On the other hand, if the cone biopsy has not cleared the lesion, either repeat conization or hysterectomy must be employed. In properly performed conization this should occur in no more than 5-10% of instances.

Cervical Conization

Conization of the cervix has two indications — diagnostic and therapeutic. In some cases — however, a diagnostic conization becomes therapeutic, particularly in the young individual.

The technique of conization, as well as the amount of tissue excised, depends on the indications for the procedure and the extent of the disease. For example, if a patient is to have a diagnostic conization followed by hysterectomy, the amount of tissue excised will depend on the answers to two questions: (1) has colposcopy been carried out for ectocervical disease, and (2) how much disease is present within the endocervical canal? If colposcopy has not been performed, it is necessary to excise all Schiller positive or iodine negative tissue on the ectocervix and as much of the endocervical canal as possible. On the other hand, if colposcopy has been performed and invasive cancer has been excluded on the ectocervix, only the canal need be sampled for proper diagnosis (Fig 2-4). When hysterectomy is carried out, however, it is important that all remaining abnormal epithelium on the ectocervix be excised. A vaginal cuff is necessary only when the disease extends onto the vagina.

If conization is to be used as a therapeutic technique, the area of the cervix that harbors the abnormal epithelium must be excised. When the disease is only on the ectocervix, only ectocervical epithelium need be removed and the canal may be ignored (Fig. 2-5). On the other hand, if there is disease on the ectocervix and in the canal, then all ectocervical disease and as much canal as necessary must be removed (Fig. 2-6). In some instances, usually in older patients, only the canal harbors disease. In these cases the conization is long and narrow (Fig. 2-7).

Although the technique of conization appears simple, it is proving to be one of the more difficult and hazardous procedures in gynecology. We have utilized all of the various methods and strategems to reduce the complication rate of conization without any significant impact.

The patient should be hospitalized and given general anesthesia. The vagina is then thoroughly prepped. We are not concerned with the problem of disturbing the ectocervical epithelium, since we already know what type of neoplasia is present on the cervix. Next the cervix is fully visualized with retractors, and Lugol's solution is

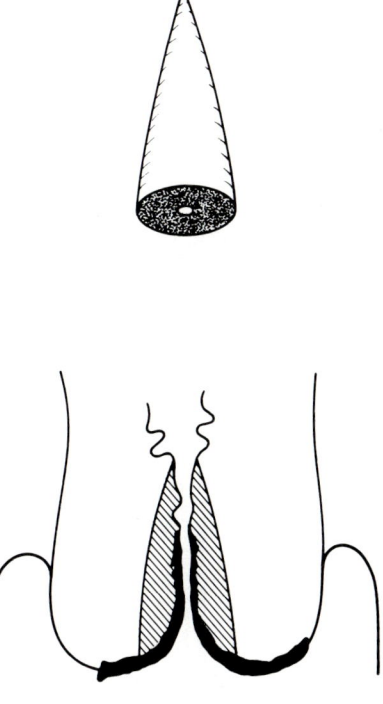

Fig. 2-4 Diagnostic conization, to be followed by hysterectomy. Disease on ectocervix and in canal; colposcopy has excluded invasive cancer on ectocervix.

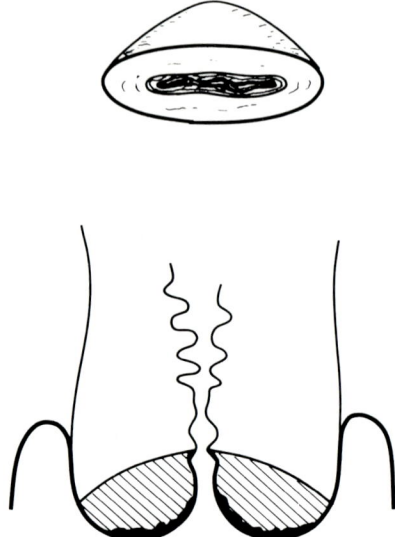

Fig. 2-5   Therapeutic conization: disease confined to ectocervix.

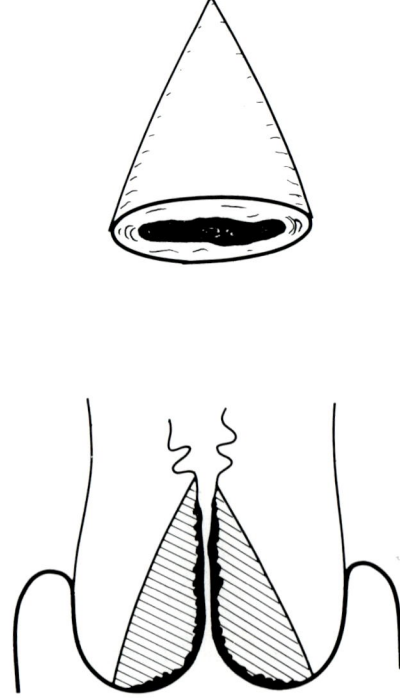

Fig. 2-6   Therapeutic conization: disease on ectocervix and in endocervical canal.

20

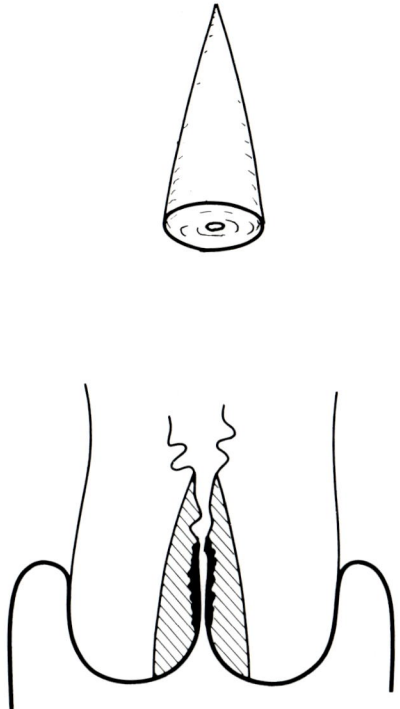

Fig. 2-7 Diagnostic conization: disease confined to endocervical canal.

literally poured into the vagina. The extent of Schiller positive or iodine negative tissue is correlated with the colposcopic picture if colposcopy has been performed. If colposcopy has not been performed, it is mandatory that iodine staining be carried out immediately before the conization. The anterior and posterior lips of the cervix are grasped with a tenaculum and brought toward the introitus. Hemostatic sutures are placed at 3 and 9 o'clock. (We often place them after the conization has been performed.) These sutures are usually located about 1½-2 cm superior to the extermal os. With a No. 15 scalpel blade, an incision 1-3 mm deep is made, defining the limits of the ectocervical incision. In a therapeutic conization, all non-iodine-staining tissue or colposcopic abnormal epithelium must be removed. If the conization is to be diagnostic, a hysterectomy is planned, and colposcopy has been performed, it is not necessary to excise all the iodine negative tissue on the ectocervix. (When the hysterectomy is subsequently performed, however, all abnormal epithelium must be removed.) The incision is then carried 2-3 mm deeper, and the scalpel is directed toward the endocervical canal. This should reduce the chance of perforation or transection of a cervical branch of the uterine artery. This tapering is continued as the conization is extended further up the cervix. If the endocervical canal is entered during the conization, one must return to this point and reexcise any endocervical gland tissue that was missed, particularly if neoplastic tissue is present in the canal. The incision is continued superiorly and is completed with either a scalpel or scissors. When incising with the scalpel, one should carve rather than saw the tissue. When the scalpel is used in a sawing fashion, control is poorer and complications are increased.

After the cone specimen has been removed, the endometrial cavity and any remaining portions of the endocervix are separately curetted. Sturmdorf sutures are placed at 12 and 6 o'clock. The pathology report is available in 24 hours*; if hysterectomy or other major therapeutic measures are planned or prove necessary, they are initiated at this time. On the other hand, if conization is therapeutic, the patient is informed of the results of the cone and is usually discharged 1 or 2 days post-operatively. Frozen section conizations have been used in some institutions with a high degree of success.

Whenever hysterectomy is performed 24 hours after conization, prophylactic antibiotics should be used to reduce infectious morbidity. If repeat conization is required, it is not carried out for 6-8 weeks to permit the cone bed to heal.

When the conization is therapeutic, regular sounding of the cervix should be done in order to lessen the chance of stenosis. This is begun as soon as the cervix heals (i.e., 6-8 weeks) and is done every 3-6 months.

Cryosurgery for Dysplasia and Carcinoma in Situ

Before performing cryosurgery, a careful gynecologic history is taken. Emphasis is placed on intermenstrual bleeding, menorrhagia, quality and character of discharge, salpingitis, and the date of the last menstrual period. Cryosurgery is best performed within 1 week after the cessation of the last menstrual period. This will avoid freezing a patient with an early pregnancy and will permit the most active phase of regeneration to take place before the onset of the next menses.

Treatment is performed in the office or clinic without anesthesia or analgesia. Nitrous oxide is the preferred refrigerant for dysplasia and carcinoma *in situ*. A speculum as large as the patient will tolerate is inserted, and the blades are fully extended, thus providing optimum visualization of the cervix as well as reducing the chance of freezing vaginal epithelium. All mucous and cellular debris is removed from the vagina and cervix with cotton balls soaked with 3% acetic acid. The extent of the disease to be treated is determined colposcopically. Once the area has been carefully outlined, the cervical probe that best approximates the anatomical configuration of the cervix is attached to the unit. If the lesion is more than 1½-times greater than the surface area of the probe tip, the lesion should be subdivided and each segment individually frozen. The tissue is thoroughly moistened with saline to ensure proper heat transfer. The probe tip at room temperature is firmly but gently positioned so that the greatest extent of the lesion is covered. A tenaculum is not used to stablize the cervix since this will cause excess bleeding and unnecessary pain.

Once the probe has been positioned, the refrigerant is circulated. Ice crystallization initially forms on the back of the probe tip and then spreads laterally from the edge of the probe. The lateral spread of the iceball usually begins within 10-15 seconds after the refrigerant has been circulated. If timing is to be conducted, it is initiated at the time of the lateral spread of the iceball. However, it is more important to make certain that the ice extends at least 4mm onto colposcopically normal appearing epithelium. Although the actual duration of freezing is less important, we have noted, when timing has been conducted, that the duration of the average probe position is about 2-3 minutes. During the freezing process it is unnecessary to know the probe tip temperature. If there is rapid

---

*The 24 hour cone-hysterectomy interval utilized at our institution avoids the problem of delayed bleeding and a second admission for hysterectomy.

lateral spread of the iceball, there will be adequate tissue necrosis. If a small portion of the vagina should become attached to the probe during the freezing process, no serious sequelae will occur. However, if a large area of the vagina becomes attached to the probe, the tip should be defrosted and reapplied. Once the area or areas have been adequately treated, the probe is defrosted and removed. The cervix is carefully inspected to make certain that the iceball has extended the necessary 4mm onto apparently normal epithelium. Any areas that do not appear to be adequately frozen at this time should, if possible, be retreated.

If multiple freeze applications are required, it is important that the iceballs overlap. Only a freeze-thaw cycle is used when nitrous oxide is the refrigerant. If liquid Freon or carbon dioxide gas is used, a freeze, partial thaw, refreeze cycle must be employed to achieve satisfactory tissue necrosis.

Posttreatment side effects and complications for CIN are not serious; they have been detailed in numerous publications. Follow-up of patients is important, and the following regimen is recommended.

At 6 weeks after freezing, cytology and colposcopy are performed. At 12 weeks after therapy, cytology, colposcopy, and curettage of the canal are carried out. Curettage is important since the squamocolumnar junction is frequently placed well within the endocervical canal. From the results of these examinations, success or failure of the cryosurgery is determined. If the patient had mild dysplasia before freezing and has two consecutive Pap tests showing mild dysplasia or worse and/or a tissue diagnosis of mild dysplasia or worse, she is considered a treatment failure. It is important, however, to carefully review the mild dysplasia material since actively regenerating epithelium may be confused with mild atypia. If a patient had moderate dysplasia or worse as a pretreatment diagnosis, she must have two consecutive Pap tests of moderate dysplasia or worse and/or a tissue diagnosis of moderate dysplasia or worse to be judged a treatment failure. An isolated abnormal Pap test, regardless of severity, does not qualify the patient as a freeze failure.

We have treated over 500 patients with CIN. Of this group more than 200 had either severe dysplasia or carcinoma *in situ*. Cryosurgery is proving effective in over 90% of the patients treated. Of the freeze failures, about 35% occurred in patients where the lesion was so extensive that the initial freezing session was inadequate. Moreover, additional treatment of these patients at the initial freezing sessions could not be completed because of the length of time that had elasped, with resultant discomfort. Although it might be argued that these patients should not be considered freeze failures, they have been included because freezing is being compared with other treatment techniques involving a single therapeutic session. Of the freeze failures, 15 have been retreated and all but 1 are free of disease after a second treatment session. The one exception underwent a third treatment session and has now been free of disease for 3 years.

The longest duration of follow-up in this patient population is 7 years. Almost 60% of the patients have been followed for over 3 years. This latter percentage is important since 85% of the treatment failures are uncovered the first year and 95% by 18 months after therapy. No recurrences have appeared in patients who have been free of disease 24 months after therapy. Follow-up of the total population is approximately 75%. Of course, longer follow-up is necessary in order to state conclusively that cryosurgery has permanently eradicated the lesion. However, even if the patient develops recurrent or new disease, she has enjoyed a disease-free interval when she could bear children—and many have done so. In comparison to hot cauterization, cryosurgery is as effective and is associated with fewer complications. Although not as effective as conization for CIN, it is more economical, is less hazardous, and poses less risk to the reproductive ability of the patient.

Cryosurgery for CIN, as well as any other outpatient technique, should be performed only by experienced colposcopists or in cases where consultation with such individuals is readily available. Freezing must be restricted to patients in whom the disease is confined to the visible portions of the cervix. Whenever disease extends well up into the canal, conization must be performed.

2-2 BASIC RADIOLOGIC-PHYSICS FOR GYNECOLOGISTS

Nuclear Particles and Radiation of Medical Interest

Symbol	Name	Atomic Mass Units	Charge
p	Proton	$1.00759(1.673 \times 10^{-24}\,g)$	+1
n	Neutron	1.00898	0
α	Alpha	4.00278	+2
e^-, β^-	Electron	$0.00055\ (9.1 \times 10^{-28}\,g)$	−1
e^+, β^+	Positron	0.00055	+1
x	X-ray	0 (photons)	0
γ	Gamma	0 (photons)	0

X-rays and gamma rays are photons. They can be considered as either waves or particles without mass. Their velocity is constant (3×10^{10} cm/second), but their energy varies.

A particle is radioactive when the nucleus is unstable and it emits particles and/or energy in the decay process to a more stable element.

Definition of Terms

Atomic number Z—number of protons in the nucleus.

Atomic weight, A—sum of neutrons plus protons in the nucleus.

Dosimetry-measurement and calculation of dose that the patient receives.

Electron volt, EV—energy of motion acquired by an electron accelerated through a potential difference of 1 volt.

Gamma rays—electromagnetic radiation emitted from within an excited nucleus. X-rays are similar photons originating outside the nucleus. The gamma rays from an isotope will have one or several sharply defined energies, whereas x-ray emissions will result in a spectrum of energies.

Half-life—time required for one half of the atoms of radioactive species to disintegrate.

HVL (half-value layer of a beam of x-rays or gamma rays)—thickness of a given material that will reduce the radiation intensity by one half.

Inverse square law—the intensity of radiation from a point source varies inversely as the square of the distance from the source. Thus the dose rate at 2 cm from a source is one fourth of that at 1 cm. At 3 cm the dose rate is one ninth that at 1 cm.

Ionization—removal of an electron from an atom, leaving a positively charged ion.

Ionizing radiation—radiation capable of causing ionization.

KeV—1000 eV.

MeV—1,000,000 eV.

Maximum permissible dose—a whole body dose of 5 (N—18) R, where N is the age in
  years.

Tumor dose—dose in the tumor volume considered for the dose prescription, usually the
  minimum dose within the tumor.

X-rays—continuous x-rays are the electromagnetic radiation that occurs when high-speed
  electrons are decelerated by interactions with matter.

X-ray and Gamma Ray Interactions with Matter (Fig. 2-8)

X-rays and gamma rays interact with tissue, giving rise to fast electrons that in turn ionize
and excite thousands of atoms in the cell before coming to rest. At each point of
ionization or excitation, radicals are formed which quickly become involved in chemical
reactions and biologic damage.

From the biologic viewpoint, the mechanism of cell injury is varied. It may proceed
through inactivation of enzyme systems, changes in permeability of cell membranes, or
disruption of the normal configuration of the genetic material. The effects of such
changes may become manifest at different time intervals after the primary event,
depending on the type of intracellular target affected and the time at which a certain
chemical constituent is called upon to perform.

Thus, with the same injury by ionization, a mature cell in a state of low metabolic
activity may be grossly unaffected whereas an actively growing cell may be destroyed.
Cells in the act of division may be more vulnerable than those resting between mitoses.
Lowered oxygen tension, dehydration, freezing, and the presence of chemical reducing
agents may protect cells from radiation injury to a certain extent. There seems to be a
tendency to recover from injury if certain key molecules are not completely destroyed
directly and if, after the primary event, they can be protected for an adequate period
before the cell's metabolic cycle is disturbed.

Microscopic changes associated with radiation injury include swelling of the cells,
vacuolization of the cytoplasm, giant cell formation, and fragmentation or partial
separation of the chromosomes at the time of division. In an exposed field some cells may
appear normal despite the obvious injury and death of adjacent cells. The nature of this
relative resistance is the basis for the response to radiation at the tissue level. From the
histologic point of view, the changes seen after radiation injury are similar to those
produced by other traumatic agents. They may be some distance from the site of
introduction because of the penetrating ability of the agent, and they may occur some
time after the traumatic event. Furthermore, there may be great variation in the degree of
reaction, depending on the intensity and site of the injury as well as the nature of the
tissue exposed.

The usual local reaction is nonspecific, however, and is a typical inflammatory
response. There occurs, after a latent period, evidence of cell death with loss of nuclear
and cytoplasmic structure. Edema, capillary dilation and proliferation, infiltration of
round cells, and a fibroplastic response are present. This immediate reaction is followed

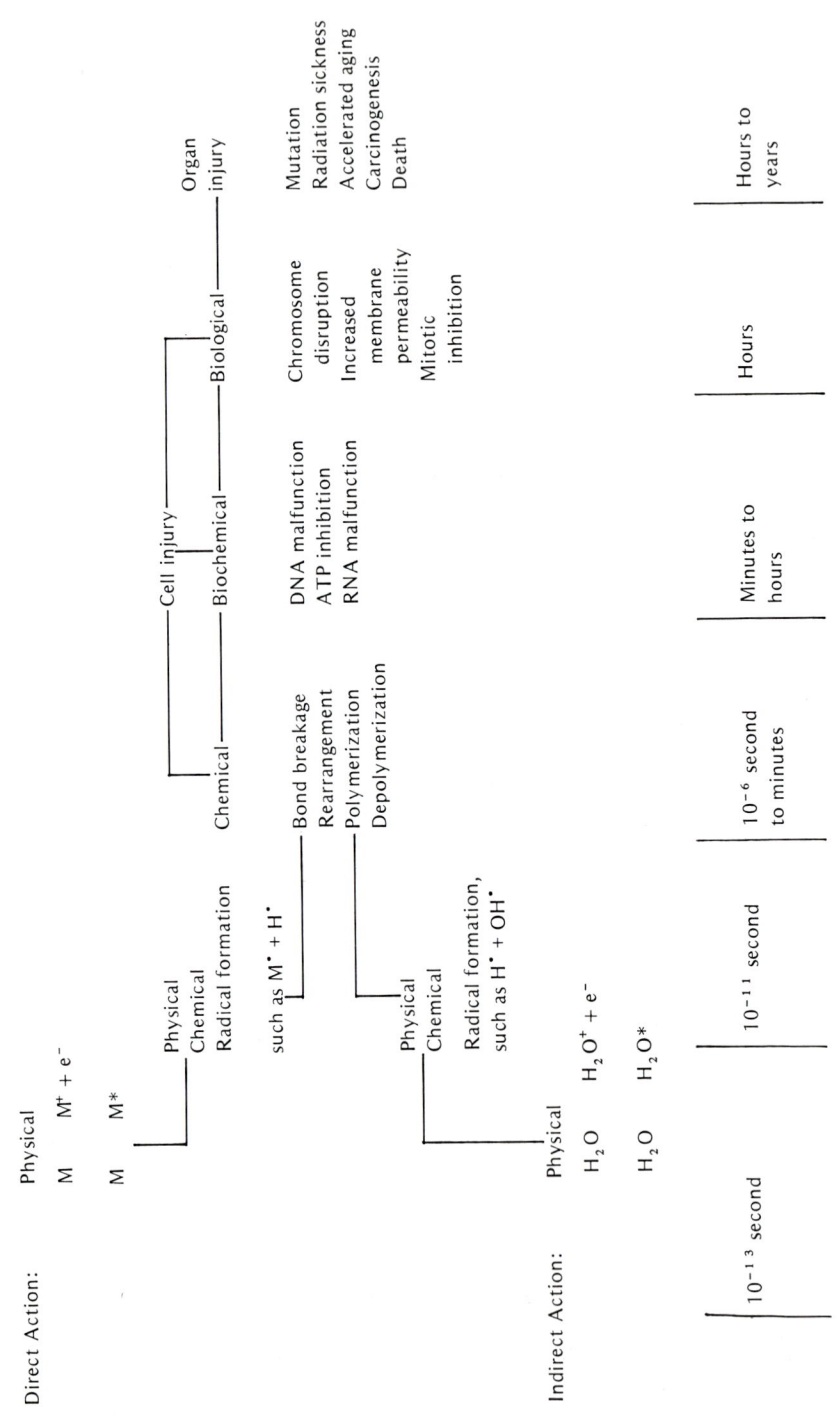

Fig. 2-8 Action of ionizing radiations on living tissue.

by gradual fibrosis, avascularity, and a walling-off of the injured area. Very late changes are scarification and contracture, with occasional inelastic dilated blood vessels pinched off by an essentially avascular stroma.

Grossly, irradiated areas whether benign or malignant, show changes that are similar to those resulting from trauma but may vary in time of appearance and in intensity. An irradiated area may become erythematous in from 1 to 2 weeks after exposure. If severely injured, there may be epidermitis and surface loss. Later, epilation and loss of pigment may occur. After such an acute phase, with gradual fibrosis extending over a period of months, scarification and contracture become evident. The injured area remains avascular, but may show dilation of surface blood vessels typical of telangiectatic radiation injury. If the local injury is especially intense, there may be deep necrosis. Cell death may occur weeks or months after the injury and be concomitant with attempts at repair. If vascularization of the area is inadequate, partial healing, further breakdown, and, again, attempts at repair will result. Severely injured tissues may eventually respond by malignant change years after the injury.

Ine normal tissues in the area of injury are vitally involved in the reparative processes. In the treatment of cancer, great dependence is placed on these structures. If they are vulnerable to excessive injury because of infection, desmoplasia, or natural radiosensitivity, ultimate healing will not occur. This may result not only in extensive local necrosis but also in the persistence of undamaged tumor cells, which may thrive in an anoxic tumor bed (see section 2—6).

The Electromagnetic Spectrum

Radiowaves	10^{-10} to 10^{-4} eV	Wavelength 3×10^5 to 1 cm
Infrared	0.01 to 1 eV	Wavelength 0.01 to 10^{-4} cm
Visible	2 to 3 eV	Wavelength 7000 to 4000 Å
Ultraviolet	3 to 124 eV	Wavelength 4000 to 100 Å
X-ray	124 eV to 124 MeV	Wavelength 100 to 0.0001 Å

1 angstrom = Å = 10^{-8} cm

Units of Radiation Measurement

1. *The Roentgen* (R). The roentgen is the quantity of x-rays or gamma radiation such that the associated corpuscular emission per 0.001293 g of air produces, in air, ions carrying 1 esu of electricity of either sign.

2. *The Rad.* The absorbed dose of any ionizing radiation is the amount of energy imparted to matter by ionizing particles per unit mass of irradiated material at the place of interest. It is expressed in rads. The rad is the unit of absorbed dose and is 100 ergs/g.

3. *The Relative Biological Effectiveness* (RBE). The RBE of a radiation is the ratio of the dose of a standard radiation to the dose of another radiation required to produce the same biological effect. The RBE is related to the rate of energy loss along the track of the ionizing particle.

Isotopes Commonly Used in Radiation Therapy

Isotope	Gamma Energy	Half-Life
Cesium-137	0.662 MeV	30 years
Cobalt-60	1.173, 1.332 MeV	5.3 years
Gold-198	0.411 MeV	2.69 days
Iridium-192	0.47 MeV av.	74 days
Phosphorus-32	(beta emission only)	14.28 days
Radium-226	0.8 MeV av.	1620 years
Radon-222	0.8 MeV av.	3.83 days
Tantalum-182	1.18 MeV av.	115 days

Radium-226, cesium-137, iridium-192, and tantalum-182 are suitable for temporary implants; radon-222 and gold-198, for permanent implants that remain in the patient; Cobalt-60 has some uses in intracavitary therapy.

Dosimetry for Radium

1. *Direct Measurements*. With "hot loaded" techniques and applicators, direct measurements with a probe type scintillation counter can be made in the operating room to quickly identify a geometry that delivers too much radiation to the bladder or rectum. If bladder or rectal readings are too high, the therapist can repack around the radium while the patient is still under anesthesia. Doses exceeding 3500 R to the bladder and 3000 R to the rectum (per radium insertion when there will be two insertions) are considered too high, and the radium geometry should be changed to decrease this dose.

2. *Lateral Throw-off*. Isodose curves for the tandem and ovoids are combined to show where the patent will receive 3500 R on completion of treatment. The dose is also assessed at centimeter intervals lateral to and through the internal os (2 cm—point A, 5 cm—point B). The plane of calculation is formed by a line passing through the internal os and the center of the ovoids. This can be determined by manual or computer methods.

Radiation Machines

Orthovoltage X-Rays (150-500 kv) (Figs. 2-9a and 2-9b)

The voltage across an x-ray tube is developed by a transformer that steps up the incoming voltage to the desired level. Electrons are accelerated from a filament in a vacuum; these bombard a target substance, and x-rays are emitted.

Mega- or Supervoltage (1—40 MeV)

1. *Linear Accelerator* (Fig. 2-10). An electromagnetic wave moving down a circular tube that has an axis parallel to the electric field of the wave provides a steady accelerating field for a particle which keeps in step with a suitable part of the field. The usual energies of these machines for radiation therapy are 6-8 MeV; however, energies of 35-40 MeV are possible for therapy.

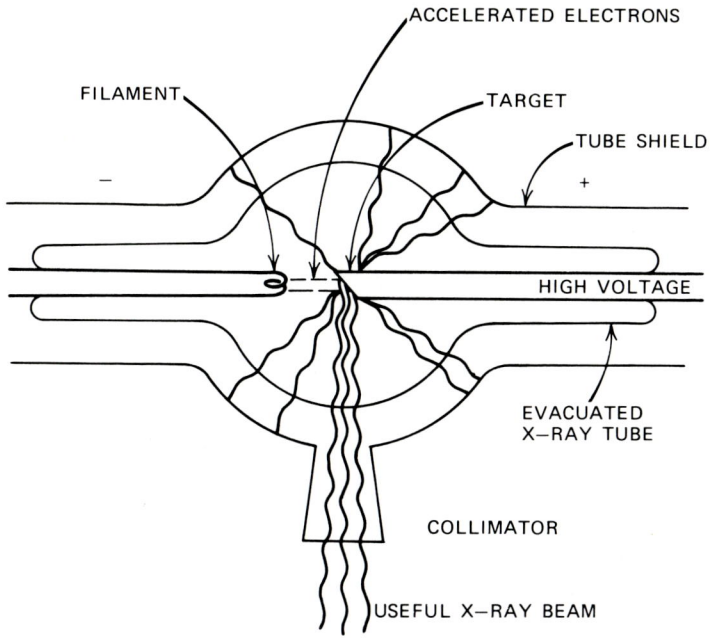

ACCELERATED ELECTRONS

FILAMENT

TARGET

TUBE SHIELD

−　　　　+

HIGH VOLTAGE

EVACUATED
X−RAY TUBE

COLLIMATOR

USEFUL X−RAY BEAM

X−RAY TUBE

Fig. 2-9a Orthovoltage x-rays (150-500 kV).

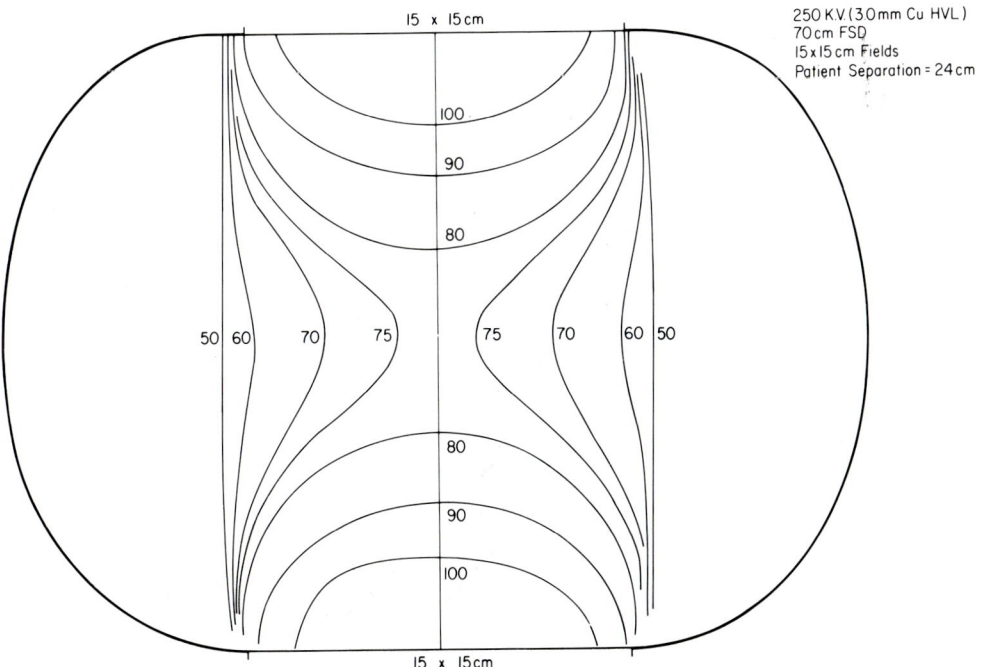

15 x 15 cm

250 K.V. (3.0 mm Cu HVL)
70 cm FSD
15 x 15 cm Fields
Patient Separation = 24 cm

100
90
80

50　60　70　75　　75　70　60　50

80
90
100

15 x 15cm

Fig. 2-9b Two field isodose curves—250 k.v. Isodose curves are normalized so that the point of maximum dose is 100%.

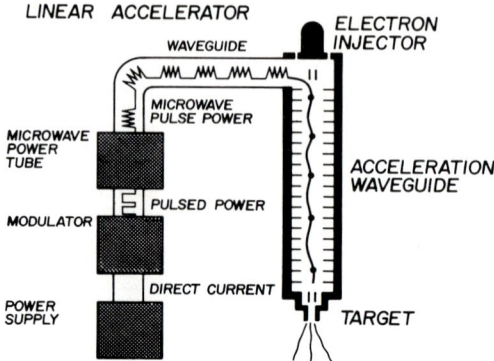

Fig. 2-10   Linear accelerator.

2. *Betatron* (Figs. 2-11*a*, 2-11*b*, and 2-11*c*). In this device for accelerating electrons up to several hundred volts, the electron travels in a circular orbit, gaining velocity during each revolution. For therapy, betatrons operating at 20-40 MeV are common. Use can be made of the electron beam or of the x-ray beam produced by bombardment of a target.

3. *Teletherapy Unit* (Figs. 2-12*a* and 2-12*b*). Teletherapy units make use of a radioactive material (cobalt-60, cesium-137, etc.) as the source of radiation. The source has a reasonably long half-life and emits gamma rays having nearly the desired energy. The advantage of the teletherapy type unit is its electrical simplicity.

4. *Cost of Units.* The cost of supervoltage unit runs from about $80,000 to $250,000. In addition, radiation protection must be provided for the rooms housing the units—1-4 feet of concrete wall, floor, and ceiling.

Comparison of Depth Doses for Various Radiation Machines
(Figs. 2-13*a* and 2-13*b*)

The dose on the central axis from the point of entry into the patient can be calculated from study of the isodose curves. For practical therapeutic purposes the principal

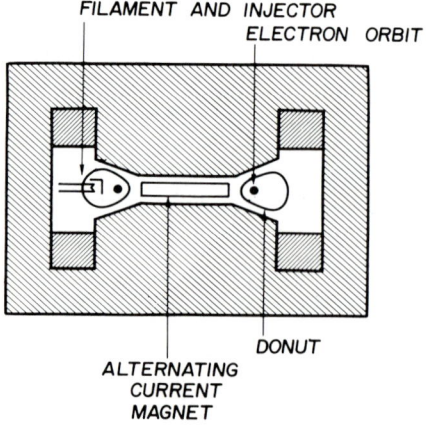

Fig. 2-11*a*   Betatron.

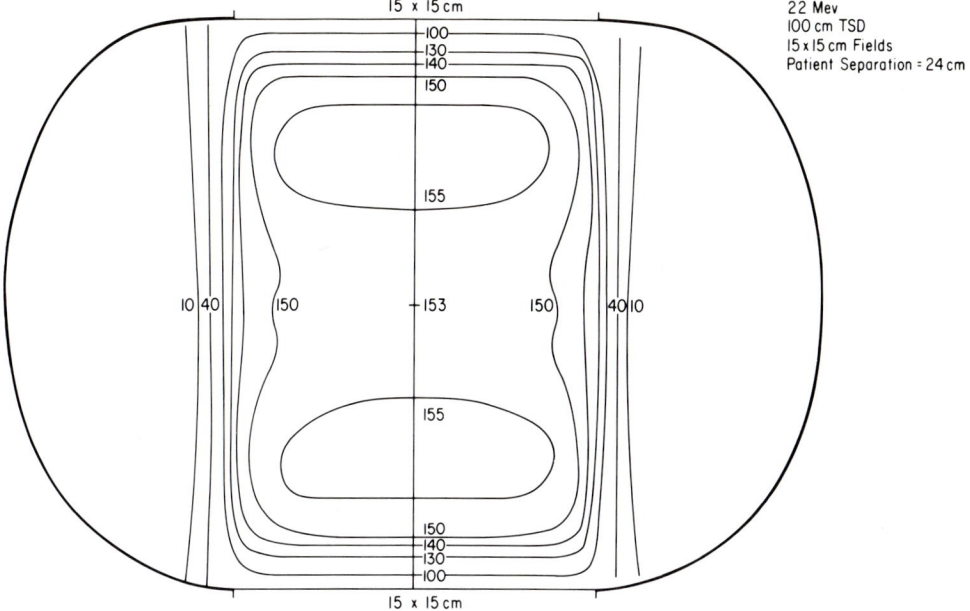

Fig. 2-11b Two field isodose curves—22 MeV betatron.

difference between the various kinds of beams is the difference in depth dose distribution. The low dose at the point of entry, zero depth, and the similarity of energy absorption in muscle and bone are advantages of the higher energy beams.

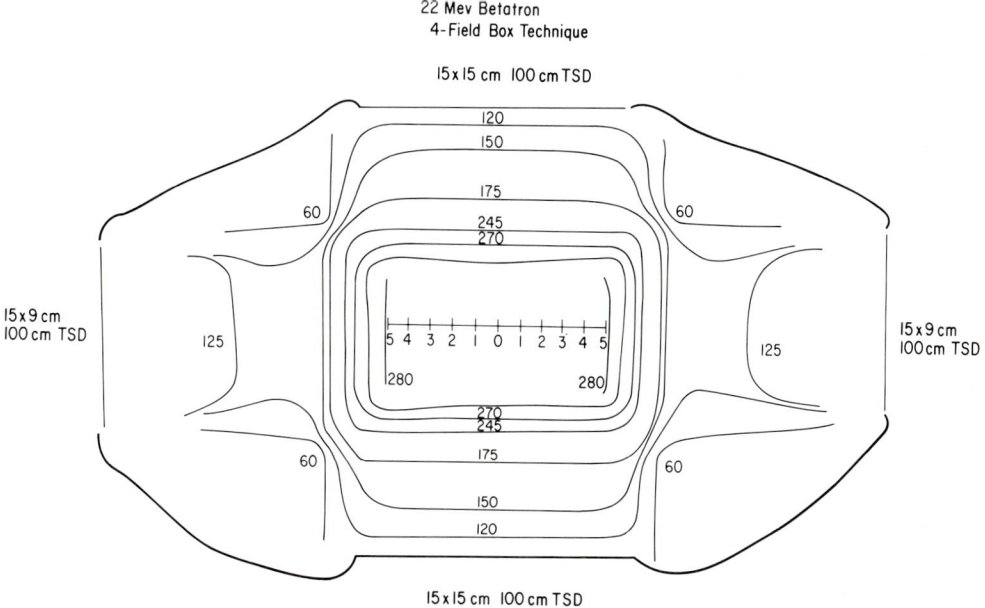

Fig. 2-11c Four field isodose curves—22 MeV betatron.

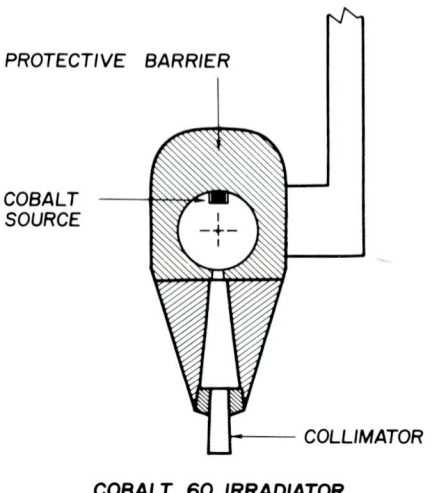

COBALT 60 IRRADIATOR

Fig. 2-12*a*   Cobalt-60 irradiator.

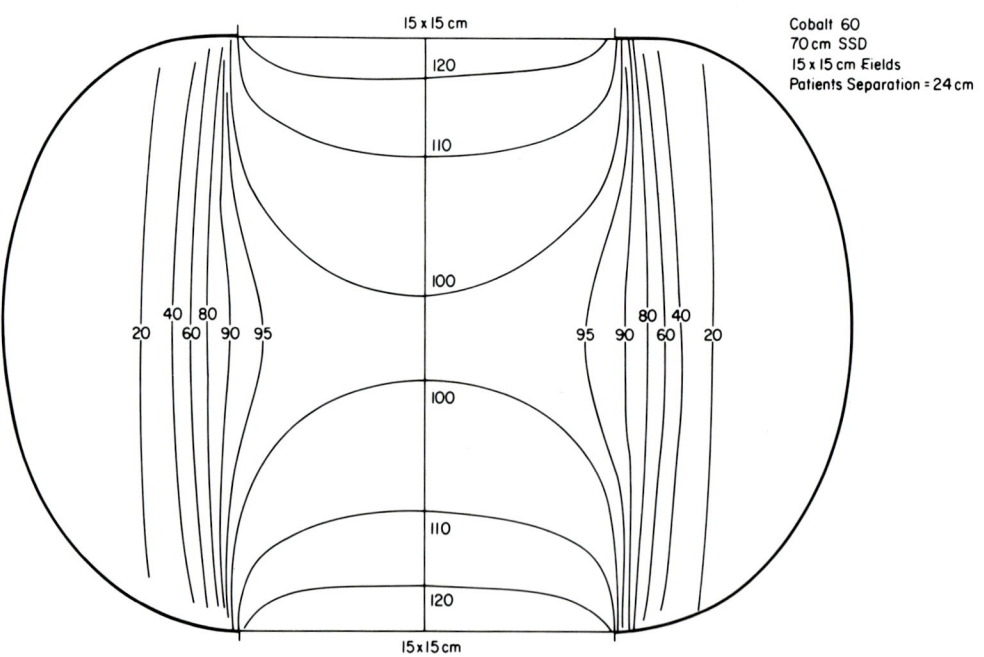

Fig. 2-12*b*   Two field isodose curves—cobalt-60.

Protection Considerations in Using Intracavitary Sources in Gynecology

1. *Limiting the Time of Exposure.* Working efficiently and spending as little time as possible in the vicinity of the patient will reduce personnel exposure to the radiation. The dose received is proportional to the time of exposure. Afterloading techniques, in which the sources are loaded after the procedures in the operating room are completed, also reduce the radiation exposure.

2. *Increasing the Distance from the Source.* The radiation dose rate is inversely proportional to the square of the distance from the source. Increasing from 1 meter to 2 meters reduces the dose to one fourth; at 3 meters the dose rate is one ninth of that at 1 meter.

3. *Interposing Absorption Barriers.* Lead or concrete barriers reduce the dose from a source. The half-value layer in lead for radium gamma rays is 1.2 cm. Thus 1.2 cm of lead reduces the dose to one half; 2.4 cm (about 1 in.) reduces it one fourth; 3.6 cm reduces it to one eighth.

Concept of Rad Equivalent Therapy

Ellis (1967) has introduced a new expression of the biological effect of irradiation called the rad equivalent therapy (RET). Here an attempt is made to calculate a dosage schedule

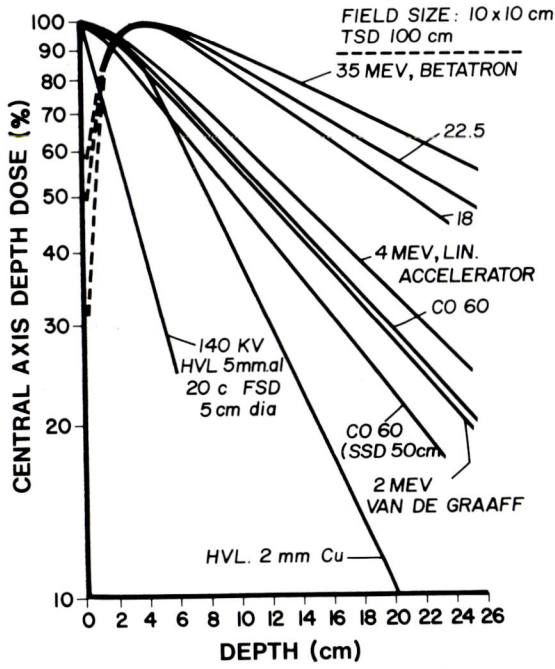

Fig. 2-13a Graphic illustration of central axis depth dose for photons of varying strengths

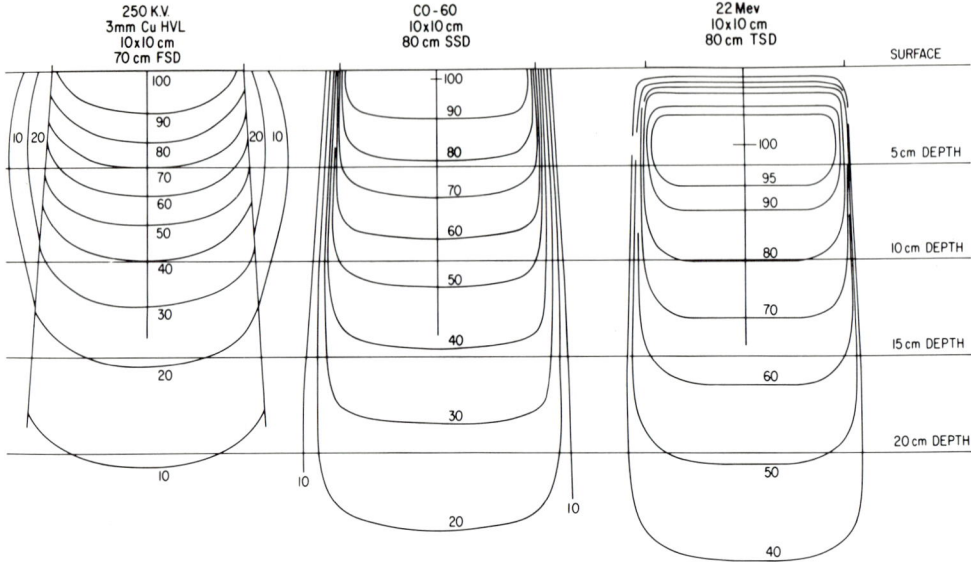

Fig. 2-13*b* Comparison of isodose curves (single field) from three sources of external irradiation.

that can be related to one figure expressing its biologic effect. This offers the obvious advantage of providing simple comparison techniques in the same center and between centers, and the further advantage of comparison with the added effects of two different types of treatment, such as intracavitary radium and external beam irradiation. The Ellis formula is as follows:

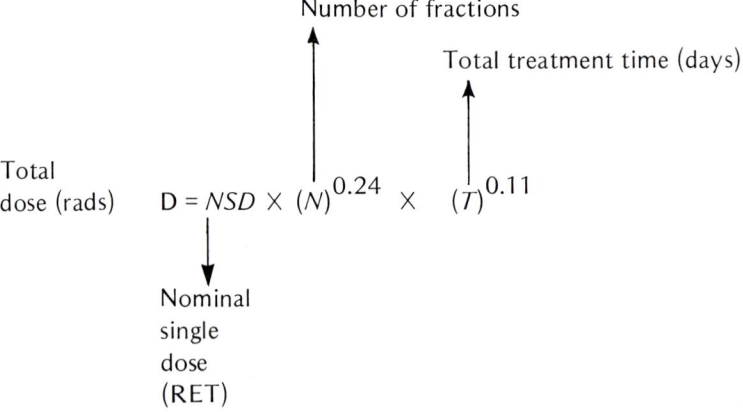

This allows one to calculate the nominal single dose, which we have referred to as RET. Ellis' calculations when compared with clinical situations consistently demonstrate that the normal tolerance of human connective tissue is between 1800 and 1900 RETs. Therefore, since Ellis takes into account both fractionation and total treatment time, as well as total rads given, one can always calculate a treatment plan to maximum tissue tolerance, regardless of the method of fractionation or even possible interruptions in therapy. Similar calculations can be made for intracavitary radium, and the tolerance to any point (e.g., point A or B in gynecologic radiotherapy) can be calculated and added to the sum of the RETs given by external beam. We thus have a method of more accurately adding the biologic effect of intracavitary radium to that of external beam irradiation and this has obvious advantages in gynecologic radiotherapy.

Genetic Effects

The genetic effects of radiation are complex and varied. It suffices here to mention that mutations are an inevitable consequence of radiation and that all such mutations are harmful. In the human being there is no evidence that subsequent generations will be damaged by radiation mutations, as they are in the fruitfly, the mouse, and other experimental subjects. Nevertheless, this possibility must be recognized, and appropriate effort made to avoid unnecessary exposure of the gonads. In the case of diagnostic radiation, this may be of great importance. In cancer therapy, however, the objective is to eliminate the lesions, and the radiation doses needed are sufficiently high that sterilization is an inevitable result; hence the reappearance of damaging mutations in subsequent generations need not be considered.

On the basis of extrapolation from damaging radiation mutations in experimental animals, it has been suggested that for the human being a total dose of 10 R of man-made radiation to the gonads, either in a single dose or in divided doses, probably has insignificant genetic effects. Larger doses are thought to be potentially harmful. Accordingly, the Committee on Genetics of the Atomic Energy Commission has recommended that no individual from conception to the age of 30 years be subjected to more than 10 R of man-made radiation to the gonads. Cosmic radiation, estimated to total approximately 4 R in this same span of years, is not included in this 10 R permissible dose.

With appropriate shielding to prevent scatter, improved x-ray film, image intensifiers, and the like, it is possible to obtain satisfactory x-ray visualization of internal structures with reduced exposure. The average doses of radiation to the gonads in some common diagnostic techniques are shown in Table 2-1. Although each technique, except gastrointestinal fluoroscopy, produces only a small dose to the gonads, the use of many films and repeated diagnostic tests may produce a considerable cumulative dose.

2-3 CLINICAL RADIOBIOLOGY

The whole basis of radiotherapy is the capacity of ionizing radiation to destroy certain types of malignant growths without causing irreversible damage to the tissues in which the tumor is growing and which necessarily receive a full dose of irradiation. Thus it is differential radiosensitivity that makes radiation therapy possible. Many speak of a therapeutic ratio, which is defined as the ratio between the lethal tumor dose and the tissue tolerance. Obviously it is high for very radiosensitive tumors such as seminomas, and it is low when there is a relatively small difference in radiosensitivity, as in adenocarcinomas and squamous carcinomas of the cervix, bowel, and lung. The therapeutic ratio can be negative when a tumor is more radioresistant than the supporting structures; an example would be most fibrosarcomas.

It must be understood that "radiosensitivity" and "radiocurability" are not identical in

TABLE 2-1 MEAN DOSE OF RADIATION TO
GONADS FROM COMMON DIAGNOSTIC PROCEDURES

	Mean Dose per Examination (mR)	
	Female	Male
Chest, heart, lung x-ray (excluding mass miniature radiography)	5.4	5.5
Abdominal x-ray following barium meal	333	448
Abdominal x-ray (scout film)	183	281
Abdominal x-ray (obstructive series)	367	723
Intravenous pyelography	585	843
Pelvimetry	745	885
Pelvis, lumbar spine, lumbosacral joint x-ray	392	536
Hip, upper femur x-ray	102	154

Modified from *Trans. N.Y. Acad. Sci.* **25**: 195, 1962.

meaning. Relatively radioresistant tumors accessible to high dose localized radiotherapy are curable, whereas radiosensitive tumors that are, at the start of therapy or shortly thereafter, widely metastasized can only be controlled locally. An excellent example of a relatively radioresistant tumor is squamous cell carcinoma of the cervix. Yet this malignancy remains one of the most curable human tumors because of its accessibility to a high dosage of radiation and the relatively radioresistant nature of the normal tissues of the cervix and vagina. The ability to place radium in juxtaposition to the tumor allows one to administer a superlethal dosage of irradiation to the malignancy with tolerable doses to the surrounding normal tissue.

Tissues with a rapid rate of cell replication (e.g. bone marrow and reproductive organ) are the most radiosensitive, and those with a moderate degree of cell replacement (e.g., the skin and mucous membrane) are moderately radiosensitive. Tolerance can be defined as the inverse of radiosensitivity. The tolerance of a particular tissue or organ not only is a function of its specific sensitivity but also relates to the volume irradiated. With the same dose in time, the severity of skin reaction increases with an increase in the area irradiated. If we can assume that the reactions of normal skin to irradiation parallel the reactions of other normal tissues, abundant experimental evidence shows that tolerance to irradiation is a function of the total dose, the volume irradiated, the number of fractions utilized, and the length of time over which the therapy proceeds. A dose of 2000 R in one treatment to a 3 x 3 cm field is well tolerated in the actual therapy of many skin cancers, but the same does given over a 10 cm field would produce an unhealing, necrotic ulcer. A total dose of 4000 R to a pelvic field approximately 15 X 15 cm over 4 weeks' time is well tolerated. However, if the volume of tissue treated is increased by irradiating the whole abdomen, one finds that 4000 R is very poorly tolerated. Finally, whereas 4000 R whole pelvis through a 15 X 15 cm field is very well tolerated over 4 weeks' time, such a dosage given within 1 week would be completely intolerable.

The generalizations made above apply to all tissues and organs of the body. For example, long segments of sigmoid or small bowel are subject to complications when they are adherent in the pelvis and daily exposure to irradiation is unavoidable. When a large volume of bowel is irradiated to a dose of 4000 or 5000 rads, the incidence of complications rises sharply as compared to the normal irradiation of the same organs during routine treatment. The difference lies in the volume of a particular organ that is irradiated. As a practical consequence, although one would wish to irradiate all potentially involved areas of malignancy, one must choose to limit irradiation to the more probable or the clinically evident diseased area; otherwise, the tumor dose has to be reduced below the level of effectiveness. That cervical cancer has the potential for spread to the periaortic as well as the pelvic nodes is well established, and thus it would be ideal to irradiate the periaortic areas in every patient. However, to embark upon such a treatment plan, one may have either to reduce the total dose given or to incur an unacceptable complication rate. It then becomes a philosophical question as to whether a high irradiation therapy complication rate is justified to salvage an unknown number of patients with microscopic metastasis in the lymph nodes above the pelvic fields.

The tolerance of tissues is often a function of the vascularization and therefore the oxygen tension (Fig. 2-14). It has been demonstrated in the treatment of soft tissue sarcomas that, if one applies a surgical tourniquet to a limb and irradiates after anoxia has been achieved, the tolerance of normal tissues is approximately doubled. This technique has been used recently in the treatment of soft tissue sarcomas under the hypothesis that many such sarcomas have multiple anoxic areas at the outset; these tumors increase in size very rapidly and apparently outgrow their blood supply. It has been suggested that the failure rate (local recurrence) is a function of these anoxic areas, which are relatively radioresistant. The application of a tourniquet equalizes the oxygen tension between the anoxic areas of the tumor and the normal tissue; thus the radiosensitivity of the tumor is at the same level as that of the normal tissue. Before the application of the tourniquet, the anoxic areas of the tumor were far more radioresistant than normal tissue.

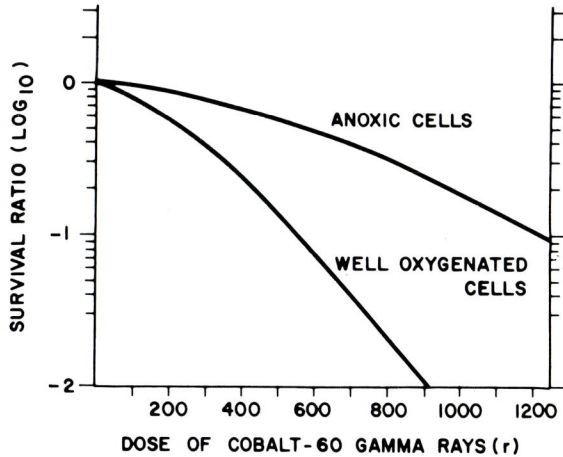

Fig. 2-14 Survival curves for anoxic cells versus well oxygenated cells.

Radiosensitivity of Tumors

The radiosensitivity of tumors depends on four factors:

1. The histologic type.
2. The degree of differentiation.
3. The tumor bed and the oxygen tension.
4. The clinical variety.

As a rule, tumors share the radiosensitivity of the parent tissue. For instance, seminomas are very sensitive whereas chondrosarcomas and fibrosarcomas are highly radioresistant. Squamous cell carcinomas and adenocarcinomas are epithelial tumors which lie somewhere between the above extremes. Experimental and clinical evidence suggests that adenocarcinoma and squamous cell carcinoma have approximately the same radiosensitivity. The reason for the apparent discrepancy in the survival results with irradiation therapy alone for cervix cancer may lie in the different routes of spread and other factors ("the barrel-shaped" lesion) that are not directly related to the radiosensitivity of the tumor. It has been stated for many years that anaplastic tumors are more radiosensitive than well differentiated ones. In the last decade this hypothesis has come under question, and considerable recent evidence suggests that there is no difference between the radiosensitivities of anaplastic and well-differentiated malignancies. The truth probably lies somewhere between the two views, and there is undoubtedly a certain amount of variation within any classification of malignancy. Whereas the degree of differentiation of bronchogenic carcinoma of the lung may not correlate with its radiosensitivity, the radiosensitivity of well-differentiated adenocarcinoma of the endometrium appears to be greater than that of undifferentiated carcinoma of the endometrium.

It is reasonably well established that anoxic cells are approximately 2 to 2½ times more radioresistant than normal oxygenated cells (Fig. 2-15) and that there appear to be foci of anoxic cells in many tumors. This is particularly true of cancers that (1) are infiltrative, (2) have been long in existence, with connective tissue reaction and poor vascularization, (3) have larger foci of anoxic cells, such as rapidly growing tumors, or (4) have recurred after a course of radiation therapy, with marked fibrosis surrounding these foci. The exophytic tumors, which are friable and well vascularized with fewer anoxic cells, are clinically more radiosensitive. In several centers throughout the world this problem of tissue oxygenation and radiosensitivity has been approached by attempts to bring the patient's oxygen tension up to the maximum level. Patients are placed in hyperbaric oxygen tanks where the oxygen tension is at 3-4 atm, and the daily radiation treatment is carried out with the patient in this environment. Although similar studies done with animals have shown improved curability, to date the trials carried out with human cancer patients have not been very impressive.

Time Factor as It Relates to Radiosensitivity

The time factor has three subfactors:
1. Overall time of treatment.

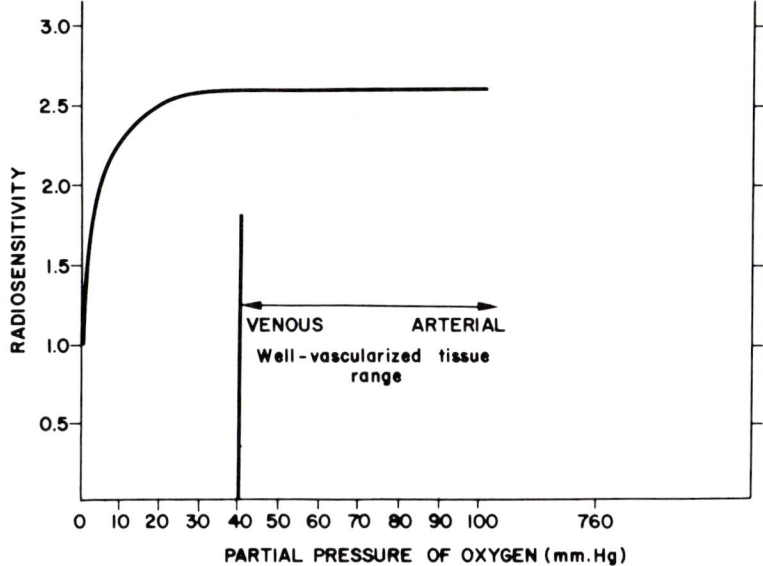

Fig. 2-15 Radiosensitivity of cells as a function of oxygen tension.

2. Fractionation.
3. Dosage rate.

The "overall time" extends from the first day to the last day of treatment. The same dose given in a shorter time is more effective. For external beam, the treatment period may be 3-7 weeks, depending on the total dose given. This may then be followed by one or two radium insertions, which can be given 1-3 weeks apart, resulting in an overall time of treatment that extends up to 3 months.

The "fractionation" is the number of treatments and is usually four or five on as many days a week for external radiation. The "dosage rate" is the quantity of irradiation given in each fraction, usually expressed as the dose per week. The biologic effect is quite dependent on the fractionation and dosage rate. As an example, one can administer 1000 R per week with five daily treatments of 200 R each for a total of 6000 R in 6 weeks, but a treatment plan of 1000 R as a single weekly pulse for 6 consecutive weeks could not be tolerated by the patient and would be associated with severe complications. Treatments 3 times a week produce more reaction than treatments 5 times a week, with probably a difference of approximately 10%. The same dose of radium produces more reaction in one insertion than when spread over two or three insertions. With the present Manchester technique, administering 10,000 mg-hours over 144 hours consecutively would produce considerably more reaction than giving 72 hours and 2 weeks later giving another 72 hours.

Whenever a radiation treatment plan is reviewed, the reviewer must know (1) the overall time of treatment, (2) the fractionation technique, (3) the total dose given, (4) the dosage rate, and (5) the volume irradiated, in order to properly assess the biologic effect of the treatment.

2-4   INVASIVE CARCINOMA OF THE CERVIX

General Remarks

Twenty-five per cent of all malignant disease in women arises in the genital tract, and half of these malignancies arise in the cervix. Next to cancer of the breast and colon, cervical carcinoma is the most frequent cancer to which womankind is subject; it is estimated that 3% of women will be afflicted with cancer of the cervix before the age of 80. Between 30,000 and 40,000 cases of cervical cancer are discovered each year in the United States alone. In recent times half of this number have been diagnosed as carcinoma *in situ.*

The unique accessibility of the uterus for cell and tissue study, as well as for direct physical examination, has led to advances in diagnosis and treatment that have resulted in some of the best cure rates of any human malignant neoplasm. The annual death rate for cancer of the cervix has fallen steadily over the past 40 years, from 20 per 100,000 in 1930 to 8 per 100,000 in 1970. This drop has been due to the introduction of diagnostic techniques such as the Pap smear and improved procedures in surgery and radiotherapy. Nevertheless, in spite of improved diagnostic and therapeutic modalities, the estimated death rate from cervical cancer remains at approximately 8000 cases per year in the United States.

The age of patients with carcinoma *in situ* is on the average, 10 years less than average age of patients with invasive cancer of the cervix. In most series, patients with carcinoma *in situ* have an average age of 35; those with invasive disease of 45. There are, however, many exceptions, and in the past two decades an increasing number of patients in their late teens and early twenties have been reported with carcinoma *in situ* as well as invasive disease. Whether all invasive carcinomas begin as *in situ* lesions is unknown, but Peterson (1956) reported that in one third of 127 untreated patients invasive carcinoma developed subsequently to carcinoma *in situ* at the end of 9 years. Masterson (1957) found that 28% of 25 untreated patients demonstrated invasive carcinoma at the end of 5 years.

The 5 year survival rate for invasive cancer of the cervix varies as shown below. Of the untreated cases 5% showed disease 5 years later. Of those treated (at all institutions) 40-60% were without disease at 5 years.

		Stockholm		M.D. Anderson Hospital	
	Univ. of			Ortho-	Supervoltage Era
	Tenn.	Heyman	Kottmeier	voltage Era	Late 1950s
Stage	1950s	1940s	1950s	Early 1950s	and 1960s
I	68	78	89	90	94
II	38	44	53	70	79
III	22	28	34	37	47
IV	2½	4	8	5	16
All Stages	38		50.5	59	64

Microinvasive Carcinoma of the Cervix

Microinvasive carcinoma of the cervix has presented itself over the past 10 years as a rather confusing subject. Contradictions and conflicts between the results of different investigators, incomplete information in the data presented, erratic interpretation of findings, and even erroneous use of the material reported can occur with such frequency as to confuse the most learned academician. A review of the literature shows that even the name of the disease itself varies greatly among authors. "Microinvasive carcinoma" has been the most frequently used term, but 14 other designations are also employed. Some authors, seemingly unable to come to a decision, refer to the disease by several different terms in the same article.

Attempts have been made to eliminate some of the confusion. In August, 1974, the Cancer Committee of the International Federation of Gynecology and Obstetrics classified these lesions as Stage Ia and defined them as early stromal invasion. This definition is, of course, quite vague, and others have specified that the depth of invasion should be no greater than 3-5 mm. Many authors have used the 3mm rule, and others the 5 mm rule. In January 1973 the Society of Gynecologic Oncologists accepted the following statement on microinvasion in cancer of the cervix uteri: (1) cases of intraepithelial carcinoma with questionable invasion should be regarded as intraepithelial carcinoma: and (2) a micoinvasive lesion should be defined as one in which neoplastic epithelium invades the stroma in one or more places to a depth of 3 mm or less below the base of the epithelium and in which lymphatic or vascular involvement is not demonstrated. This definition was submitted to the executive board of the American College of Obstetrics and Gynecology for consideration, with the recommendation that it be approved and forwarded to the International Federation of Gynecology and Obstetrics.

In our opinion, "microinvasion" should be defined as invasion to a depth of no more than 3 mm with no confluent tongues and no areas of lymphatic or vascular invasion. The bulk of the invasive process is probably the key to predicting the behavior of the disease. The physician should review the histologic sections himself; and if indeed there are only isolated tongues of invasion (Fig. 2-16), the patient may be managed by simple hysterectomy. On the other hand, if multiple confluent tongues of invasive disease (Fig. 2-17) are noted, the patient should be considered under risk of lymphatic involvement and, even though this is not seen on the microscopic sections, should be treated with a radical hysterectomy with pelvic lymphadenectomy.

Several prospective studies are under way at this time, including one by the Gynecologic Oncology Group in which 25 member institutions are participating in an effort to clarify this dilemma. Creasman and Parker (1973) reported 1 of 19 patients with invasion of 5 mm or less had a positive pelvic node, an incidence of 5.2%. Others have reported an incidence of positive nodes in "microinvasion" of between 2 and 5%. These figures include, of course, lesions with bulky invasion relative to the 5 mm depth.

Clinically Invasive Cancer

Increased knowledge and experience in the application of radiation techniques to the treatment of carcinoma of the cervix have resulted in steady improvement of the survival and control rates.

Three techniques for the application of irradiation to the cervix have found continuing favor. The most successful systems for radiation treatment of these lesions have evolved from (1) the Stockholm technique, which utilized high intensity radium applications of relatively short duration, repeated in 2-3 weeks, (2) the Paris technique, which employed low intensity radium treatments of up to 1 week's duration, and (3) the Manchester

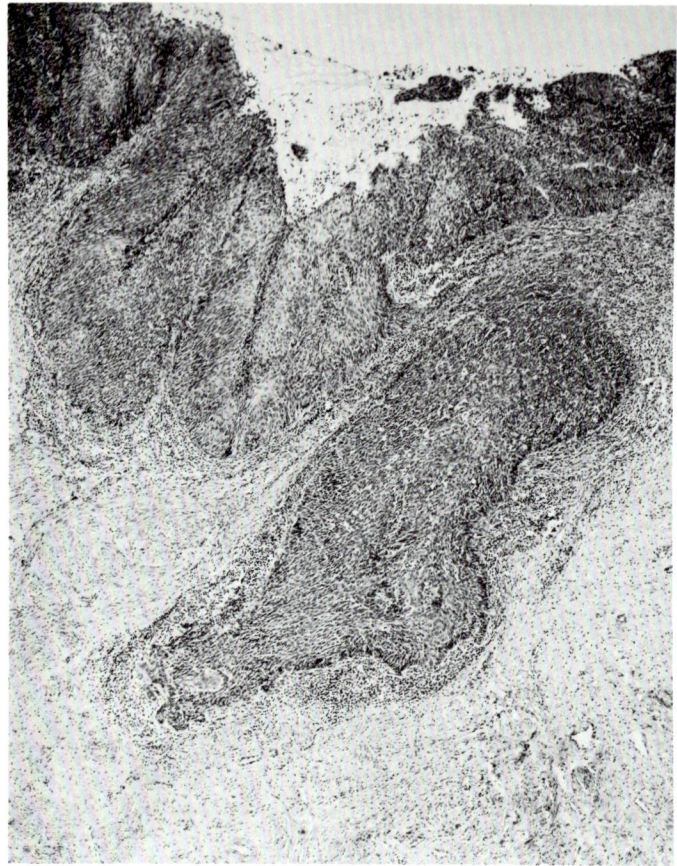

Fig. 16 Early stromal invasion (true microinvasion). Note an isolated tongue of invasive cancer (with budding projections to a depth of 2 mm) surrounded by heavy lymphocyte infiltrate. (Courtesy of William Creasman, M.D., Director of Gynecologic Oncology, Duke University, School of Medicine.)

modification of the Paris technique, which attempted to improve treatment by delivery of predetermined doses to fixed points within the pelvis. Modification of the Manchester system by refinements in radium and external radiation techniques has resulted in the highest control rates yet known. The purpose here is to review the techniques currently used at Los Angeles County-University of Southern California Medical Center, which are modifications of those employed by the M. D. Anderson hospital and Tumor Institute under the direction of Gilbert H. Fletcher, M. D., Director of the Department of Radiotherapy, and Felix N. Rutledge, M. D., Head of the Section of Gynecology.

Clinical Varieties (Gross Lesions)

The clinical appearance of carcinoma of the cervix varies widely, depending on the nature of its growth pattern and mode of regional involvement.

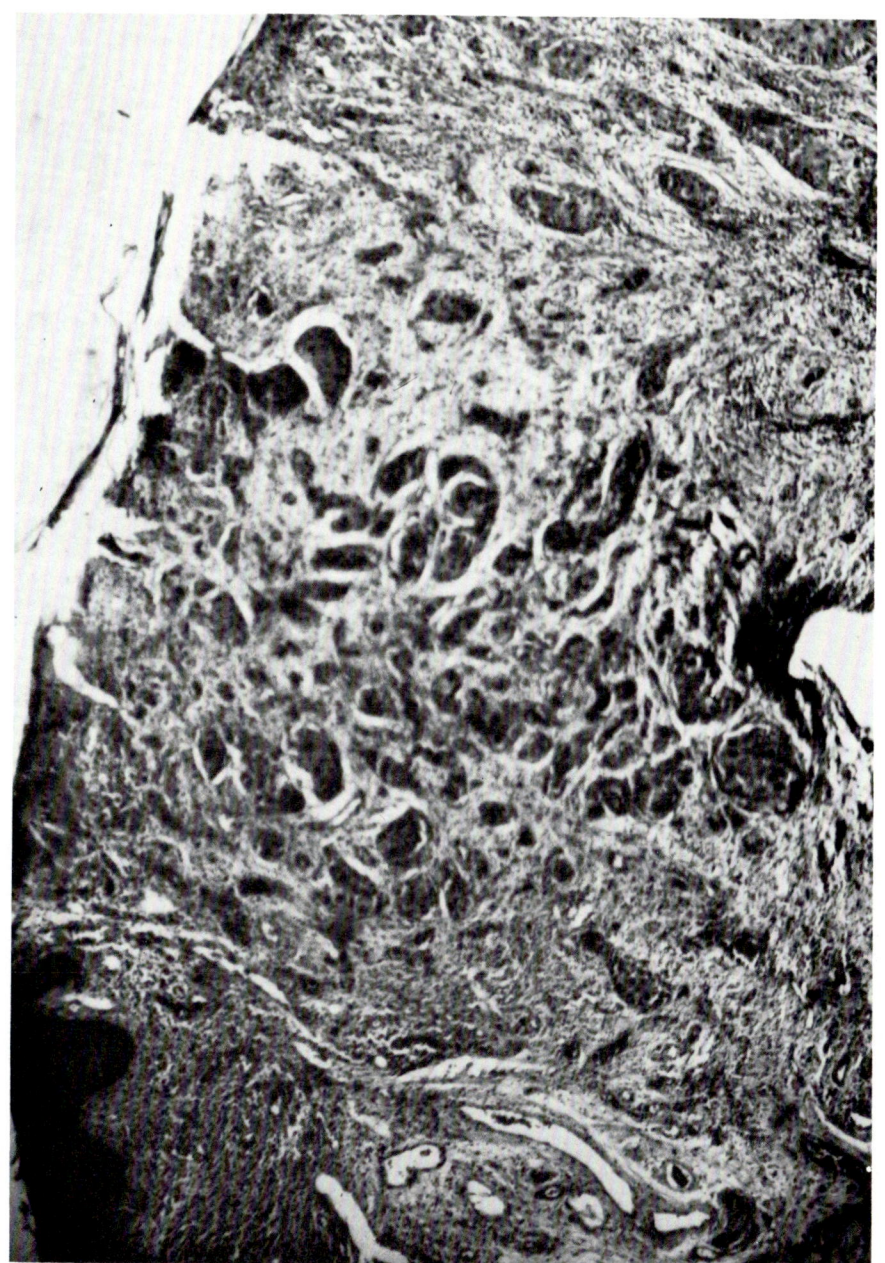

Fig. 2-17 Carcinoma of the cervix with invasion limited to 3-4 mm but with confluent tongues of disease. This should be considered true invasion and not treated conservatively. 40x

43

1. *Exophytic lesions* originating on the portio vaginalis often grow to form large, friable polypoid masses (Fig. 2-18). Such tumors arising in the endocervix produce a concentric enlargement of the cervix, which may reach enormous proportions and fill the entire pelvis. These endocervical masses are more likely to result in residual pelvic disease and distant metastases than are other clinical varieties.

2. *Infiltrative tumors* tend to show little visible ulceration but may present as a stony hard cervix, which regresses very slowly under external radiation.

3. *Ulcerative lesions* can erode the entire cervix, replacing the cervix and upper vaginal vault by a large crater (Fig. 2-19) associated with infection and discharge.

Routes of Spread (Fig. 2-20)

The main routes of spread of carcinoma of the cervix are as follows:

1. Into the vaginal mucosa, extending microscopically down beyond visible or palpable disease.

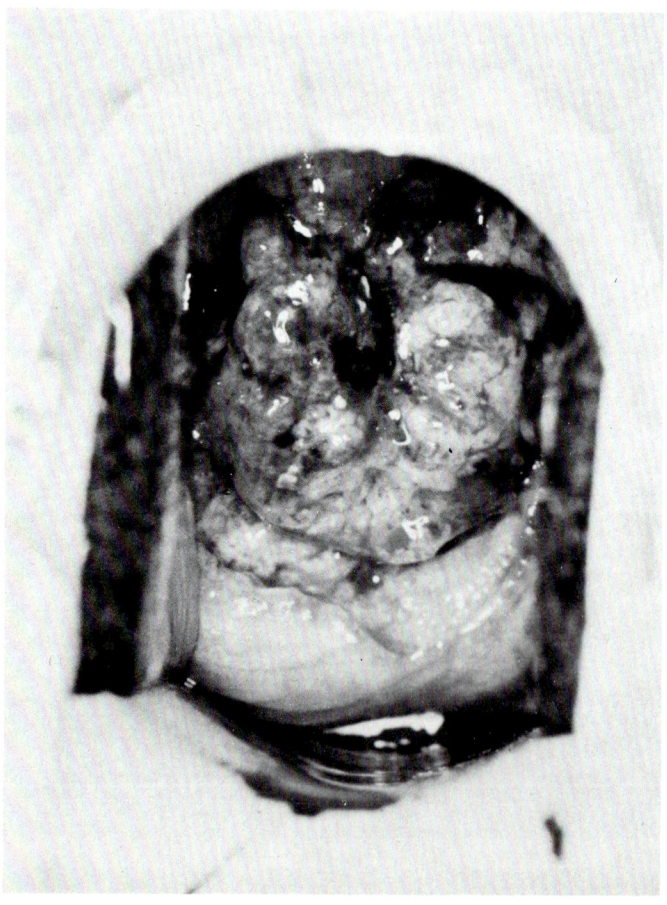

Fig. 2-18 Large exophytic squamous cell carcinoma of the cervix. (Courtesy of William Creasman, M. D., Director of Gynecologic Oncology, Duke University, School of Medicine).

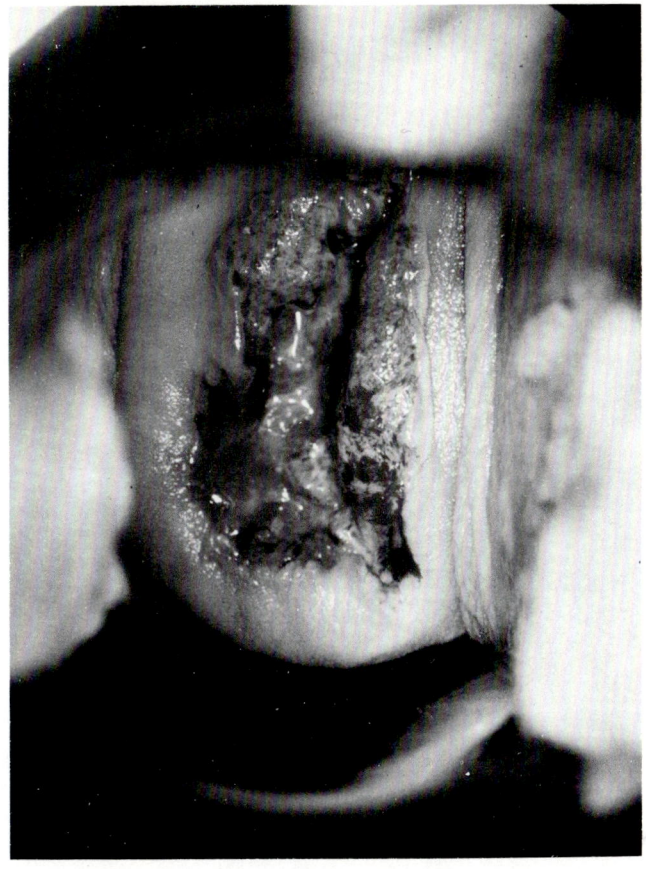

Fig. 2-19 Ulcerative squamous cell carcinoma of the cervix. (Courtesy of William Creasman, M.D., Director of Gynecologic Oncology, Duke University, School of Medicine.)

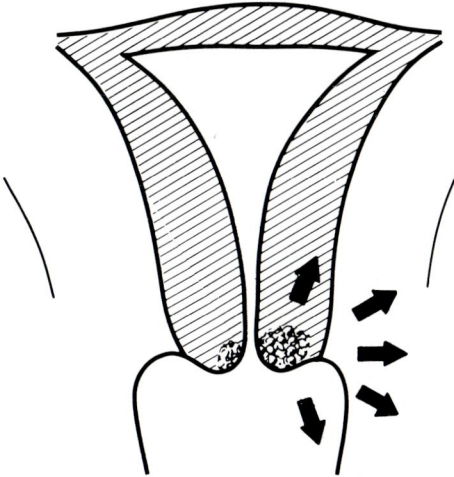

Fig. 2-20 Routes of spread of cervical cancer to myometrium, parametrium, and vagina.

2. Into the myometrium of the lower uterine segment and corpus, particularly in lesions originating in the endocervix (Fig. 2-21).

3. Into the paracervical lymphatics and from there to the most commonly involved lymph nodes (Figs. 2-22 and 2-23). Two groups have been described by Henriksen.

Primary Group

a. The parametrial nodes, which are the small lymph nodes traversing the parametria.

b. The paracervical or ureteral nodes, located above the uterine artery where it crosses the ureter.

c. The obturator or hypogastric nodes surrounding the obturator vessels and nerves.

d. The hypogastric nodes, which course along the hypogastric vein near its junction with the external iliac vein.

e. The external iliac nodes, which are a group of six to eight nodes that tend to be uniformly larger than the nodes of the other iliac groups.

f. The sacral nodes, which are originally included in the secondary group of nodes.

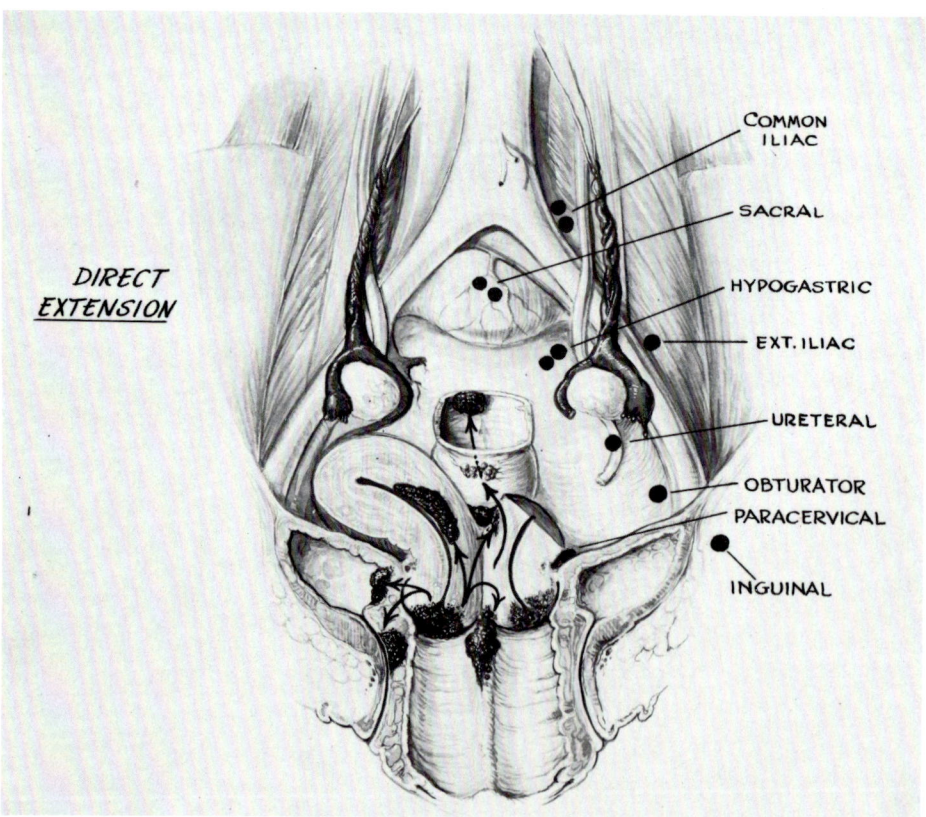

Fig. 2-21 Pathways of direct extension of cervical cancer. (Courtesy of E. Henriksen, M.D., Clinical Professor of Ob/Gyn, University of Southern California School of Medicine, Lymph nodes and lymph channels of pelvis, in *Surgical Treatment of Cancer of the Cervix*, Grune & Stratton, New York, 1954.)

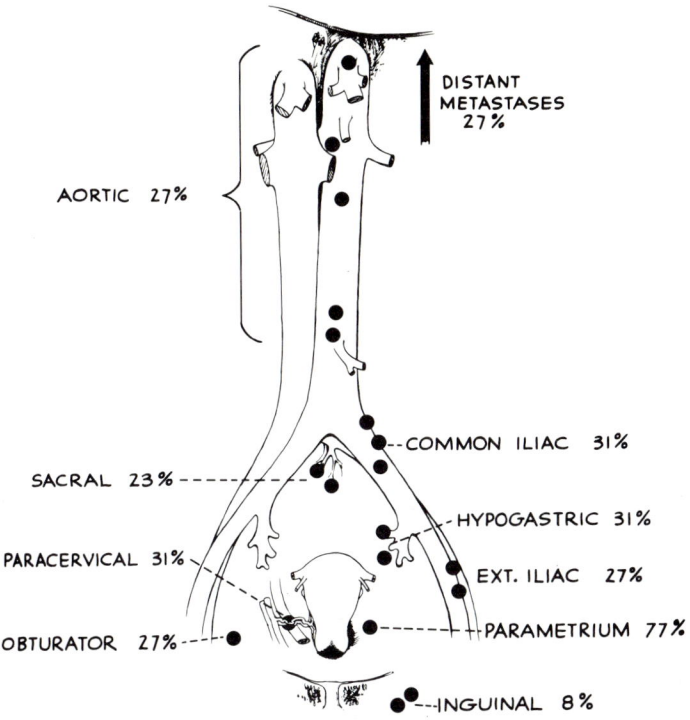

Fig. 2-22 Percentage involvement of regional lymph nodes in untreated patients with carcinoma of the cervix. (Courtesy of E. Henriksen, M.D., Clinical Professor of Ob/Gyn, University of Southern California School of Medicine, The lymphatic spread of Carcinoma of the cervix and of the body of the uterus, *Am. J. Obstet. Gynecol.* **58:**924, 1949.)

Secondary Group

    a. The common iliac nodes.

    b. The inguinal nodes, which consist of the deep and superficial femoral lymph nodes.

    c. The paraaortic nodes.

    4. Direct extension into the parametria, which may reach to the obturator fascia and the wall of the true pelvis.

Pathology

Carcinomas of the uterine cervix are squamous in about 90% of the cases and are generally moderately undifferentiated tumors. Less than 10% of cervical lesions are adenocarcinomas. These probably have a radiosensitivity similar to that of squamous carcinomas, although hysterectomy has often been added to radiation therapy because of the propensity of adenocarcinomas to spread into the corpus of the uterus and the myometrium at the level of the uterine isthmus.

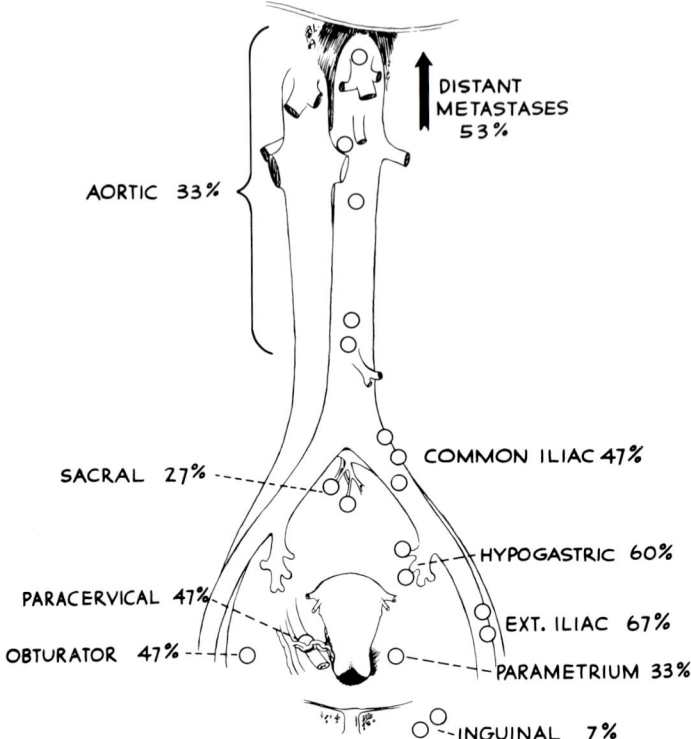

Fig. 2-23 Percentage involvement of regional lymph nodes in treated patients with cancer of the cervix. (Courtesy of E. Henriksen, M.D., Clinical Professor of Ob/Gyn, University of Southern California School of Medicine, The lymphatic spread of carcinoma of the cervix and of the body of the uterus," *Am. J. Obstet. Gynecol.* **58**:924, 1949.)

Lymphatics

One of the major routes of spread is into the paracervical lymphatics and from there through lymphatic pathways to the regional lymph nodes (Fig. 2-24). Only the obturator (principal) node lying at the pelvic wall near the obturator nerve, and the hypogastric nodes clustered around the hypogastric artery actually lie within the true pelvis. Commonly involved regional nodes include the external and common iliac nodes along the distribution of the external iliac and common iliac arteries, presacral nodes, and low para-aortic nodes. Lymph nodes lying in the obturator canal are very rarely involved.

   The incidence of involved regional nodes is directly related to the bulk of the tumor. *Early* Stage I tumors show a frequency of less than 5% nodal involvement, whereas large Stage III tumors may have lymph node involvement in 40-50% of the cases. In a series of over 400 patients at the M. D. Anderson Hospital, pelvic lymphadenectomy after radiation therapy revealed 3% positive nodes in Stage I and under 20% in Stage III. This striking decrease indicates the efficacy of external radiotherapy in the control of involved lymph nodes. Lymphadenectomy after irradiation was not found to be useful in the control of positive lymph nodes and was abandoned because of its high morbidity.

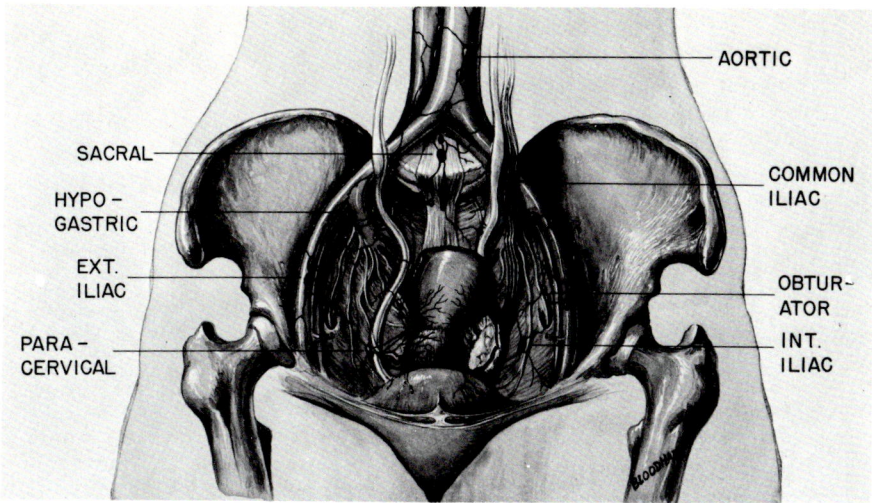

Fig. 2-24 Lymphatic drainage pathways of the cervix. (Courtesy of E. Henriksen, M.D., Clinical Professor of Ob/Gyn, University of Southern California School of Medicine, Distribution of metastases in Stage I carcinoma of the cervix, *Am. J. Obstet. Gynecol.* **80**:919, 1960.)

International Classification of Cancer of the Cervix

Stage 0   Carcinoma in situ, intra-epithelial carcinoma.

Cases of Stage 0 should not be included in any therapeutic statistics.

Invasive carcinoma

Stage I   Carcinoma strictly confined to the cervix (extension to the corpus should be disregarded).

Stage Ia   Microinvasive carcinoma (early stromal invasion).

Stage Ib   All other cases of Stage I (Fig. 2-25). Occult cancer should be marked "occ".

Stage II   The carcinoma extends beyond the cervix but has not extended on to the pelvic wall. The carcinoma involves the vagina, but not the lower third.

Stage IIa   No obvious parametrial involvement. (Fig. 2-26)

Stage IIb   Obvious parametrial involvement. (Fig. 2-27)

Stage III   The carcinoma has extended on to the pelvic wall. On rectal examination there is no cancer-free space between the tumour and the pelvic wall.
The tumour involves the lower third of the vagina.
All cases with a hydro-nephrosis or non-functioning kidney.

Stage IIIa   No extension on to the pelvic wall. (Fig. 2-28)

Stage IIIb   Extension on to the pelvic wall and/or hydro-nephrosis or non-functioning kidney. (Fig. 2-29)

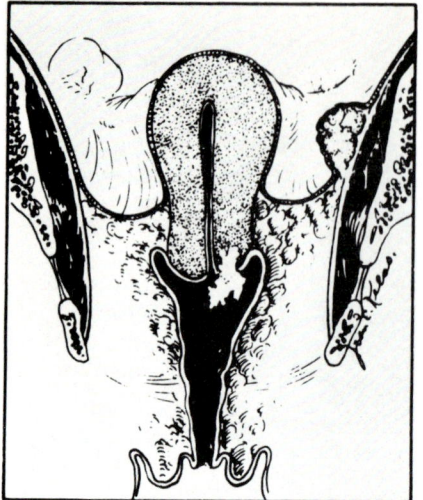

Fig. 2-25 Cancer of the cervix, Stage Ib.

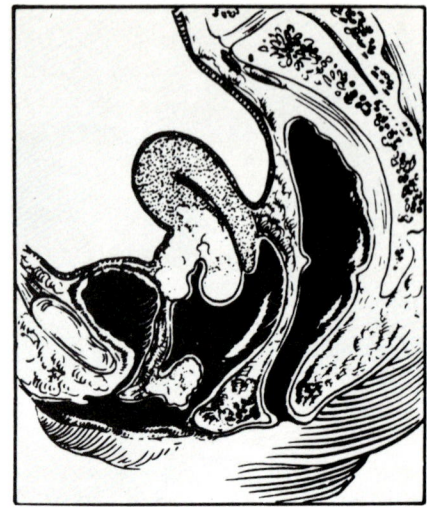

Fig. 2-26 Cancer of the cervix, Stage IIa.

Stage IV   The carcinoma has extended beyond the true pelvis or has clinically involved the mucosa of the bladder or rectum. A bullous oedema as such does not permit a case to be allotted to Stage IV.

Stage IVa   Spread of the growth to adjacent organs. (Fig. 2-30 and 2-31)

Stage IVb   Spread to distant organs.

Diagnostic Studies

Diagnostic studies permitted in staging include clinical examination, examination under anesthesia where indicated, colposcopy, hysteroscopy, cystoscopy, proctosigmoidoscopy,

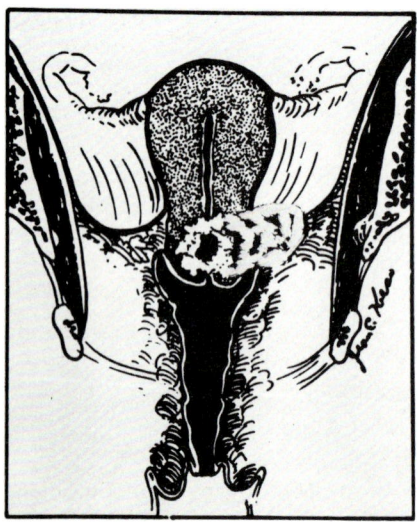

Fig. 2-27 Cancer of the cervix, Stage IIb.

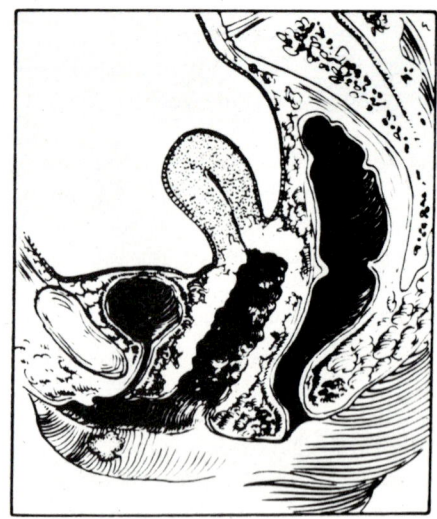

Fig. 2-28 Cancer of the cervix, Stage IIIa.

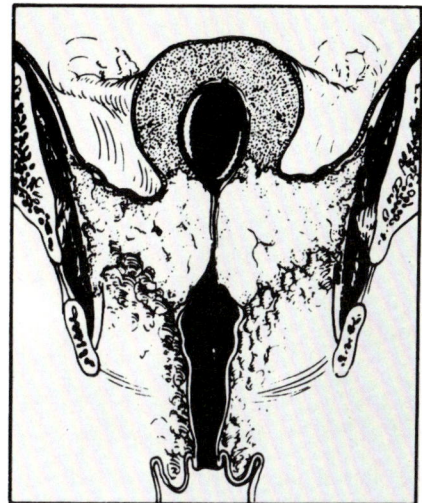

Fig. 2-29 Cancer of the cervix, Stage IIIb.

routine x-ray examination (chest, IVP, metastatic series), and cervical biopsies even as extensive as cervical conization.

Routine Studies for Patients with Cervical Carcinoma

1. Laboratory studies
   CBC, platelet count, BUN, creatinine, protein, SGOT, SGPT, bilirubin
   If patient over 35, ECG
   Pap smear

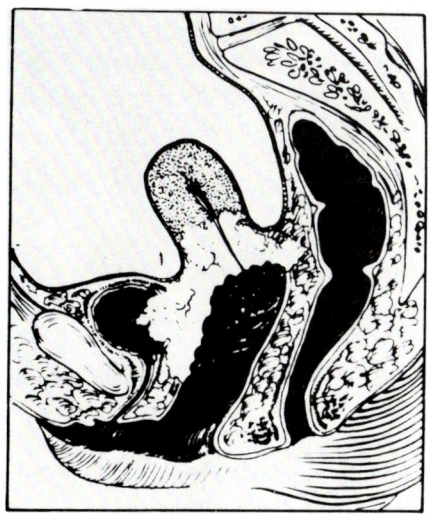

Fig. 2-30 Cancer of the cervix, Stage IVa (bladder involvement).

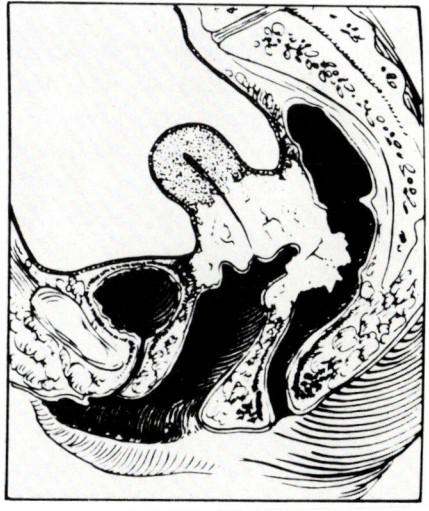

Fig. 2-31 Cancer of the cervix, Stage IVa (rectal involvement).

2. X-ray studies
   Chest (posterior-anterior and lateral)
   IVP
   Lymphangiogram on patients with bulky Stages I-IV
   (This test should not be ordered for patients with severe diabetes, severe pulmonary disease or during pregnancy)
3. Other studies
   Cystoscopy
   Sigmoidoscopy
   Adequate biopsies of ectocervix and endocervix
   Careful pelvic examination
   Colposcopy

Clinical staging cannot be altered once treatment has begun or after the exact extent of the tumor has been surgically determined, since this would prevent intercomparison of techniques between institutions. The patient may, however, be treated in whatever manner is appropriate in view of all the findings.

Treatment Planning

The patient is initially seen by the radiotherapist and gynecologist together, and treatment is planned. The patient's general condition is brought as nearly as possible to the normal state by correction of nutritional deficiencies, anemia, and associated diseases.

Lesions of limited extent in Stages I and IIa are considered locally radiocurable and are primarily treated by intracavitary radium therapy. Parametrial irradiation is added only when the incidence of regional node metastases warrants such treatment, and when it is desirable to augment the dose to the paracervical triangle.

Larger lesions, Stage IIb and greater (or large Stage Ib), are treated initially by external radiotherapy. Shrinkage of large exophytic or endocervical lesions by external radiotherapy renders subsequent intracavitary radium more effective. Radium therapy should be fractionated over several weeks in order to provide (a) maximum tumor shrinkage, (b) optimum dose distribution, and (c) improved normal tissue tolerance.

External radiotherapy is also useful in the presence of distorted local anatomy, such as the following:

1. Narrow vaginal vault.
2. Asymmetric fornices.
3. Tumor invasion of fornices and/or vaginal wall.
4. Asymmetric lesions, such as those confined to one cervical lip or cases where the cervix is retracted laterally to one fornix.

Guidelines to combination of external radiotherapy and radium are given in Table 2-2. Massive tumors may require the taking of greater risk in order to control them.

Radium Techniques and Dosimetry

1. The steep fall-off in the radiation intensity surrounding the radioactive sources (described by the inverse square law) precludes the selection of one or two points in the pelvis to specify the dose.

2. A minimum tumor dose must be deliver to *all portions* of the tumor, with as much contribution to the paracervical tissues and regional lymphatics as is possible.

3. Point A (Fig. 2-32) is not superimposed on any definite pelvic structures and is an unreliable guide to radium therapy. The original description states that point A is located 2 cm from the midline of the cervical canal and 2 cm superior to the lateral vaginal fornix; point B is 3 cm lateral to point A, or 5 cm from the midline along the same lateral axis. Since the exact position of the lateral vaginal fornix cannot be assigned on x-ray films, the point at which the tandem enters the external os is usually the source from which 2 cm can be measured superiorly to calculate the lateral axis line. The external os can usually be identified on x-ray films since a flange or other metal device is set there at the time of vaginal packing. Here the difficulty with the concepts of points A and B lies in the necessity of calculating dosages with regard to the radiopaque applicators and not the cancer itself. These points fall mathematically in a predetermined arrangement around the applicators, which may have little if any relevance to the actual distribution of the malignancy. In bulky lesions or cone-shaped vaginal vaults in which the radium system has been displaced downward, point A may be in the paracolpos instead of the paracervical triangle.

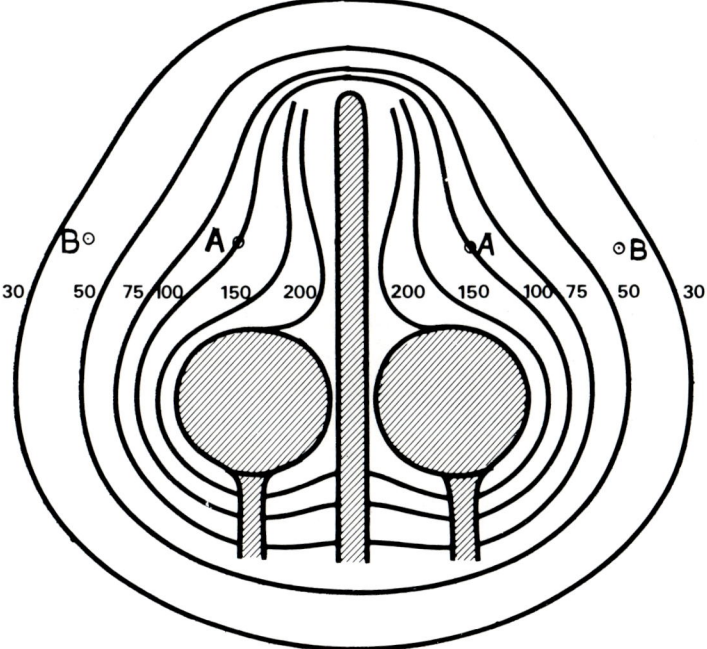

Fig. 2-32   Isodose curves surrounding a typical Manchester type radium applicator with points A and B noted.

4. The dose at point B is representative only of the obturator node dose, and then only with radium systems high in the pelvis.

5. The dose at points A and B is not closely correlated to bladder and rectal complications.

6. Milligram-hours is used as the variable in arranging the table of maximal doses for treatment since the dose on the periphery of a 10 cm sphere centered on the center of gravity of the radium system approximates the radium contribution to the pelvis, with which external radiation is combined. This dose is approximated by the relationship

$$\text{Dose} = \frac{(\text{milligram-hours})\,(8.25)}{25}$$

in which milligram-hours is the only variable.

7. Combinations of milligram-hours of radium and external radiotherpy (Table 2-2) are developed empirically by analyses of results and complications with this system (Fletcher, 1973), and cannot easily be applied to different systems of vaginal-uterine applicators.

8. Localization films (Figs. 2-33 and 2-34) taken after each radium insertion provide the basic data for a hand-drawn isodose curve in a plane passing through the internal os and the center of the colpostats, which provides dose information regarding the lower uterine segment and paracervical area.

9. Computer dosimetric calculations are helpful to evaluate the adequacy of the radium insertions and assist in adjusting external therapy to compensate for defects in the radium application.

10. The contribution of the radium system to the regional lymph nodes may be determined more accurately from a lymph node plane especially chosen to correspond to the position of the external iliac, common iliac, and low para-aortic lymph nodes as determined by lymphangiography and surgical exploration.

11. The following facts have been determined from computer dosimetry and comparative direct measurements made at laparotomy:

a. Most of the dose to the hypogastric, iliac, and lower aortic nodes comes from the uterine tandem.

b. The vaginal radium, if located high in the fornices, may contribute significantly to the obturator and external iliac nodes but not to the common iliac nodes.

c. The younger the patient, the roomier the vault, and the more distensible the tissues, the higher the radium system lies within the pelvis and the better the contribution to the iliac, hypogastric, and low aortic nodes.

Radium Applicators (Figs. 2-35a and 2-35b)

Experience in the design and use of intrauterine tandems and vaginal applicators has shown that flexibility is desirable in order to adapt the radium to various anatomical and clinical situations.

1. Long intrauterine *tandems* can be used to correct ante- or retroflexed uteri. The high and posterior position increases the dose to the iliac, hypogastric, and low common

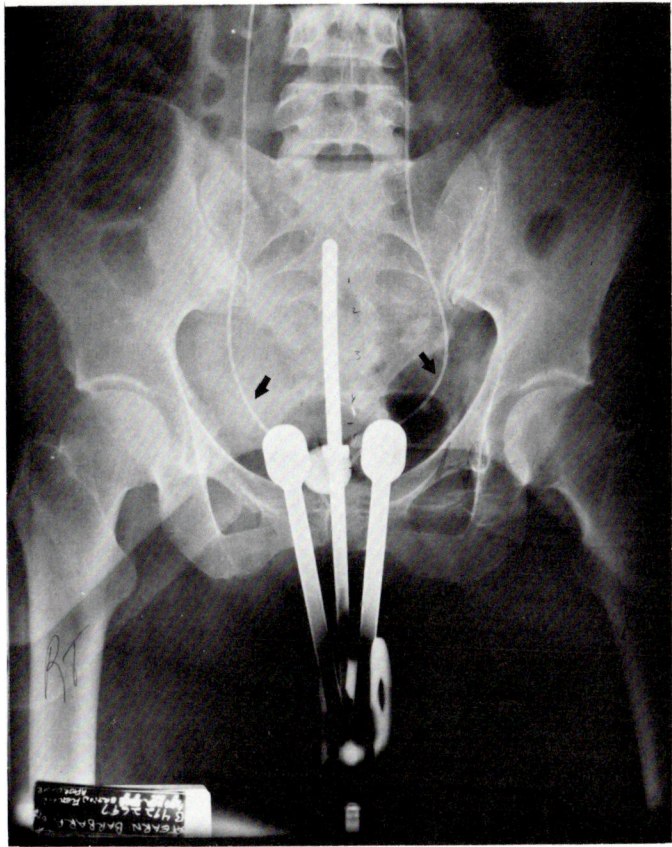

Fig. 2-33 Anterior-posterior view of the abdomen in a patient with a Fletcher-Suit radium system in place along with ureteral catheters (arrows). Hypaque has been placed in the Foley catheter balloon, and the silver seeds can be seen at a depth of 0.5 cm with the cervix. This provides information about the anatomical relationship of the ureters and bladder to the radium system. (Courtesy of A. Robert Kagan, M.D. Chief of Department of Radiotherapy, Southern California Permanente Medical Group.)

iliac lymph nodes. The entire uterine canal should be lined with radium sources to increase the contribution at any given point in the paracervical triangle.

2. *Vaginal colpostats* should be as large as will comfortably fit, since this increases the dose at a distance from the applicator without giving an abnormally high surface dose.

3. Other varieties of vaginal applicators may be of use in special situations, such as plastic vaginal cylinders fitted over the long tandems so the sources can be placed longitudinally in the vaginal part of the tandem, or specially designed applicators to treat the entire vagina.

4. At the time of the radium insertion, silver seeds are placed in the cervix to visualize it on localization radiographs. The tandem should be equidistant from the vaginal ovoids and bisect their height. To avoid any local cold spot, the distal end of the endocervical source should not overlap the edge of the ovoids. If the ovoids are widely separated, an additional 5 mg source may be placed in the tandem between them. A keel is placed on

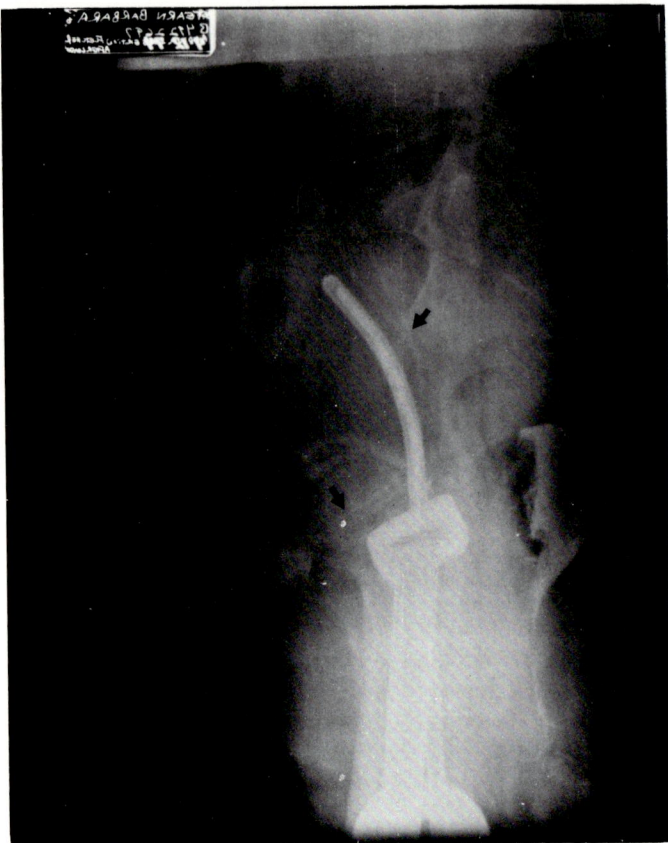

Fig. 2-34 Lateral view of the abdomen, again illustrating the relationship of the bladder and ureters (arrows) to the radium system. Barium is within the rectum and emphasizes its proximity. (Courtesy of A. Robert Kagan, M.D. Chief of Department of Radiotherapy, Southern California Permanente Medical Group.)

the long tandem and fits between the ovoids so that, when vaginal packing is completed, the system is stabilized. For several years, in some institutions, both the intrauterine tandem and the colpostats have been afterloaded, thus affording the operating personnel ample time to carefully place the applicators. The active radium sources are loaded into the applicators on the ward after the localization films have been carefully checked. Since the actual loading takes only about 30 seconds, exposure to personnel is at a minimum.

5. The usual radium loading for tandems are 15-10-10 or 15-10 mg, although these may be modified according to the clinical situation. Endocervical tumors commonly have increased uterine radium loading, such as 15-15-10 or even 20-15-10 mg.

6. Vaginal ovoids are loaded with 15-15, 20-20, and 25-25 mg for 2.0, 2.5, and 3.0 cm sizes, respectively (Fletcher-Suit system), although these loadings may also be varied according to the clinical situation.

7. Two 72 hour radium insertions separated by 2 weeks to allow for tumor shrinkage and improved normal tissue tolerance are usual. Supplementary external irradiation to the parametria is given between and after radium insertions.

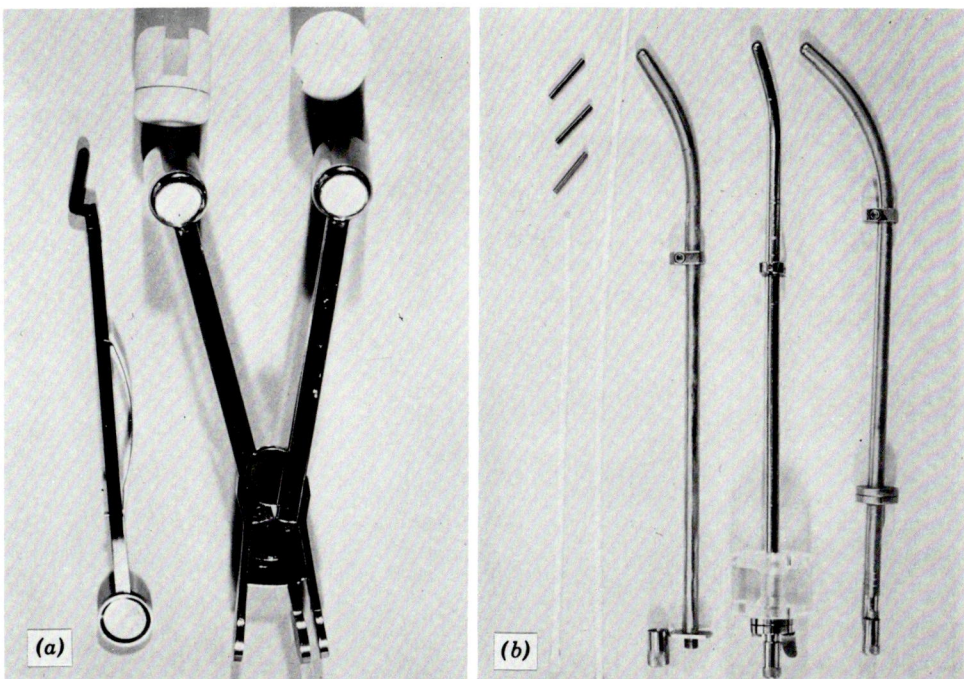

Figs. 2-35a and 2-35b Fletcher-Suit radium applicators, afterloading type. Note the Lucite caps to increase the size of the ovoids should the vagina accommodate them and the varying curves on three different tandems.

8. Guidelines to radium treatment are shown in Table 2-2 but must be modified according to such factors as patient age, tumor anatomy, and vaginal vault.

9. With the use of afterloading long tandems, severe ante- or retroflexion of the tandem is avoided, and accordingly direct measurements of bladder and rectal doses with microsources are not necessary. Careful evaluation of the localization films will reveal a malposition or perforation if it has not been detected at the time of insertion of the applicator.

External Radiotherapy

1. *Whole pelvis irradiation* (Fig. 2-36) with supervoltage equipment utilizes a 15-18 × 15-18 cm portal to cover the primary tumor and regional nodes. The height of the portal is always at least 15 cm, although it may be extended if there is lymphangiographic evidence of involved iliac or low para-aortic lymph nodes.

A radiopaque marker can be utilized in the taking of portal films to provide an adequate inferior margin around the tumor.

For bulky tumors, whole pelvis external radiotherapy is used before radium treatment to shrink them and provide better dose distribution from radium therapy. In situations of poor geometry due to a narrow vaginal vault or asymmetric massive tumors, such external radiotherapy may be the mainstay of the treatment, and in some Stage IIIb and Stage IV lesions it is used entirely alone.

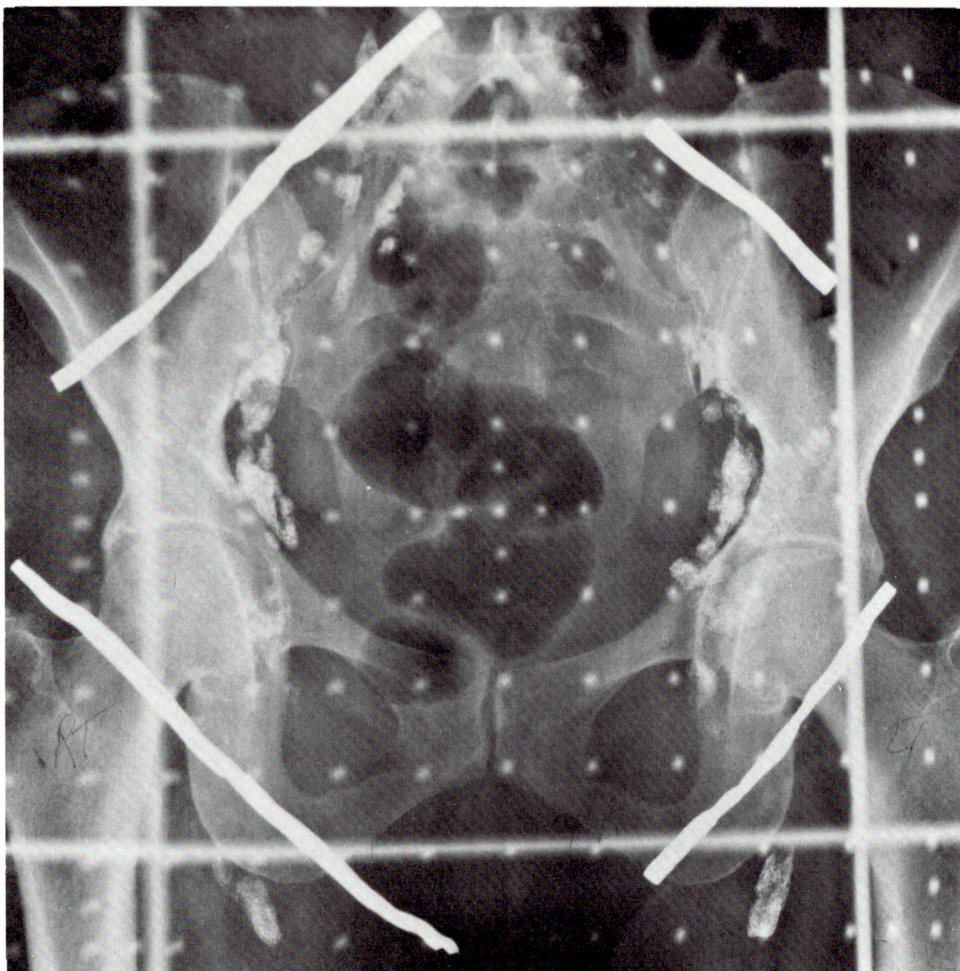

Fig. 2-36 Whole pelvis field on a simulator. Note that the corners are excluded to reduce volume. The patient received a lymphangiogram before therapy, and the pelvic nodes are visible.

2. *Supplementary parametrial irradiation* (Fig. 2-37) is used to augment the radium dose to the regional lymphatics and paracervical area. Supervoltage machines are utilized with approximatedly a 15 × 15 cm field. A 10 cm high lead shield is placed in the midline to protect the bladder and rectum or is shifted laterally according to the position of the radium. The width of this shielding at midpelvis is either 3 or 4 cm, depending on the isodose distribution of the radium insertion.

Hemorrhage

1. Transvaginal cone radiotherapy with 140-250 kV is of use to halt hemorrhage in exophytic lesions and to initiate rapid shrinkage of the lesion before starting on whole pelvis irradiation. The usual dose is 1000 rads, given in two daily fractions of 500 rads each.

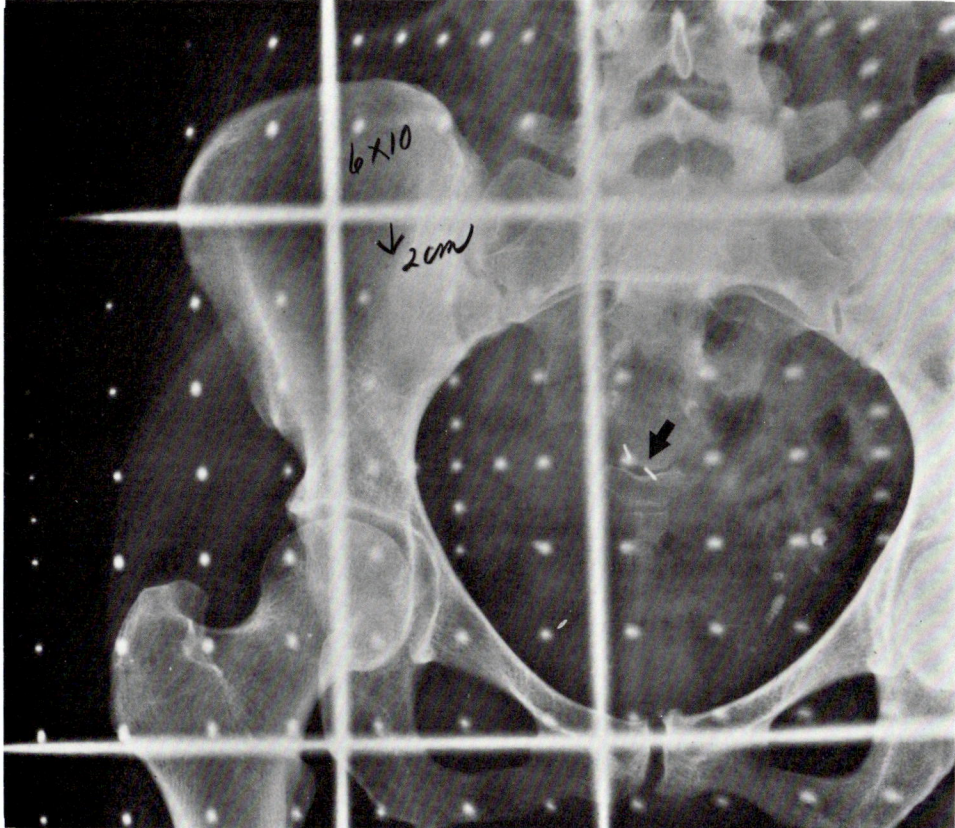

Fig. 2-37 Parametrial fields can be used to supplement the dose on one side of the pelvis, where bulky disease may exist. Silver seeds (arrow) identify the cervix and the general area of the bladder and rectum.

2. If transvaginal irradiation is not available, three daily pulse doses (megavoltage-external irradiation) of 400 rads each through a reduced pelvic field (10 × 10 cm) directed at the midline will produce a similar effect. Whereas the transvaginal dose may be disregarded in calculating the sum dose, this external radiation must be considered in the determination of bladder and rectal tolerance.

Adenocarcinoma

1. Myometrial invasion is probably the cause for the alleged radioresistance of adenocarcinoma of the cervix. Enlargement of the endocervix places disease in the myometrium too far from the radium sources for adequate dosage. After myometrial invasion adenocarcinoma spreads through the wall of the uterus to the serosa and thence to other pelvic structures.

2. Lesions limited to the cervix are treated similarly to squamous cell carcinomas. Local radium therapy is accentuated because of the endophytic nature of these lesions.

3. For larger lesions, radiation treatment is reduced slightly and a conservative hysterectomy added to remove residual cancer in the myometrium.

Cancer of the Cervix and Pregnancy

Carcinoma of the cervix complicates pregnancy in from 0.005 to 0.2% of cases, depending on which report is reviewed. The extent of the cancer and the duration of the pregnancy must be considered in the management of cervical carcinoma complicated by pregnancy. Despite many tales to the contrary, the effect of pregnancy on cancer of the cervix has never been demonstrated to be very great. The suggestion that pregnancy accelerates the growth of the tumor has not been substantiated. Trauma at parturition may squeeze viable cells into the vascular system and thereby increase metastatic spread, but again, this has not been documented in the literature. Metastases depend more on the biologic quality of the disease than on the pregnant state.

The treatment of cancer of the cervix in the pregnant uterus will depend on several factors, including stage of disease, duration of pregnancy, religious conviction of patient and family, desire of the mother for a child, and background of the physician, as well as medical problems. During any trimester a radical surgical procedure is, of course, applicable to Stage I and early Stage II cases. Desire for preservation of the pregnancy often requires waiting several weeks to ensure reasonable viability of the fetus. It is usually not recommended, however, that patients in the first and early second trimester be allowed to continue the pregnancy.

Before 24 weeks of gestation, treatment with irradiation therapy can begin immediatedly after the diagnosis is made. The pregnancy is disregarded, and whole pelvis irradiation is begun. This usually will cause demise of the fetus and a resulting abortion by the fourth or fifth week of treatment. If abortion is not induced, excision of the cancer by means of an extended hysterectomy or surgical evacuation of the uterus is indicated. Once the uterus is evacuated, radium therapy can commence.

After the 24th week of gestation, therapy is usually delayed until fetal viability is reached. Cesarean section can be carried out as soon as is consistent with pediatric and obstetric indications. If a radical hysterectomy with pelvic lymphadenectomy is not performed at the time of the cesarean section, whole pelvis irradiation begins immediately after the surgical wound has healed. These patients later can receive intracavitary radium upon completion of whole pelvis irradiation. In general, patients in whom cesarean section has been carried out can follow the same basic treatment plans used for cancer of the cervix in a nonpregnant patient.

Complications

1. In an anaysis of 1331 Stage I and Stage II lesions (from M. D. Anderson Hospital) treated by irradiation only, there has been a very low incidence of complications. Eighty-three patients showed some type of complication, of which only 21 were severe (fistulae, sigmoiditis, ileitis, or fatal vault necrosis). Of these 21 patients, 15 received 4000 rads or more whole pelvis irradiation because of extensive central tumors.

2. Previous analysis of 831 patients from the same institution receiving 4000 rads or more of whole pelvis irradiation revealed 46 severe bowel complications (fistulae or severe sigmoiditis). The incidence of bowel complication increases proportionately with a greater amount of external irradiation. Experience has shown that the incidence of complications may rise rapidly with small increments in dose.

3. Ureteral strictures secondary to radiation alone are rare, as are marked cystitis or bladder ulcers.

TABLE 2-2   RADIATION TREATMENT OF INVASIVE
CERVICAL CANCER—SUGGESTED MAXIMA

Stage	Whole Pelvis (rads)	Radium (mg-hours)	Parametrial (rads)
Ia microinvasive	0	8,000 (2 appl.)	0
Ib (small)	2,000	8,000 (2 appl.)	2,000
Ib (large)	4,000	6,000 (2 appl.)	0
IIa	2,000	8,000 (2 appl.)	2,000
IIb	4,000	6,000 (2 appl.)	0
IIIa	4,000	7,000 (2 appl.) or 4,000 (1 appl.) and interstitial implant	0
IIIb	5,000—6,000	4,000 (1 appl.) 5,000 (2 appl.)	Possible 1,000 rad boost on involved side
IVa	6,000	4,000 (1 appl.) 5,000 (2 appl.)	Possible 1,000 rad boost on involved side
IVb	1,000 rad pulse 2 times, 1 week apart	Palliation	

Modified from Fletcher, 1973.

4.   Rectal ulcers have rarely occurred except when protruding sources in the vagina and afterloading tandem were heavily loaded in the presence of extensive vaginal disease. Separate tandem and ovoid insertions are now used.

5.   Very rarely, vault necrosis is noted; this usually heals with conservative treatment. Occasionally this may be severe in the presence of extraradical treatment given for massive central disease.

A more detailed discussion of radiation injuries is given in Section 2-6.

Summary

1.   Carcinoma of the cervix is locally radiocurable. Before radioresistance can be claimed, treatment techniques must be carefully analyzed to show that local treatment was adequate.

2.   Radiosensitivity of carcinoma of the cervix depends on the size and vasularity of the tumor. Exophytic lesions with good tissue oxygenation are controllable by radiation. Large massive tumors or infiltrating tumors with central anoxia may be more resistant.

3.   Because of the steep dose gradient with radium therapy, correlation of exact tumor dose with tumor control is difficult. A recent analysis by Castro et al (1970) of 108 cases treated entirely by external radiotherapy shows a dose response curve in lesions of

moderate extent with the highest local control at 7000 rads. Massive, advanced tumors, on the other hand, show a similar control rate at a dose of 6000 or 7000 rads.

4. Evaluation of any treatment for carcinoma of the cervix must include consideration of the following facts:

    a. Basic dosage determination.
    b. Beam charcteristics.
    c. Precise description of tumor dose determinations.
    d. Dose-time fractionation schedule.
    e. Irradiated tissue volume.
    f. Exact position of portals.

Thus critical analysis of the radiation treatment plan is needed in order to establish basic treatment techniques, compare local control and survival rates, and evaluate radiation tolerance and complications. Established guidelines of combinations of external and intracavitary radiation have been found to represent normal tissue tolerance limits in various situations according to the extent of disease. These must not be followed in a regimented fashion since careful individualization of each case will result in the best treatment plan. Radical alteration of established therapy techniques must be avoided, however, since the threshold of complications as well as tumor recurrence is extremely close.

2-5 SURGERY VERSUS RADIOTHERAPY IN THE TREATMENT OF INVASIVE SQUAMOUS CELL CARCINOMA OF THE CERVIX

Stage I lesions are of particular importance in cancer of the cervix because with better detection techniques and wider use of the Pap smear they are now found in more than one half of the cases in the country. In 1959, for example, in New York State, excluding New York City, there were 749 cases of invasive cancer of the cervix. Of these, 424 or 57% were Stage I. Although advanced lesions are quite common at university hospitals where large numbers of indigent patients are seen, in general, early lesions are detected.

Many institutions consider radiotherapy to be the standard treatment for this disease. However, surgery is used in various localitites for any of the following reasons: (1) under the impression that results are as good as they are with radiotherapy; (2) in the hope that surgery will control the disease in those who cannot be cured by radiotherapy; (3) in an effort to obtain anatomical information about the disease; and (4) as a surgical exercise or educational measure.

Let us examine some of the comparative figures in terms of 5 year cure rate, applicability of the technique, and complications.

Cure Rate

Unfortunately, no control series is available in which radiotherapy or surgery alone has been randomly assigned to patients with Stage I lesions in the same clinic. Twombly and Taylor (1954) compared the results of treatment with radiation plus surgery to those for radiation alone in Stages I and II, randomly assigned, obtaining 5 year salvage rates of

58% (25 of 43) and 79% (31 of 44), respectively. Newton (1954) compared 15 surgical patients with 15 matched irradiated patients and found 13 living and well in each group at the average follow-up of 26 months.

We are, therefore, left with the task of comparing the results of treatment of this disease by equally competent surgical and radiotherapeutic teams in different institutions. Currie (1971) reported the results of 552 radical operations for cancer of the cervix in a 35 year period at his institution. His 5 year survival rates were as follows:

Stage I	189 cases,	86.3%
Stage IIa	103 cases,	75.0%
Stage IIb	78 cases,	58.9%
Other stages	41 cases,	34.1%

It is interesting to compare these figures with the results for patients treated by radiotherapy at M. D. Anderson Hospital and Tumor Institute in Houston, Texas. For 2000 patients treated in a 25 year period, the 5 year cure rates are as follows:

Stage I	91.5%
Stage IIa	83.5%
Stage IIb	66.5%
Stage IIIa	45.0%
Stage IIIb	36.0%
Stage IV	14.0%

Applicability

It must be stated at this point that in all surgical series there is selectivity. Obviously there are many patients who, for medical or other reasons, are not candidates for a radical operative procedure. Radiotherapy on the other hand, takes all comers and most radiotherapeutic series are unselected; this difference must be kept in mind at all times when comparing survivals.

Thus virtually all Stage I cases can be treated by irradiation; however, surgery cannot be applied to those whose general condition (too old, fat, or infirm) rules out this technique. Some series, such as that reported by Meigs (1954), show an operability rate for Stage I as low as 45-60% in the years reported.

The Case for Surgery

It is evident that surgical intervention is the most decisive means of cure, whereas radiotherapy has a wider range of effective application. If the malignant tumor can be removed entirely along with a margin of normal tissue, then obviously it cannot recur. With radiotherapy there is some chance that viable cancer cells will remain. However, operation ensures control of the primary growth only for patients whose lesions are small enough to be encompassed along with an extra margin of normal tissue. Both the physician and the patient feel more secure if the site of disease is excised and the pathologic examination indicates that the boundaries are free of cancer cells.

The true state of spread, which is determined by study of the operative specimen, is never known when irradiation is the treatment. When the true state of the disease is known, the treatment can be prescribed more accurately. Operation identifies both early and late disease with a precision not possible by clincial study of the patient without laparotomy. Lacking this knowledge, the radiotherapist is doubtful in some cases and may use higher doses than necessary, thus subjecting the patient to needless risk of radionecrosis. Clinical examples are the postinflammatory changes caused by prior surgery, salpingitis, or endometritis. Fibrosis and adhesions pull the tube and ovary low, where they can be fixed behind the broad ligament and produce induration and nodularity of the parametrium, which simulate cancer extension. The radiotherapist will treat such patients intensively as if they had cancer, unless laparotomy is performed in advance to correct the mistake.

A radical hysterectomy performed on an otherwise healthy young woman whose postoperative course is uneventful is, in terms of recovery from disease, a rewarding experience for both the physician and the patient. The patient is rid of her cancer and recovers sooner than if treated by irradiation. The ovaries continue to function, and her vaginal membrane is unaltered.

Complications

Obviously the frequency of severe complications is related to the clinical material, the method employed, and the skill of the therapist. The mortality with radiotherapy is in the range of 1%; deaths are due mostly to pelvic sepsis,urinary tract infection, bowel damage, or hemorrhage. From 1936 through 1955 radiotherapy at the Radiumhemmet had a complication rate of less than 2%. Radical surgery has carried a high morbidity in some series. For example, the morbidity rate from urinary tract fistulae ranged to as high as 15% in the early series by Meigs (1954). Presently, the surgical mortality rate is in the range of 1-2%, but the rate of fistulae continues to be approximatedly 2-5%. The morbidity from surgery can be considerably reduced by diminishing the radicality of the operative procedure. Obviously, however, when this is done, one compromises the overall cure rate and certainly limits the applicability of the procedure to advanced cases.

The Controversy

Proponents of surgical treatment of cervical cancer have argued as follows:

1. Tumor radioresistance prevents control of the local disease in some patients.
2. Delayed or late recurrence of the disease in or about the cevix occurs in some patients because of regrowth of the cancer or development of a new malignancy.
3. Irradiation fails to cure metastatic cancer within the pelvic lymph nodes.
4. Irradiation injury rate is high.

The radiotherapist answers these accusations as follows. The problem of tumor resistance and local failure has recently been solved by high voltage irradiation. The megavoltage era has brought a central control rate with radiotherapy that appears very encouraging. At M. D. Anderson Hospital, Stage I and Stage II squamous cell carcinomas of the cervix had less than a 3% local recurrence rate. The proper utilization of intracavitary irradiation along with megavoltage external beam radiotherapy has essentially refuted the argument based on tumor radioresistance.

The argument related to late recurrence is best answered by suggesting that an individual who develops a lesion of the same histologic type 10, 15, or 20 years after primary treatment with irradiation probably has a new tumor. Some patients are predisposed to develop cancers in many sites along the genital tract at different times. Irradiation of the first cancer site that appears does not stop the slow development of new cancers.

Failure of radiation to cure lymph node cancer has long been a strong argument for surgical removal of these nodes. For many years the radiotherapist's defense against this argument was limited to statistical evidence. Recent findings reported by Rutledge (1965) suggest very strongly that irradiation therapy is capable of sterilizing positive pelvic lymph nodes. In a series of 500 patients who received pelvic lymphadenectomy after full dose irradiation therapy, the number of positive nodes was one third of that found in the surgical series, stage for stage. This large number of patients with such an impressive difference in the number of positive nodes suggests strongly that irradiation therapy is capable of sterilizing positive nodes.

The high rate of irradiation injury remains controversial because the undesirable effects of irradition, like those of operation, vary with the skill of the therapist and the technique and the facilities used for application. The surgeon's impression of the severity and frequency of irradiation injury will be affected by his personal experience. Residents and other physicians in training tend to remember patients with severe irradiation injuries, who are often subject to prolonged hospitalizations. However, with new megavoltage equipment and careful use of radium techniques, especially those with afterloading, the number of patients who are subject to radiation injury is quite small. This is especially true of patients who receive irradiation therapy for a Stage I lesion. These patients receive only moderate irradiation, and the rate of morbidity is much less than 2%. In cases of advanced disease of the pelvis (Stage III), the dosages of irradiation are optimized and the morbidity is increased. However, the morbidity is accepted in these patients in the hope of a higher cure rate. Again, this is not the case in the irradiation of Stage I and Stage II squamous cell carcinoma of the cervix.

Conclusion

There probably is no significant difference in the cure rates of Stage I squamous cell carcinoma of the cervix treated by surgery versus irradiation. The applicablity of irradiation is superior to that of surgery, for about one fifth of the patients who for some reason are usually found to be inoperable. The mortality rates for the two procedures do not differ significantly. However, the morbidity from surgery is at least twice as great as that from radiotherapy. For these reasons, radiotherapy is the obvious treatment of choice and must remain so until unequivocal evidence to the contrary is presented.

2-6   RADIATION INJURY

The success of radiation therapy in the treatment of malignant disease is contingent on an exploitable gradient of susceptibility to injury in favor of normal tissue. Ideally this gradient should be of sufficient magnitude to permit eradication of the malignancy without serious or permanent injury to normal tissues. In reality, however, most malignant tumors are only marginally more sensitive to irradiation than is normal tissue, and radiation dosages are limited by complication rates rather than cure rates. In any biologic system individual variations can be anticipated. Consequently, radiation dosages that have been determined empirically to be safe will occasionally result in serious injury to an uncommonly sensitive tissue. To obtain a maximum number of cures a modicum of complications is inevitable.

This variation in susceptibility to actinic injury is a natural phenomenon observed at the cellular as well as the tissue level. Within any field of irradiation the most sensitive tissue will determine the dosage limitation, provided that injury to this tissue would result in significant morbidity. In gynecologic oncology the vast majority of radiation injuries result from treatment of cervical carcinoma and largely involve structures within the pelvic field of therapy. The dose limiting normal tissues in the pelvis are the rectosigmoid, bladder, and small bowel, particualrly the terminal ileum. Extension of the treatment field to the abdomen in the management of ovarian carcinoma, and to the aortic region in cervical carcinoma, requires even more restrictive dose limitations because of the intolerance of the liver, kidneys, and small bowel to radiation. Proliferating tissues are more susceptible to radiation injury than are static tissues. Consequently epithelial and parenchymal cells are more liable to injury than connective tissue cells.

Pathology

The acute reaction to radiation consists of a rapid cessation of mitotic activity, followed by cellular swelling and, if the injury is lethal, dissolution. Small vessel edema appears with endothelial swelling and thrombosis. The connective tissue becomes edematous and congested with dilated lymphatics and small vessels. If the injury is severe enough, focal necrosis may be seen. Subsequent changes include intimal thickening with obliteration of the small vessels, fibrosis and hyalinization of vessel walls and connective tissue, and permanent reduction of the epithelial and parenchymal cell population. The extent to which these changes occur is dependent on the degree of injury.

Significant pathophysiologic effects of these changes are reduction in the microcirculation (both vascular and lymphatic), loss of parenchymal tissue, and proliferation of fibrous tissue. These changes are progressive and may continue for many years. Consequently irradiated tissue loses in varying degrees the specific function of its parenchymal component. Furthermore, because of the impaired blood supply, the tissues are poorly supplied with oxygen and other nutrients, including the humoral and cellular arms of the immune defense system. All of these changes in combination produce an increased susceptibility to any type of injury, a reduction in the tissue's capacity to repair itself, and an increased vulnerability to bacterial infection. In these tissues, any injury may result in a vicious, self-sustaining cycle of necrosis and infection. Bacterial proliferation in the necrotic tissue leads to invasion of the viable tissue at the perimeter, producing additional stress that results in a further advance of the necrotic and infectious process.

Acute Radiation Reactions

A number of side effects from irradiation are commonly seen during the course of treatment, but these are usually transient and do not lead to permanent injury. A study by Buchler et al (1971) suggests that individuals who show the most severe reactions during irradiation have an increased probability of a delayed radiation complication. The skin reactions so important in the orthovoltage (Fig. 2-38) era are seldom a limiting effect of radiation therapy with high energy machines unless the beam is striking the skin tangentially, as may occur over the vulva and natal crease. Folliculitis and moist desquamation may develop. The symptoms of cystitis are usually well controlled with urinary analgesics, antispasmodics, and increased fluid intake. When there is evidence of bacterial infection, antibiotics are also indicated.

Actinic proctosigmoiditis, manifested by tenesmus, diarrhea, and cramps, usually responds well to a low residue diet, antispasmodics, and steroid suppositories. Belladonna

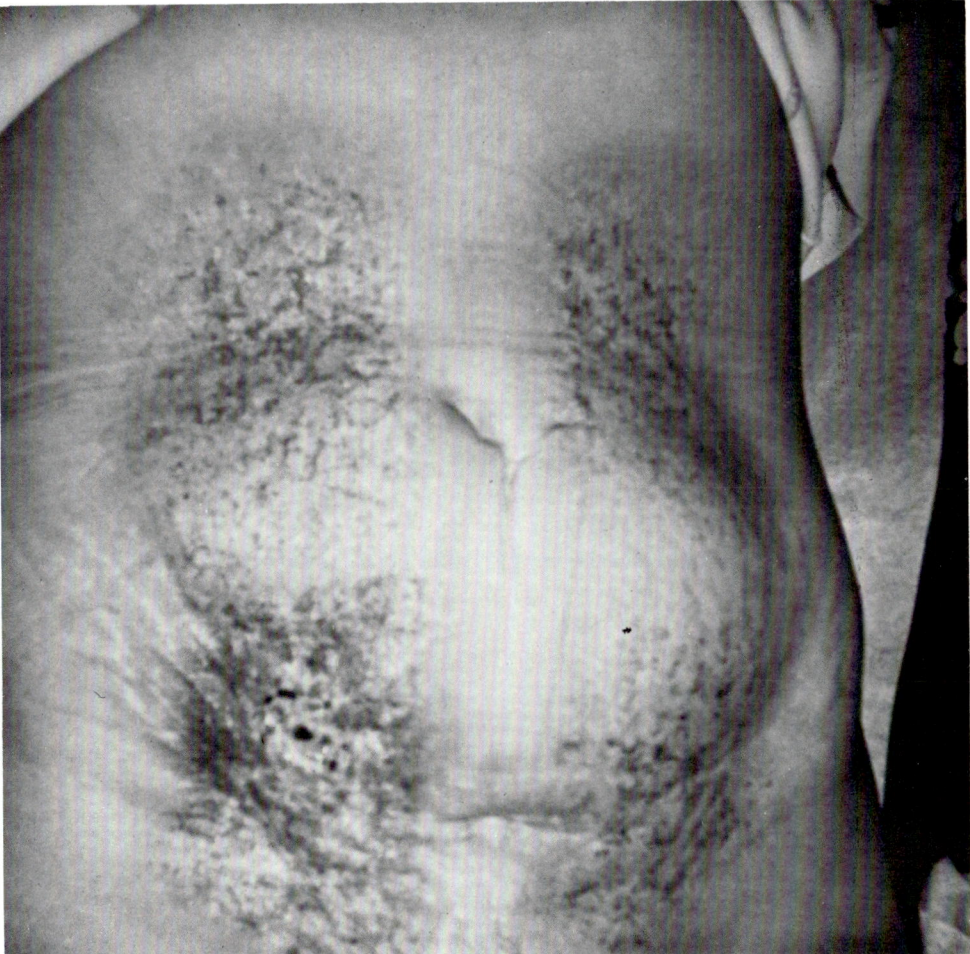

Fig. 2-38 Telangiectasia of the skin, noted in a patient treated with whole abdomen irradiation on orthovoltage equipment.

and opium (B and 0) suppositories are also very effective. Enteritis may be a problem, particularly in irradiating the abdomen or the para-aortic area for ovarian or cervical cancer. Usually associated are nausea, cramps, and diarrhea. Antispasmodics and antiemetics generally produce satisfactory control of the symptoms. Occasionally a patient who is very susceptible to the effects of irradiation may develop severe bowel symptoms necessitating discontinuation of therapy, at least temporarily. Acute severe radiation enteritis may produce a prolonged paralytic ileus simulating a small bowel obstruction.

The effects of pelvic irradiation on bone marrow function are usually not clinically significant, although some depression of the white cell count or platelet count may be noticed. Bone marrow suppression is a more important problem when irradiating the abdomen and pelvis. Serious bone marrow toxicity is particularly likely when irradiating a patient who has previously received myelosuppressive chemotherapy.

Delayed Radiation Reactions

Proctitis

The majority of serious injuries from pelvic and abdominal irradiation are not manifest until 6-24 months after completion of therapy. Proctitis is usually seen in combination with sigmoiditis as part of a pelvic field injury. The close spatial relationship of the rectum to the upper vagina and cervix makes it especially vulnerable to radium injuries or to a combination radium and external therapy injury. The symptoms of proctitis with or without ulceration include pain, tenesmus, intermittent diarrhea and constipation, and rectal bleeding. The symptoms may be mild with ulceration persisting for years, or they may be severe and require vigorous therapy. The management includes low residue diet, Metamucil, antispasmodics, and mild analgesics. Steroid enemas and B and 0 suppositories may also be useful. When medical management fails to relieve the symptoms or excessive bleeding is a problem, a diverting colostomy is indicated.

When rectal bleeding occurs proctosigmoidoscopy and barium enema should be performed because of the possibility that a primary bowel carcinoma may have developed. However, a radiographic contrast study must always be undertaken with the utmost caution because the injured rectosigmoid is vulnerable to perforation, and barium-fecal peritonitis is always fatal. In other cases, if the symptoms do not respond to medical management, the severity of the injury and the degree of obstruction can be evaluated by studies of the types mentioned. Rectal ulcers are invariably located on the anterior rectal wall at the level of the cervix and have a punched out appearance with a dirty gray membrane covering the crater. Biopsies should be carried out cautiously since the trauma may result in fistula formation.

Rectovaginal fistula is one of the most common complications of pelvic irradiation requiring surgical intervention. If it is associated with vault necrosis, a proximal diverting colostomy should be performed as soon as possible. Even what seems to be an obvious rectovaginal fistula may represent multiple fistulae from other sections of the large bowel or small bowel, so that a barium enema, a small bowel examination, and a vaginogram should be performed before the colostomy. Occasionally a very small fistula may heal spontaneously after diversion of the fecal stream. Surgical repair of the fistula will always require the bringing of a new source of blood supply (omentum, bulbocavernosus, gracilis muscle) into the area. Before repair is attempted, the margins of the fistula should be clean and free of necrosis. After surgical repair the colostomy should not be taken down for at least 6 months to permit adequate healing of the fistula. The success of surgical repair would be expected to be much greater when the injury has been produced by radium, since such an injury is focal as compared to the field injury resulting from large volume external radiation therapy.

Progressive fibrosis resulting from actinic injury of the rectum may result in a stricture severe enough to require diverting colostomy. This stricture can usually be felt on rectal examination. It may not appear until 5-10 years after therapy.

Sigmoiditis

Clinically significant radiation sigmoiditis increases in severity and frequency as the dose of external whole pelvis irradiation is raised. It is an infrequent problem when the external therapy is limited to 4000 rads in 4 weeks. However, the sigmoid is still subject to radium injury because of its relatively fixed position in the hollow of the sacrum and its close association with the uterine fundus. Factors contributing to sigmoiditis, other than a high dose of external therapy, include age, inflammatory disease, and a posterior location of the radium system in the hollow of the sacrum (Strockbine et al, 1970). As with isolated proctitis, the symptoms of sigmoiditis include "crampy" pelvic pain, alternating diarrhea and constipation, and rectal bleeding. If the injury is severe, the pain may be disabling and associated malaise, anorexia, and chronic weight loss are evident. This combination of severe, intractable pain and weight loss may be tragically misinterpreted as recurrent or persistent unresectable carcinoma.

Milder forms of sigmoiditis may be managed medically using low residue diet, Metamucil, mineral oil, and antispasmodics. The use of laxatives and enemas must be interdicted. When there are severe symptoms or moderate symptoms unresponsive to medical mangement, or when evidence of obstruction or serious bleeding occurs, a proximal diverting colostomy is necessary. Undue delay must be avoided because of the constant threat of necrosis and perforation, which will produce generalized peritonitis, a condition uniformly fatal in an irradiated individual. Preoperative evaluation with a colon contrast radiographic study carries the risk of perforation, and this risk may be increased by the use of enemas and laxatives. As a rule, sigmoidoscopy is not possible because of rectosigmoid fixation at the peritoneal reflection. In the case of a segmental injury to the sigmoid in a patient who has had less that 5000 rads whole pelvis, serious consideration should be given to a segmental resection and anastomosis at the time the diverting colostomy is performed. The colostomy must be done outside the field of radiation, preferably in the right transverse colon. The colon should be completely divided to assure total diversion of the fecal stream. Patients with higher doses of external irradiation will have more diffuse injury of the sigmoid colon, and reestablishment of intestinal continuity is seldom feasible.

Small Bowel Injury

The small bowel is not as commonly injured as the large bowel by radiotherapy, although its dose tolerance is usually less than that of the sigmoid colon. However, because of its mobility the small bowel is able to move in and out of the field of irradiation, and thus it generally receives less than a full dose. The terminal ileum is the most common site of small bowel injury for the reasons that it is usually fixed just proximal to the cecum, it has a relatively poor blood supply, and it is the narrowest portion of the small bowel. Furthermore, it is the portion of the small bowel most likely to be adherent in the pelvis as a result of previous surgery (supracervical hysterectomy, cesarean section, adnexal surgery) or inflammatory disease such as chronic salpingitis, appendicitis, endometriosis, granulomatous inflammations of the bowel, and diverticulitis. When the whole pelvis external irradiation has been less than 4000-5000 rads in 4-5 weeks, a clinically significant injury to the small bowel is usually due to radium as a result of a perforation or the presence of a loop of small bowel adherent to the uterus. This injury from the radium is focal. It can produce progressive narrowing, resulting in obstruction or necrosis, and perforation may result.

The symptoms of small bowel injury are usually those of an incomplete bowel obstruction with delayed postprandial cramping, nausea, and vomiting that relieves the pain and bloating. Diarrhea and progressive weight loss are often prominent symptoms of chronic, incomplete small bowel obstruction. The high energy x-ray generators have permitted higher depth doses with the capability of producing small bowel damage. Doses of 5000-7000 rads can cause such extensive injuries that malabsorption may result, leading to wasting with or without evidence of obstruction. These patients usually have intermittent or constant "crampy" abdominal pain, diarrhea, anorexia, and periodic episodes of bloating. The clinical picture often suggests recurrent advanced carcinoma and hence may result in nonintervention of a surgically curable disease state. Radiation reduces the inflammatory response of the peritoneum and bowel wall to ischemia, necrosis, and infection (Fig. 2-39), thus masking the occurrence of these events. The patient may have a florid peritonitis without the anticipated signs of abdominal rigidity

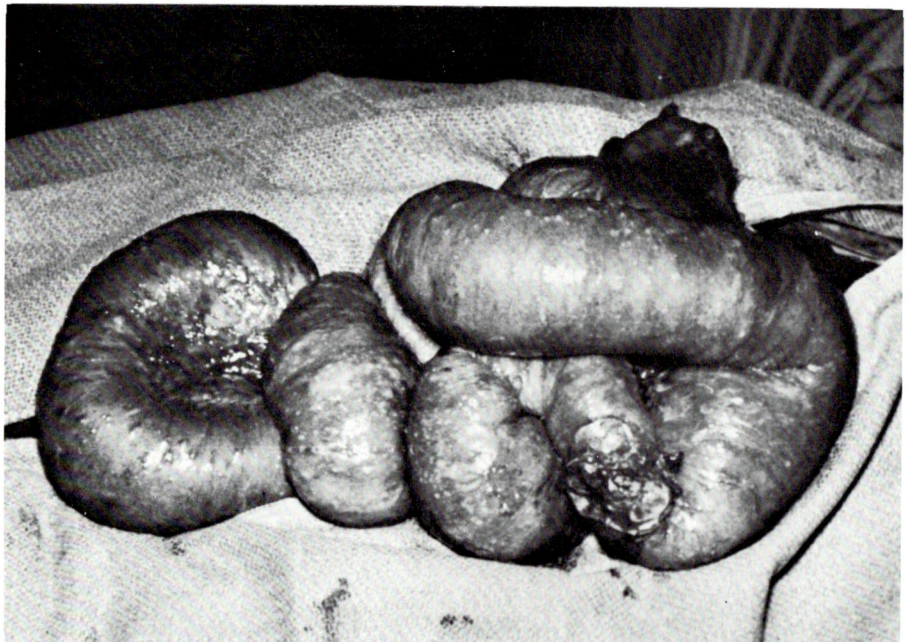

Fig. 2-39 Radiation injury to the small bowel. Note the thickened, edematous wall of the bowel, accompanied by the whitish sheen usually seen in this condition.

or rebound tenderness. There may be no elevation of the temperature or white blood count. As stated previously, generalized peritonitis in an irradiated patient is invariably fatal since the tissues are unable to heal. Treatment should be aggressive since bowel necrosis and perforation are much more likely to occur than in the nonirradiated bowel and at an earlier point in time relative to the symptomatology. Furthermore, the usual warning symptoms are obtunded in any irradiated abdomen. Hence, surgical intervention should be undertaken as soon as the diagnosis is suspected. An upper gastrointestinal radiographic series may demonstrate the injury but should not be relied on if negative.

The management of radiation small bowel injuries is complex and requires fine surgical judgment. In the presence of generalized peritonitis, exteriorization of the proximal and distal loops should be accomplished and the patient maintained on hyperalimentation and antibiotics until the peritonitis resolves. A bowel anastomosis will not heal in the presence of peritonitis. Reestablishment of bowel continuity can be achieved at a later date. When necrosis and perforation with a localized infection are present, resection and anastomosis (ileo-ileostomy) may be carried out, provided that relatively normal proximal and distal bowel is available. This is true of short or long segment injuries if there is adequate mobility. Frequently, however, there is obstruction related to extensive interloop adhesions and adhesions to structures in the pelvis. In these cases or in patients where the distal ileum would be involved in the anastomosis, it is better to do a sidetracking end-to-side or side-to-side anastomosis with the ascending or transverse colon (Figs. 2-40 and 2-41). Resection of small bowel requiring dissection of adhesions from the pelvis is foolhardy, since the remaining small bowel will fall into the pelvis and form new adhesions and obstructions. Such complex adhesions should be left undisturbed. Not uncommonly both the terminal ileum and the sigmoid colon have been injured, and the symptoms of one injury mask the presence of the other. This possibility should always be kept in mind, and both areas assessed preoperatively as well as at surgery (Fig. 2–42).

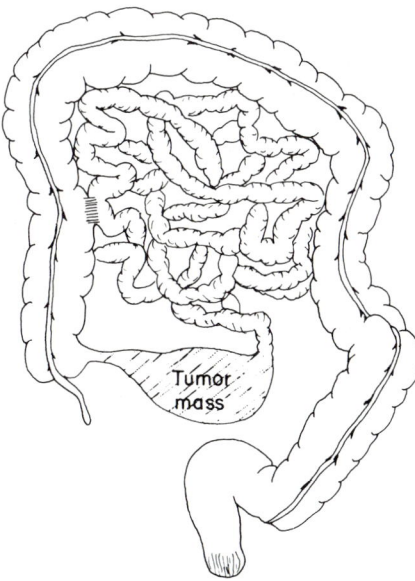

Fig. 2-40 Partial obstruction of terminal ileum; side-to-side ileoascending entero-colostomy as a diversion. Obstruction may be radiation injury and/or tumor.

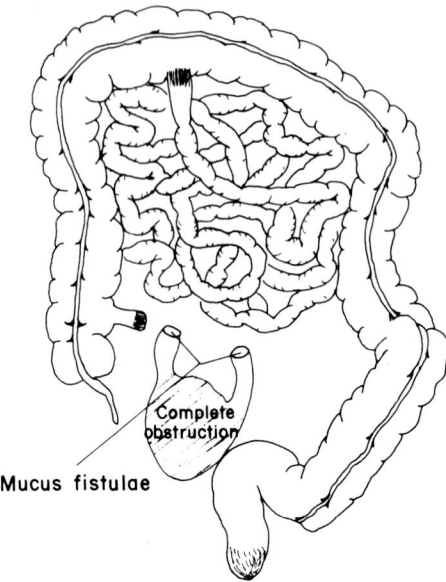

Fig. 2-41 Complete obstruction of terminal ileum; end-to-side ileo-transverse entero-colostomy as a diversion. Stump of terminal ileum turned in, and two mucous fistule are constructed.

Preoperatively, in all patients suspected of having small bowel radiation injury a long tube should be passed for decompression and for splinting loops of bowel to prevent postoperative adhesions, as well as postoperative decompression and protection of the anastomosis.

Vault Necrosis

Development of vault necrosis may be attended by severe pain unresponsive to narcotic analgesics and associated with extreme malaise, anorexia, progressive weight loss, and

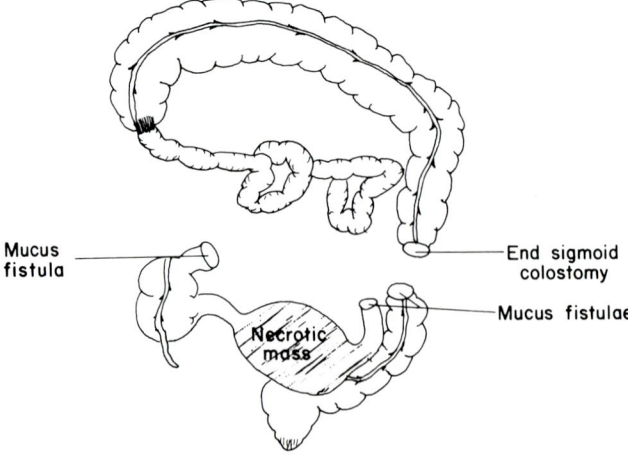

Fig. 2-42 Necrotic mass involving terminal ileum and rectosigmoid. Diversion accomplished with end sigmoid colostomy and end-to-end ileoascending entero-colostomy. Three mucous fistulae are produced.

psychological withdrawal. Fistulae of the bowel or urinary tract may develop. Occasionally life threatening hemorrhage will result. The clinical syndrome often exactly reproduces that of advanced, terminal carcinoma, including the mythical "smell of cancer." Although it is difficult to determine whether cancer is or is not persistent in the presence of such extensive tissue necrosis, a helpful clue may be the severity of the pain, which is usually more insufferable in the presence of radiation necrosis than extensive recurrent disease. These patients often are so exquisitely tender that examination is impossible without anesthesia.

In the presence of urinary or fecal fistulae, the necrosis, pain, and infection cannot possibly be controlled and immediate diversion is indicated. Management includes hospitalization and bedrest. The most important phase of treatment other than diverting the fistulae is utilization of full strength hydrogen peroxide douches several times daily. Dibridement of the necrotic tissue is also helpful, but many patients cannot tolerate this. Systemic antibiotics are administered only during the early phase of management. Biopsies should be taken, but this can be delayed until the pain is controlled and the necrosis cleared up. Care must be observed always in biopsying irradiated tissues, particularly in the region of the bladder and rectum, because of the threat of initiating fistulae. Untreated, these patients may die from inanition or sepsis despite the fact that the process is reversible and there may be no persistent disease.

CASE REPORT. R.B., a 27 year old white female, was seen in consultation because of pelvic necrosis and advanced recurrent cancer. She was 9 months postirradiation for Stage I "occ". squamous cell carcinoma of the cervix. During the prior 3 months she had been hospitalized because of intractable pelvic pain requiring meperidine and morphine around the clock for palliation. Weight loss in the same time interval amounted to 60 lbs. She had recently developed vesicovaginal and rectovaginal fistulae. Examination disclosed extensive necrosis of the upper vagina with a gray-green shaggy membrane. There was nodular induration, extending to both side walls, which was palpably indistinguishable from cancer. A sigmoid conduit and end-descending colostomy were performed to divert the urine and fecal stream, after which peroxide douches and hyperalimentation were initiated. She was discharged from the hospital 1 month later with mild pain controlled by oral analgesics. The vault necrosis was almost entirely cleared up. During the ensuing 6 months, she gained 60 lbs., the vaginal vault necrosis healed completely, and the large vesicovaginal and rectovaginal fistulae were clean and pink. She felt entirely, well, and there was no evidence of recurrent disease.

Such a response to diversion and peroxide douches should not be considered extraordinary, although not every patient will respond so dramatically. Exenteration, recommended by some authors, seems to be an extreme means of controlling pelvic necrosis.

Miscellaneous

Other types of radiation injury include atrophy and telangiectasia of the skin, which result only from orthovoltage irradiation; the high energy machines have a skin sparing effect. With low megavoltage therapy units (Co^{60}) subcutaneous fibrosis, which may produce a rock-hard mass in the abdominal wall, occurs occasionally. Radiation injury to large vessels, for which arteriosclerosis may be a predisposing factor, may occur. Reports are on record of bilateral iliofemoral occlusion following pelvic irradiation.

Hemorrhagic cystitis is an uncommon complication of pelvic irradiation and tends to appear later (10-20 years after therapy) than the bowel complications. It is usually mild and associated with a bacterial urinary tract infection. Most cases of hemorrhagic cystitis can be managed by appropriate antibiotics, urine cultures, and bladder irrigation utilizing ¼% acetic acid or dilute silver nitrate solutions. In the presence of more extensive hemorrhage, removal of the clots and light electrocautery of the bleeding points at the time of cystoscopy may be very helpful. In all patients cystoscopy is indicated. Often a dirty, gray shaggy ulcer is visualized. A biopsy should be performed but must be done with caution, realizing that there is a risk of producing a fistula. Occasionally a urinary conduit is required because of recurrent, severe or intractable hemorrhage.

Vesicovaginal fistulae due to radium injury may be successfully repaired in properly selected cases. A new source of blood supply is always necessary. Fistulae associated with high dose external beam therapy are best managed by conduit diversion.

There are numerous and important differences in the consideration of surgery on the irradiated and the unirradiated patient. The risks of surgery rise logarithmically as the dose of irradiation increases. The reason largely revolves around the diminished blood supply and the resultant limited capacity of these tissues to repair injury and combat infection. Skin incisions should never be crossed and parallel incisions should never be utilized within the field of radiation because necrosis and infection invariably result.

Prophylactic antibiotics are recommended since a wound infection in an irradiated area will cause necrosis and long-term morbidity. Debridement and peroxide irrigations are the mainstays in the care of these wounds. Irradiated tissues are often friable and easily torn or injured. This is especially true of the small bowel. Any surgery, even a "simple hysterectomy," may be followed by cuff necrosis and fistulization in a patient who has previously had pelvic irradiation. Any injury to the rectosigmoid necessitates a diverting colostomy outside the radiation field. Abdominal wounds should always be closed with some form of retention suture, using a permanent material. The recommended method is the internal retention suture of "Tom Jones" (Jones et al, 1941).

2-7 RECURRENT CERVICAL CARCINOMA

Despite the fact that squamous carcinoma of the cervix is one of the most curable human malignancies, treatment is unsucessful in nearly one half of the cases. Persistent or recurrent carcinoma of the cervix, the consequence of treatment failure, is by comparison a devastatingly malignant disease with a 1 year survival rate of 15% and a 5 year survival rate of less than 5%. The common occurrence of cervical carcinoma combined with the frequency of treatment failure makes the diagnosis and management of recurrent cervical carcinoma one of the foremost challenges in gynecologic oncology.

Since most treatment failures occur in the more advanced stages of disease, the discussion in this chapter will be directed toward recurrence or persistence after irradiation. Few treatment failures are anticipated after primary surgical therapy because the modality is largely reserved for cases in which the tumor is confined to the cervix. Treatment failure after primary surgical therapy is usually managed by irradiation.

Recurrence Time and Survival

Characterizing the patterns of recurrence provides a sound basis for planning a posttherapy surveillance program aimed at the early detection of treatment failure. Approximately 50% of recurrences will develop during the first year of follow-up, and 75% within 2 years after treatment. This recurrence pattern varies from stage to stage until the 5 year mark, after which the patterns by stage are nearly indentical. The curves constructed for deaths from recurrent disease are nearly congruent with those for recurrence. About 95% of all deaths due to treatment failure for cervical carcinoma will have occurred by 5 years after therapy. Hence, for cervical carcinoma, the 5 year survival rate is a fairly accurate measure of curability. Survival time after recurrence is not as dependent on the interval since therapy as it is on the location of the recurrence, that is, whether or not the disease is localized and resectable.

Location

In addition to the pattern of recurrence it is useful to examine the recurrence tendencies by site, recalling that this disease spreads almost exclusively by contiguous growth and lymphatic metastases. The incidence of central failure (cervix, vagina, bladder, rectum, and parametrium) after irradiation in Stages I and II is quite small. Paunier et al (1967) reported that only 2.5% of 1341 Stage I and Stage II cases demonstrated active central disease with or without disease in other areas within the first 5 years after treatment. When isolated active central disease was considered, the figure dropped to less than 1%. The incidence of central failure increased to 7% and 38% in Stages IIIb and IV, respectively. Few of these cases have disease limited to the central pelvis.

Other frequent sites of recurrence are the pelvic wall, the para-aortic nodes, the peripheral lymph nodes, the lungs, the lower vagina, especially the suburethral region, and the axial skeleton (Table 2-3).

Symptoms

In about 15% of individuals followed on a regular basis after irradiation for cervical carcinoma, recurrence will be diagnosed from examination (Fig. 2-43) or laboratory

TABLE 2-3 CERVICAL CARCINOMA
COMMON SITES OF RECURRENCE
AFTER RADIOTHERAPY

1. Central (vagina, cervix, uterus, parametrium, bladder, rectum)
2. Pelvic wall
3. Para-aortic nodes
4. Peripheral lymph nodes (supraclavicular, inguinal)
5. Lung
6. Lower vagina
7. Axial skeleton

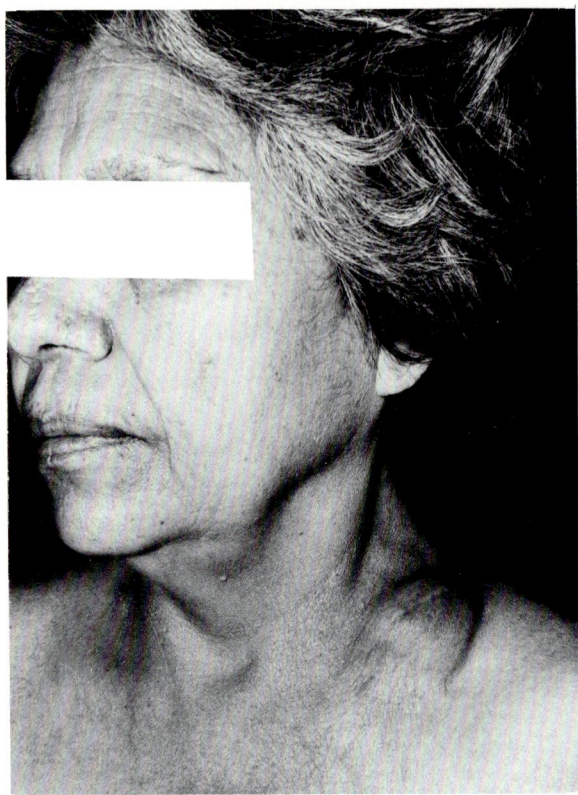

Fig. 2-43 Patient with a left supraclavicular mass appearing 4 years after primary treatment for Stage I squamous cell carcinoma of the cervix.

studies before the appearance of any symptoms. A very insidious, but frequent, indication of persistent or recurrent tumor is weight loss. However, in the months immediately after treatment, weight loss is an unreliable index of disease activity because of the catabolic effects of irradiation and its complications. Another common presenting symptom is pain (Table 2-4). Although sciatic pain frequently is identified as characteristic of pelvic recurrence, this is probably not the most common type of pain resulting from pelvic disease. The patient may describe pain in the groin, leg, hip, buttocks, vagina, pelvis, pubic area, and so on. Persistent pelvic pain is highly suggestive of recurrence, but does not necessarily indicate unresectable disease. Occasionally such an ominous symptom is due to irradiation fibrosis or necrosis. Vertebral metastases, para-aortic nodal disease, and obstructed ureters (Fig. 2-44) are all capable of producing back pain. Abdominal pain is an uncommon complaint usually associated with intra-abdominal or para-aortic disease. At any rate, pain, wherever and whenever it occurs, must be investigated in these individuals. Pulmonary metastases produce cough, hemoptysis and/or chest pain. Vaginal bleeding is a widely publicized but infrequent first symptom of recurrent cervical carcinoma. It is especially important, however, because it is highly suggestive of centrally recurrent cancer or may herald the development of endometrial carcinoma. A malodorous, watery, or purulent vaginal discharge may signal the appearance of centrally recurrent cervical cancer, but often it is symptomatic of irradiation necrosis with or without recurrence. Occasionally the first evidence of treatment failure is leg edema from progressive lymphatic obstruction or occlusion of the iliofemoral vein system.

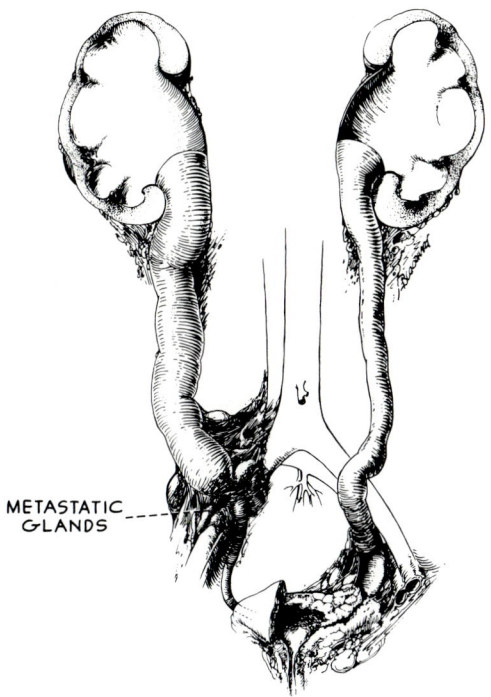

METASTATIC
GLANDS

Fig. 2-44 Obstructed ureters: on the right, secondary to common iliac node metastases, on the left, parametrial extension of recurrent disease has obstructed the ureter. (Courtesy of E. Henriksen, M.D., Clinical Professor of Ob/Gyn, University of Southern California School of Medicine.)

None of these symptoms per se is diagnostic of recurrent cancer. Each can be due to such benign causes as irradiation necrosis, irradiation bowel injury, irradiation fibrosis, or thrombophlebitis. There is a myriad of other symptoms that any patient with cervical

TABLE 2-4 CERVICAL
CARCINOMA SYMPTOMS OF
RECURRENCE AFTER RADIOTHERAPY

1. Weight loss
2. Pain (pelvic, back, abdomen)
3. Cough, hemoptysis, chest pain
4. Vaginal bleeding
5. Watery foul, or purulent vaginal discharge
6. Leg edema (thrombophlebitis)

cancer may experience when tumor recurs. It must be kept in mind that any symptom in the patient treated for cervical cancer may be due to recurrence; it is equally important to remember that no symptom is uniquely diagnostic of recurrence, and that patients who have had cancer may also develop other disease.

Diagnosis

Very few recurrences are detected by Pap smear because it is exceptional when a centrally recurrent tumor is shedding cells in the vagina at a time when the upper vault and cervix appear normal. Usually, when the Pap smear is positive, changes are present in the upper vagina and cervix that indicate the need for a tissue biopsy (Table 2-5). Nevertheless, cytology is at times the first clue leading to the diagnosis of recurrent disease.

When recurrence is suggested by an enlarged peripheral node or a lesion in the vagina, external genitalia, or other readily accessible area, tissue biopsy should be obtained without delay. Lesions in the vagina and cervix cannot be adequately evaluated by cytology alone. Care must be exercised in the interpretation of cervical biopsies during the first month or two after treatment since a positive biopsy during this interval does not always mean persistent viable tumor. Cystoscopy rarely reveals recurrence in the absence of other evidence of pelvic disease. Intravenous pyelogram has a very high incidence of abnormalities associated with recurrent cervical carcinoma. Tumor in para-aortic nodes, pelvic wall nodes, parametrium, or bladder may displace or block the ureters at any point between the kidney and bladder. Hydroureter and hydronephrosis are common sequelae of recurrence, and nonvisualization of the kidney may result. Bone metastases rarely appear outside the axial skeleton. Symptoms almost always precede x-ray evidence of bone involvement. Routine radiographs will usually confirm the presence of symptomatic bone metastasis; but if they are negative, a bone scan may be fruitful. The chest x-ray and IVP include all the bones that are involved by metastatic cervical carcinoma. Metastasis to the long bones or cranium is rare. Lung metastases are usually suspected because of a chronic cough, hemoptysis, or chest pain. If the posterior-anterior chest film is negative, tomograms or bronchial washings for cytology may be diagnostic. On occasion, cough precedes by several months any radiographic evidence of metastasis. Bilateral lower extremity lymphangiography can be a useful diagnostic tool, but interpretation of the findings is frequently difficult and often inconclusive.

When metastatic disease is associated with serous effusion, cytologic examination of the fluid is usually but not always positive. Other diagnostic studies that may be utilized are radioisotope scanning of the liver and brain. An inferior vena cavagram may be helpful when there is lymphatic obstruction on the lower extremity lymphangiogram. Proctosigmoidoscopy and barium enema are occasionally useful and should always be done to exclude primary bowel disease when rectal bleeding occurs. In patients who have had high doses of irradiation, findings from barium enema must be interpreted cautiously. Frequently distortion from irradiation injury and pelvic fibrosis suggests intrinsic or extrinsic malignant disease. Sigmoidoscopy may not be helpful since the sigmoidoscope can seldom be advanced more than 12-15 cm after pelvic irradiation. A similar problem of interpreting the IVP may be encountered because of bladder changes after irradiation.

When recurrent carcinoma is suspected in the pelvis clinically, cervical and parametrial needle biopsies occasionally will confirm the presence of cancer, but often the diagnosis will not be made without surgical exploration.

TABLE 2-5 DIAGNOSTIC EVALUATION
OF RECURRENT CERVICAL CARCINOMA
AFTER RADIOTHERAPY

1. Tissue biopsies
2. Cytology (vaginal, sputum, serous effusion)
3. X-ray studies
    Intravenous urography
    Chest x-ray
    Radiographs of axial skeleton
    Lymphography
4. Radioisotope scans (bone, liver, brain)
5. Exploratory laparotomy

Management

Recurrences can be considered in two categories: those that may be treated with some hope of cure, and those for which palliative treatment only is available. Potentially curable lesions include isolated central pelvic recurrences, lung metastases, and, perhaps, lower vaginal metastases. Isolated central recurrence is the most common potentially curable type, but few patients will be candidates for curative surgery because of this type of lesion. Although surgical management must be tailored to suit the patient's needs, in almost all cases of central recurrence ultraradical surgery is necessary. The role of surgery in the management of central recurrence is discussed in detail in Section 2-8.

Occasionally a patient will develop an isolated recurrence in the lower third of the vagina, usually in the suburethral area. Generally, however, a metastasis in this location indicates the presence of widespread disease. Local irradiation is the treatment of choice. The incidence of inguinal node metastasis secondary to these lesions is high, and the treatment for this type of recurrence should include therapy to the groin nodes if there is no evidence of metastasis elsewhere. Rarely a lesion in this area may be a second primary cancer.

Metastatic lung carcinoma is frequently viewed with extreme pessimism by the clinician; paradoxically the lung is one of the most favorable areas for single organ metastasis. When there is no evidence of disease in other areas of the body, and when the pulmonary lesions are not diffuse (although they may be bilateral), a surgical resection is indicated. If the surgical margin is unsatisfactory, irradiation should be administered postoperatively. Five-year survival rates of 15-30% have been reported. Most patients with pulmonary metastasis however, will not be candidates for surgical resection.

The great majority of recurrences are suitable for palliative management only. When recurrence is outside the initial treatment field, irradiation is frequently successful in providing local control and symptomatic relief. External irradiation to bone metastasis is often effective in relieving pain. Orthopedic pinning to stabilize a pathologic fracture before irradiation is desirable, and healing may result. Irradiation may provide palliation of peripheral nodal metastasis. Even when such metastases are not symptomatic, the patient may receive psychological palliation if regression of these visible tumor masses is achieved.

The most common area of treatment failure, the pelvic wall, is within the original field of irradiation. This type of recurrence is frequently associated with ureteral obstruction, leg edema, and intractable pain. This triad occurring on the same side is the only clinical syndrome of recurrent pelvic disease that is pathognomonic of unresectable cancer. It is uncommon for pelvic wall recurrences to be associated with all three of these symptoms, however. Most patients with unresectable pelvic recurrence have received therapeutic doses of irradiation to the entire pelvis and cannot be safely reirradiated even if the field size is kept small. Occasionally a localized, bulky pelvic wall recurrence will respond favorably to gold grain implants, but few cases are suitable to this form of therapy. Recurrent unresectable pelvic wall tumor associated with intractable pain is one of the most frustrating problems a gynecologic oncologist encounters. When nonnarcotic analgesics have failed and the patient has already received irradiation to the limits of normal tissue tolerance, chemotherapy may be the best recourse. Unfortunately, the palliation rate is not high and is seldom sustained for more than a few weeks. A neurosurgical procedure to achieve pain relief may become necessary.

The recurrence of disease in multiple sites may be managed by local irradiation to symptom-producing areas. When multiple areas require palliation, systemic chemotherapy may be the only practical manner of attempting to achieve relief (see Chapter 10).

Some patients develop dysplasia of the vagina after irradiation for cervical cancer. This appears several years after treatment, and there is a tendency to ignore it as a harmless, irradiation induced change. However, these lesions should be followed with Pap smears, biopsies, and colposcopy. Progression to carcinoma *in situ* necessitates surgical excision since invasive carcinoma may subsequently develop.

Post-treatment Surveillance

Because the majority of recurrences appear within the first 2 years after treatment, follow-up visits should be most frequent during that time interval. Similarly, the interval can be significantly prolonged after 5 years because of the very low incidence of recurrence thereafter (Table 2-6). At each visit the historical inquiry should include data about the patient's general health and activities since the last examination: pain, vaginal bleeding, bowel and bladder function, appearance of lumps, respiratory infections, cough, and so forth. The patient should be weighed at each visit. Although weight loss is not a specific indicator of recurrent tumor, the maintenance of weight or weight gain in the absence of fluid accumulation provides some assurance that the patient is doing well; on the other hand, progressive weight loss should alert the physician to the possibility of recurrence. Patients frequently attribute such weight loss to voluntary diet control.

Physical examination includes careful palpation of the supraclavicular and the inguinal nodes and examination of the abdomen for enlargement of the liver or kidneys, abdominal masses, ascites, and evidence of bowel obstruction. While inspecting the external genitalia, special attention should be paid to the lower vagina and suburethral areas. The vaginal tube and cervix are inspected and palpated. Adequate pelvic evaluation always includes a bimanual rectovaginal examination, noting uterine size and mobility, parametrial induration (smooth or nodular), tenderness, and masses. A Pap smear is obtained at each visit and a chest x-ray biannually as a routine. Intravenous pyelography probably should be done routinely at 6 month intervals for the first 2 years after treatment because of the high incidence of abnormal studies in the presence of recurrent tumor. In addition, a few patients will develop progressive ureteral obstruction from irradiation fibrosis, and early detection may salvage renal function.

TABLE 2-6 POST-THERAPY SURVEILLANCE
PROGRAM FOR CERVICAL CARCINOMA

1. Examination every 2 months for 2 years, then every 4 months for 3 years, every 6 months for 5 years
2. Pap smear at every visit
3. Chest x-ray every 6 months
4. Intravenous urography every 6 months for 2 years

2-8 PELVIC EXENTERATION

Introduction

"Clinical experience has established the pelvic exenteration operation for treating patients with cancer which is advanced and not suitable for conventional treatment or has recurred within the pelvis after irradiation was previously used. The pelvic exenteration carries a great risk because the margin for safety and recovery is very limited; thus, a single error in the management may cause death, result in a fruitless operation, and aggravate the patient's present misery. From the first evaluation for suitable treatment of recurrent cancer to the completion of the treatment in recovery, there are great demands upon the physician for wisdom in identifying the suitable patient, judgment in the assessment of the physical boundaries of the cancer, diligent investigation for metastases, skill in the performance of the operation with meticulous and vigilant support of the patient during the postoperative period, and concern for the ultimate outcome. The entire management course is subject to error leading to increased patient suffering, to frustration of the clinician with a futile dissipation of the energies of the staff, and even to castastrophe.

"An error of omission in the preparation of a patient may be responsible for a lost opportunity to cure even when the disease is amenable to resection. Successful exenteration depends upon (1) wisely selected patients; (2) thoroughly studied preoperatively; (3) perfect design for resection and reconstruction; (4) uneventfully executed operation; and (5) diligent and controlled postoperative support."

Felix Rutledge, M.D.

Patient Selection

Only a small portion (<5%) of patients with recurrent cancer of the cervix are suitable for this operation. To allow a futile preparation for operation to progress is an inhumane and wasteful error. Obviously any patient who has evidence of disease outside the pelvis is initially unsuitable for exploration and possible pelvic exenteration. On the other hand, although cachexia, pain, cough, severe anemia, and leg edema may seem to indicate an inoperable condition, patients with these symptoms deserve enough attention in examination to avoid the error of a premature decision. Many patients may appear inoperable by examination alone; this should be the first step in investigation but not always the sole excluding factor. Patients who have disease confined to the pelvis, as determined by both clinical and roentgenographic studies, should be considered for exploratory laparotomy and possible pelvic exenteration. The extent of the disease as estimated by pelvic (rectovaginal) examination may provide considerable indication of the possibility of resectability in a particular patient, but whether this examination should in and of itself determine whether or not the patient is acceptable for laparotomy is a very moot point. There are some patients in whom the possiblity of resection is less than 5%. The clinician must then ask himself the question: "Is it of value to explore 100 patients in order to find 5 who may be resectable?" This becomes a matter of individual judgement on the part of the oncologist.

At laparotomy the lymph nodes around the aorta become the first area of sampling if the exploration of the abdomen has revealed no evidence of disease. Usually the right paraaortic lymph node chain is excised and sent for frozen section analysis. If this is negative, a bilateral pelvic lymphadenectomy is performed. There have been very few survivors in the group of patients who have undergone pelvic exenteration with positive pelvic wall nodes. Therefore immediate pathologic review of the lymphadenectomy specimen and frozen section analysis of the suspicious pelvic wall nodes are necessary in order to determine whether the resection should continue. Positive nodes usually signal the termination of the procedure. A possible exception occurs when the parametrial nodes are positive; then the decision is based on the extent of the disease in these nodes.

In Ketcham's (1970) series of approximately 200 patients undergoing pelvic exentera-tion, only 1 patient who had a positive pelvic lymph node after irradiation therapy survived 5 years. In the series from Memorial Hospital reported by Barber (1969), 148 patients undergoing exenteration had positive nodes at the time of the procedure. All of these patients had had previous irradiation therapy for their primary lesions, and only 4 survived for 5 years, for a total of 4.7%. In all the cases reported in the literature of survivors following exenteration for recurrent squamous cell carcinoma of the cervix who had positive pelvic nodes, the nodes were positive unilaterally. There appear to be no reports of survivors in whom the nodes were positive bilaterally.

The pelvic lymphadenectomy having been completed, attention is turned to the status of the web or cardinal ligaments. The paravesical and pararectal spaces are identified and developed, and the proximity of the malignant disease to the pelvic wall is analyzed. If there is a tumor-free space between the disease and the pelvic wall, the patient is considered resectable. Care must be taken to analyze the entire web, especially the area immediately above the levator ani muscles. Often the most visible portion of the web will be free of the side wall, but subsequently the surgeon will find dense adherence of tumor to the pelvic wall low down in the pelvis, just above the levator muscles.

If the pathologic report of the lymphadenectomy specimen is now available, it is at this point that the final decision is made as to whether exenteration is possible. *Pelvic exenteration is not considered a satisfactory means of intentional palliation.* The details of the operation can be found in standard textbooks and will not be described here. The magnitude of these procedures can be appreciated, however, by study of Figs. 2-45 to 2-47.

Observations on the Preparation and Care of the Exenteration Patient

Preoperative Preparation

Preparation of the patient should start when she is first seen and includes the following measures.

Anterior Exenteration

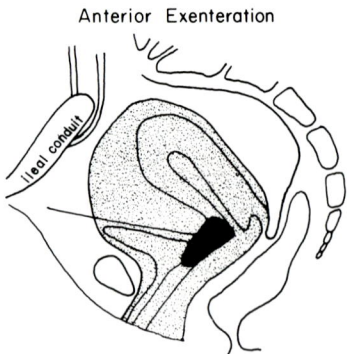

Fig. 2-45 Performance of an anterior exenteration denotes removal of the entire urinary bladder and all internal genitalia including *all* supporting structures, as well as draining lymphatics and nodes within the pelvis (shaded area above) with preservation of the rectosigmoid. Urine is diverted by construction of a conduit, usually utilizing a segment of ileum. (From DiSaia, P.J., et al, Calif. Med. 118:13, 1973.)

Posterior Exenteration

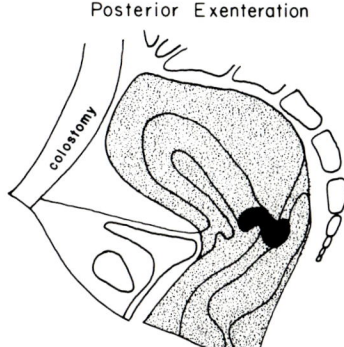

Fig. 2-46 Performance of a posterior exenteration denotes removal of the rectosigmoid with its mesentery and all internal genitalia including *all* supporting structures, as well as draining lymphatics and nodes within the pelvis (shaded area above). The fecal stream is then usually diverted by means of an end sigmoid colostomy.
(From DiSaia, P.J., et al, Calif. Med. 118:13, 1973.)

General Supportive Measures

1. The patient should be given multivitamins and iron.
2. The importance of proper diet should be stressed with all patients, including the obese. The obese patient should not be encourage to lose weight at this time. A well balanced 2000-2500 cal high protein diet is recommended.
3. The importance of discontinuing smoking should be stressed. Patients with chronic pulmonary disease should be given proper medications and receive IPPB preoperatively.

Mental Preparation

1. Continuing contact with one interested physician is important.
2. The operation should be explained in detail with all its ramifications.

Total Exenteration

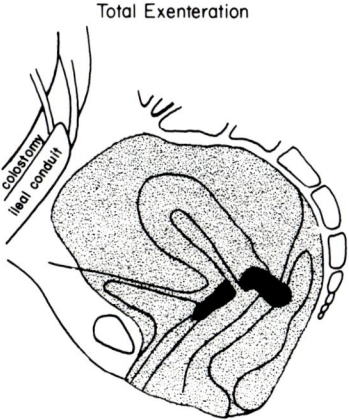

Fig. 2-47 Performance of a total pelvic exenteration denotes removal of all the pelvic organs, supporting structures, and lymphatic pathways within the pelvis (shaded area above). Varying amounts of the levator ani muscles and vulva may also be excised. Both a conduit and a colostomy are constructed. (From DiSaia, P.J., et al, Calif. Med. 118:13, 1973.)

3. It is important to stress that the minimum procedure consistent with cure will be done. Constant reassurance is necessary on this point.

4. The patient should be advised that removal of the bladder or rectum may not be necessary, thereby avoiding despair if the patient proves inoperable.

5. Length of stay, future sexual adjustment, the inevitability of some problems, which we are equipped to handle—discussion of these and other questions assures the patient of the physician's interest and gains her confidence.

6. Questions and explanations should be addressed to the patient in a confident tone.

Physical Preparation and Medication

1. The patient should be admitted to the hospital at least 3 days, and possibly 4 or 5 days, before operation, depending on her physical status.

2. Intensive pulmonary care, including IPPB or bronchodilators, may be started at this time.

3. The minimum acceptable hematocrit should be 36, and preferably 39-40. Blood transfusions should be given at the earliest possible time and should allow for adjustment of blood volume.

4. The following laboratory studies should be obtained: CBC, UA, urine culture with colony count, BUN and electrolytes, TP and A/G ratio, liver battery, coagulation profile, platelet count, skeletal survey when indicated, EKG, recent IVP, proctosigmoidoscopy and chest x-ray.

5. The patient should be started on a low residue diet and should have clear liquids for 48 hours preoperatively. A long tube may be inserted 24-48 hours preoperatively.

An alternative method which is gaining popularity is to avoid the long tube preoperatively and to insert a jejunostomy tube at surgery if it is considered necessary.

6. Adequate mechanical preparation of the bowel is essential.

7. A daily Phisohex bath should be given for several days before surgery, especially in the obese patient.

8. It is the responsible physician's obligation to review all pathology slides before the proposed exenteration.

9. The sites of the proposed urostomy and colostomy buds are best marked on the day before surgery with the patient standing.

10. A betadine douche HS should be given preoperatively for several days for an infected lesion.

11. Should the patient have poor veins subclavian catheter should be inserted before surgery.

12. Fluid and electrolyte replacement are given as necessary preoperatively.

Observation on the Postoperative Care of the Exenteration Patient

Nothing can be more reassuring to the physician in charge of the postexenteration patient than the knowledge that the operation was technically perfect and that the patient is in the best possible condition. Postoperative care starts in the operating room and should include adequate blood replacement and hemostasis, a spray plastic dressing for easier care and observation of the incision, and antibiotics during the procedure as well as for the first 24 hours postoperatively.

All the details of excellent postoperative care will not be repeated here; only the factors that apply particularly to the exenteration patient will be stressed.

1. Prophylactic antibiotics (cephalosporin) administered at intervals sufficient to maintain therapeutic tissue levels are recommended on the day of surgery beginning pre-operatively.

2. *Blood, fluids, and electrolytes:* It is extremely important to maintain the blood volume and an adequate hematocrit in the initial post-operative phase (3-4 weeks); the majority of patients show a progressive drop. This is probably related to sequestering of fluid into the large pelvic cavity, initial hemoconcentration, decreased survival of bank blood, and postoperative blood loss. The hematocrit should be maintained above 28 at all times, especially in the first 7-14 days, and perhaps higher in the face of infection or other potential complications.

Although the maintenance of· fluid and electrolyte balance is based on experience, certain guidelines can be given. Electrolytes (and BUN) should be determined on the *first*, *third*, and *fifth* days, and also on any day that was preceded by an electrolyte imbalance and at any time a complication, particularly intestinal, exists. After some experience, such studies will be necessary only one or two times in the postoperative period in the uncomplicated patient. This differs from the hematocrit, which should be obtained daily for the first 5 days and then every other day until the patient is nearly ready for discharge. Experience has shown that exenteration patients may require relatively large volumes of fluids, including salt solutions, in the early postoperative period. The amount is guided particularly by the loss of gastrointestinal fluids, the urinary output and the pulse rate. Saline should replace gastrointestinal output liter for liter.

Urinary output should be maintained at 1000-1500 cc daily. Potassium should be given cautiously, at least 40 meq daily, with the amount modified depending on the urinary output and serum potassium. Many patients will require 25-50 g of albumin daily intravenously after 2-3 days. Alternatively, hyperalimentation may be instituted to provide the necessary protein and calories to induce an anabolic state (See chapter 11).

3. Naturally, the psychiatric management is important, and encouragement, explanation, and other support are vital. The importance of rapport with the family cannot be overemphasized.

4. Movement of the legs and deep breathing are encouraged on each visit by the physician. Especially in the immediate post-operative period, IPPB should be used.

5. The pelvic pack (if used) is removed over a 1-3 day period, starting on the 3rd postoperative day. The pack should be cultured on the initial removal and the last day. Once the pelvic pack is removed, it is recommended that the pelvic cavity be irrigated with a solution of saline and peroxide every 6-8 hours. Irrigation may not be necessary if an omental carpet has been used.

6. When a pelvic pack has been used, ambulation is delayed until the 6th and possibly the 7th, postoperative day. The patient is kept flat on the day of the final removal of the pack and then ambulated once the next day and at least b.i.d. thereafter. The patient may be ambulated sooner if an omental carpet has been used and/or the levator muscles have been preserved.

7. Urostomy cultures are obtained if the patient becomes febrile or exhibits CVA tenderness.

8. Extreme conservatism is used in the management of the long tube. Constant low suction is employed for a minimum of 5 days. When the patient is passing flatus, or the colostomy begins to demonstrate function and the abdomen is soft, flat, and nontender

with good bowel sounds, the tube is clamped for 24 hours before giving clear liquids. If after 1 day of clear liquids the patient is without signs of distention, a KUB is obtained and the tube removed if there is no evidence of obstruction. The diet is increased cautiously over the next 4-5 days.

9. When normal bowel function is present, the patient is given multivitamins, and prophylactic urinary antiseptics (suggested is Mandelamine). A single IM dose of Imferon may be better if oral iron intolerance is present.

10. The colostomy irrigations may start on the 8-10th day, but are seldom necessary daily.

11. An IVP is obtained before discharge.

Complications in the exenteration patient are occasionally fulminating, and the magnitude and the nature of the surgery make this patient especially vulnerable. Therefore it is advisable to "*stay ahead*" of the patient and to anticipate complications. Liberal use of the laboratory (cultures, electrolytes, hematocrits, and x-rays) should be combined with *frequent* observation of the patient.

Survival Results

The reported 5 year cumulative survival rate after pelvic exenteration varies from 25 to 40% (Table 2-7). Reported survival rates depend on the circumstances of patient selection for exenteration. For example, where exenteration is a primary procedure, the 5 year survival rate is close to 50%. (Pelvic exenteration might be done as a primary procedure for carcinoma of the vulva extending up the vagina and into the rectum or bladder, and carcinoma of the cervix with extension into the bladder but not out to the pelvic side walls.) In contrast, the 5 year survival rate associated with exenteration after full irradiation therapy for cervical carcinoma is much less than 50% in most series. Excluding the elderly, the obese, the heavily irradiated, and other high risk patients would of course raise survival rates. Withholding exenteration if there is a positive pelvic node after pelvic irradiation also improves cumulative survival rates. In general, however, both the morbidity and mortality rates and the 5 year survival rate have steadily improved over the last decade. Mortality rates in most centers are now well below 10%, and morbidity rates are similarly lower.

The outcome for many patients is related to certain preoperative findings. In the series from M. D. Anderson Hospital, 47% of the patients who had symptoms (pain or edema) with their recurrence but were found at operation to have resectable lesions survived for 2 years, whereas 73% of the patients who were symptom-free at the time of laparotomy survived for 2 years. Of the patients who had a normal intravenous pyelogram at the time of laparotomy, 59% survived for 2 years, while only 34% in whom the IVP showed some abnormality survived for a similar period. In the group who had recurrence within 2 years of the primary treatment, 46% survived for 2 years; if recurrence did not happen until 5 years or more after treatment, 61% survived for 2 years. Therefore such factors as pyelographic findings, the presence or absence of symptoms, and the interval between primary treatment and recurrence should be considered in the preoperative assessment of the patient, but here again they should not be so weighted as to forego the chance for cure in patients with resectable lesions.

TABLE 2-7 PATIENTS TREATED FOR ADVANCED
PELVIC CANCER BY EXENTERATION OF THE PELVIC ORGANS

First Author	Institution	Number of Patients Treated	Number of Operative Deaths	Number Surviving for 5 years
J.S. Krieger (1969)	Cleveland Clinics	35	4	13
E.M. Bricker (1967)	Washington University	153	15	53
A.S. Ketcham (1970)	NCI	162	12	62
R. Symmonds (1968)	Mayo Clinic	118	14	14
R. Douglas (1957)	New York Hospital	23	1	5
L. Parsons (1964)	Pondville Hospital	112	24	24
F. Rutledge (1965)	M. D. Anderson Hospital	108	18	31
A. Brunschwig (1965)	Memorial Hospital	535	86	108
Total		1246	174(14%)	310 (25%)

As mentioned above, the survival rate after pelvic exenteration has improved
considerably over the past decade. Without question, the operation is now done with
more dexterity, resulting in better survivals and lower mortality. Nevertheless, the
morbidity associated with this operation is often severe. It varies considerably from
individual to individual. The chief enemy of the clinician who follows pelvic exenteration
patients is chronic urinary tract infection. On the positive side, psychological adjustment
to the postoperative state comes with considerably more ease than the novice would
anticipate. It is encouraging to watch a patient rally her defense mechanisms and continue
in a fairly normal life pattern after recovery from this procedure. Many times these
women become enthusiastic supporters of the procedure and constitute convincing
evidence to patients who are about to undergo similar surgery.

Summary

1. Although lesions other than carcinoma of the cervix may be treated by pelvic
exenteration, it is cervical cancer that is numerically of significance. With better use of
carefully planned radiotherapy, the number of patients who are acceptable for this
operation is small and should decrease even further.

2. In the interest of progressive reduction of mortality and morbidity and for the
accumulation of significant results, the surgery should preferably be done in areas or
hospitals where sufficient volume may be expected to provide the experience necessary
for proper selection of patients and skilled performance of the operation.

3. Pelvic exenterations should be done only by individuals with adequate training and
background who are willing to take on the responsibility of these patients as a long-term

project and to give special attention to postoperative care and rehabilitation. Under no circumstances should a physician or a team of physicians entertain thoughts of performing these operations unless they are willing to virtually live with their patients postoperatively.

4. Each patient must be assessed individually. The risks of the procedure must be weighed against the possible benefits, as in every other procedure in gynecology. The variables are so numerous that overall survival rates can be misleading.

REFERENCES

Alp, M. H., Seymour, A. E., and Grant, A. K.: Radiation enterocolitis: A report of seven cases and some aspects of pathology and management. *Aust. N. Z. J. Surg.* **40**:144, 1970.

Arneson, A. N.: Cancer of the cervix: Principles of radiation treatment. In *Progress in Gynecology*, J.V. Meigs and S.H. Sturgis, Eds. Grune & Stratton, New York, 1946.

Ashley, D. J. B.: The biological status of carcinoma *in situ* of the uterine cervix. *J. Obstet. Gynaecol. Brit. Commonw.* **73**:372, 1966.

Badib, A. O., Kurohara, S. S., Webster, J. H., and Pickren, J. W.: Metastasis to organs in carcinoma of the uterine cervix: Influence of treatment on incidence and distribution. *Cancer* **21**:434, 1968.

Barber, H. R. K.: Relative prognostic significance of pre-operative and operative findings in pelvic exenteration. *Surg. Clin. North Amer.* **49**:431, 1969.

Barber, H. R. K., and Brunschwig, A.. Gynecologic cancer complicating pregnancy. *Am. J. Obstet. Gynecol.* **85**:156, 1963.

Barber, H. R. K., and Brunschwig, A.: Definitive treatment of radiation necrosis: 5-Year results in 77 patients, *Obstet. Gynecol.* **35**:344, 1970.

Barber, H. R. K., and Jones, W.: Lymphadenectomy in pelvic exenteration for recurrent cervix cancer. *J. Am. Med. Assoc.* **215**:1945, 1971.

Barber, H. R. K., and O'Neil, W. H.: Recurrent cervical cancer after treatment by a primary surgical program. *Obstet. Gynecol.* **37**:165, 1971.

Barron, B. A., and Richart, R. M. Eds.: A statistical model of the natural history of cervical carcinoma based on a prospective study of 557 cases. *J. Nat. Cancer Inst.* **41**:1342, 1968.

Beller, F. K., and Khatamee, M.: Evaluation of punch biopsy of the cervix under direct colposcopic observation (target punch biopsy). *Obstet. Gynecol.* **28**:622, 1968.

Bloedorn, F. G., Gallaher, J. P., and Mould, L. L.: Trends in cooperative management of cancer of the cervix. In *Cancer of the Uterus and Ovary*, a collection of papers presented at the Eleventh Annual Clinical Conference on Cancer, 1966, at the University of Texas, M. D. Anderson Hospital and Tumor Institute at Houston. Year Book Medical Publishers, Chicago, 1969, pp. 195-203.

Bonfiglio, M.: The pathology of fracture of the femoral neck following irradiation. *Am. J. Roentgenol., Radium Ther. Nucl. Med.* **70**:449, 1953.

Bonney, V.: Results of 500 cases of Wertheim's operation for carcinoma of the cervix. *J. Obstet. Gynaecol. Brit. Emp.* **48**:421, 1941.

Bonte, J., and Ide, P.: Prognostic value of persistent cancer cells in vaginal smears of patients with cervical carcinoma treated by radiotherapy. *J. Reprod. Med.* **6**:51, 1971.

Boronow R. C., and Rutledge, F N.: Vesicovaginal fistula, radiation, and gynecologic cancer. *Am. J. Obstet. Gyecol.* **111**:85, 1971.

Bosch, A., and Marcial, V. A.: Carcinoma of the uterine cervix associated with pregnancy. *Am. J. Roentgenol. Radium Ther. Nucl. Med.* **96**:92, 1966.

Brack, C. B., Everett, H. C., and Dickson, R.: Irradiation therapy for carcinoma of the cervix: Its effect on urinary tract. *Obstet. Gynecol.* **7**:196, 1956.

Bricker, E. M.: Bladder substitution after pelvic evisceration. *Surg. Clin. North Am.* **30**:1511, 1950.

Bricker, E. M., Butcher, H. R. and McAfee, A.: Results of Pelvic exenteration. *Am. Med. Assoc. Arch. Surg.* **73**:661, 1956.

Bricker, E. M., and Modlin, J.: The role of pelvic evisceration in surgery. *Surgery* **30**:76, 1951.

Brunschwig, A.: Surgical treatment of carcinoma of the cervix, recurrent after irradiation or combination of irradiation and surgery. *Am. J. Roentgenol., Radium Ther. Nucl. Med.* 99:365, 1967.

Brunschwig, A.: The surgical treatment of Stage I cancer of the cervix. *Cancer* 13:34, 1960.

Brunschwig, A.: What are the indications and results of pelvic exenteration? *J. Am. Med. Assoc.* 194:204, 1965.

Brunschwig, A., and Pierce, V. K.: Necropsy findings in patients with carcinoma of the cervix: Implications for treatment. *Am. J. Obstet. Gynecol.* 56:1134, 1948.

Buchler, D. A., Kline, J. C. Peckham, B. M., Boone, M. L. M., and Carr, W. F.: Radiation reactions in cervical cancer therapy. *Am. J. Obstet. Gynecol.* 111:745, 1971.

Burns, B. C., Jr., and Upton, R. T.: Management of urinary tract complications of treatment of carcinoma of the uterine cervix. In *Cancer of the Uterus and Ovary*, Year Book Medical Publishers, Chicago, 1969, p. 257.

Calame, R. J.: Recurrent carcinoma of the cervix. *Am. J. Obstet. Gyecol.* 105:380, 1969.

Carlson, V., Delclos, L., and Fletcher, G.H.: Distant metastases in squamous cell carcinoma of the uterine cervix. *Radiology* 88:961, 1967.

Castro, J. R., Issa, P., and Fletcher, G. H.: Carcinoma of the cervix treated by irradiation alone. *Radiology* 95:163, 1970.

Chau, P. M., Fletcher, G.H., Rutledge, F. N., and Dodd, G. D., Jr.: Complications in high dose whole pelvis irradiation in female pelvic cancer. *Am. J. Roentgenol., Radium Ther. Nucl. Med.* 87:22, 1962.

Christopherson, W. M., and Parker, J. E.: A critical study of cervical biopsies including serial sectioning. *Cancer* 14:213, 1961.

Clayton, R. S.: Carcinoma of the cervix uteri: Ten-year study with comparison of results of irradiation and radical surgery. *Radiology* 68:74, 1957.

Colpitts, R. V., and Rogers, R. E.: Recurrent carcinoma of the cervix at the University of Texas, M. D. Anderson Hospital and Tumor Institute at Houston, January, 1948, to August, 1963. In *Cancer of the Uterus and Ovary*, Year Book Publishers, Chicago, 1969.

Coppleson, M., Pixley, E., and Reid, B.: Coloscopy. Charles C Thomas, Springfield, Ill., 1971.

Coppleson, M., and Reid, B., (with the assistance of E. Pixley), with a forword by J. Stallworthy: *Preclinical Carcinoma of the Cervix Uteri: Its Nature Origin, and Management*. Pergamon Press, New York, 1967.

Coppleson, M., and Reid, B.: Editorial: The etiology of squamous carcinoma of the cervix. *Obstet. Gynecol.* 32:432, 1968.

Creadick, R. N.: Carcinoma of the cervical stump. *Am. J. Obstet. Gynecol.* 75:565, 1958,

Creasman, W. T., and Parker, R. T.: Microinvasive carcinoma of the cervix. *Clin. Obstet. Gynecol.* 16:261, 1973.

Currie, D. W.: Operative treatment of carcinoma of the cervix. *J. Obstet. Gynaecol. Brit. Commonw.* 78:385, 1971.

Delclos, L.: Analysis of 19 cases of low vaginal metastases in previously treated patients with carcinoma of the cervix or cervical stump. In *Cancer of the Uterus and Ovary*, Year Book Medical Publishers, Chicago, 1969.

Delclos, L., and Carlson, V.: Treatment of distant metastases from squamous cell carcinoma of the uterine cervix. In *Cancer of the Uterus and Ovary*, Year Book Medical Publishers, Chicago, 1969.

Douglas, R. G., and Sweeny, W. J.: Exenterative operations in treatment of advanced pelvic cancer. *Am. J. Obstet. Gynecol.* 73:1169, 1957.

Durrance, F. Y., and Fletcher, G. H.: Computer calculations of dose contribution to regional lymphatics from gynecological radium insertions. *Radiology* 91:140, 1968.

Durrance, F. Y., Fletcher, G. H., and Rutledge, F. N.: Analysis of central recurrent disease in Stages I and II squamous cell carcinomas of the cervix on intact uterus. *Am. J. Roentgenol., Radium Ther. Nucl. Med.* 106:831, 1969.

Easley, J. D., and Fletcher, G. H.: Analysis of treatment of Stage I and Stage II carcinomas of uterine cervix. *Am. J. Roentgenol., Radium Ther. Nucl. Med.* 111:243, 1971.

Ellis, F.: Fractionation in radiotherapy (the NSD concept). In *Modern Trends in Radiotherapy*, Vol. 1, Ch. Z, Eds. T.J. Deeley and C.A. P. Wood, pp 34-51 (Butterworths, London) 1967.

Friedell, G. M., Hertig, A. T., and Younge, P. A.: *Carcinoma in Situ of the Uterine Cervix*. Charles C. Thomas, Springfield, Ill., 1960.

Fletcher, G. H.: The role of supervoltage therapy. In *Proceedings of the Conference on Research on Radiotherapy of Cancer*. American Cancer Society, New York, 1961.

Fletcher, G. H.: External Radiation therapy in cancer of the uterine cervix. In *New Concepts in Gynecological Oncology*, 1st Ed., Lewis, Wentz, and Jaffee, Eds. F. A. Davis, Philadelphia, 1966, p. 111.

Fletcher, G. H.: Results of radiotherapy of carcinoma of the uterine cervix. *Proc. Roy. Soc. Med.* **61**:391, 1968.

Fletcher, G. H.: *Textbook of Radiotherapy*, 2nd Ed. Lea & Febiger, Philadelphia 1973.

Fletcher, G. H., and Rutledge, F. N.: Overall results in radiotherapy for carcinoma of cervix: Modern treatment. *Clin. Obstet. Gynecol.* **5**:958, 1968.

Fletcher, G. H., Shalek, R. J., Wall, J. A., and Bloedorn, F. G.: A physical approach to the design of applicators in radium therapy of cancer of the cervix uteri. *Am. J. Roentgenol., Radium Ther. Nucl. Med.* **68**:935, 1952.

Fletcher, G. H., Stovall, M., and Sampiere, V.: Radiotherapy of cancers of the cervix uteri. In *Carcinoma of the Uterine Cervix, Endometrium and Ovary*, a collection of papers presented at the Fifth Annual Clinical Conference. Year Book Medical Publishers, Chicago, 1962, pp. 69-148.

Fluhmann, C. F.: The squamocolumnar transitional zone of the cervix uteri. *Obstet. Gynecol.* **14**:133, 1959.

Fluhmann, C. F.: Carcinoma *in situ* and the transitional zone of the cervix uteri. *Obstet. Gynecol.* **16**:424, 1960.

Fluhmann, C. F.: *The Cervix Uteri and Its Disease*. W. B. Saunders, Philadelphia, 1961.

Fluhmann, C. F.: Involvement of clefts and tunnels in carcinoma *in situ* of the cervix uteri. *Am. J. Obstet. Gynecol.* **83**:1410, 1962.

Fluhmann, C. F., and Dickmann, Z.: The basic pattern of the glandular structures of the cervix uteri. *Obstet. Gynecol.* **11**:543, 1958.

Gagnon, F.: Contribution to the study of etiology and prevention of cancer of cervix of uterus. *Am. J. Obstet. Gynecol.* **60**:516, 1950.

Gagnon, F.: The lack of occurrence of cervical carcinoma in nuns: *Proc. 2nd Nat. Cancer Conf.* **1**:625, 1952.

Gardner, H. L.: Cervical endometriosis: A lesion of increasing importance. *Am. J. Obstet. Gynecol.* **84**:170, 1962.

Glasser, O., Quimby, E. H., Taylor, L. S., and Weatherwax, J. L.: *Physical Foundations of Radiology*. Paul B. Hoeber, Medical Division of Harper and Brothers, New York, 1952.

Graham, J. B. and Abab, R. S.: Ureteral obstruction due to radiation. *Am. J. Obstet. Gynecol.* **99**:409, 1967.

Graham, J. B., and Graham, R. M.: Curability of regional lymph node metastases in cancer of uterine cervix. *Surg., Gynecol., Obstet.* **100**:149, 1955.

Greiss, F. C., Blake, D. D., and Lock, F. R.: Complications of intensive radiation therapy for cervical carcinoma, with emphasis on supervoltage radiation and supplemental radical pelvic operation. *Obstet. Gynecol.* **18**:417, 1961.

Gusberg, S. G., and Corscaden, J. A.: The pathology and treatment of adenocarcinoma of the cervix. *Cancer* **4**:1066, 1951.

Gusberg, S. G., Fish, S. A., and Wang, Y. Y.: The growth pattern of cervical cancer. *Obstet. Gynecol.* **2**:557, 1953

Gusberg, S. B., and Marshall, D.: Intraepithelial carcinoma of the cervix: A clinical reappraisal. *Obstet. Gynecol.* **19**:713, 1962.

Gusberg, S. B., and Moore, D. B.: Clinical pattern of intraepithelial cancer of the cervix and its pathological background. *Obstet. & Gynecol.* **2**:1, 1953.

Gusberg, S. B., and Rudolph, J.: Individualization of treatment for cancer of the cervix. *Proceedings of American College of Surgeons Meeting, Munich, 1968.* In press.

Halpin, T. F., Frick, H. C., II, and Munnell, E. Q.: Critical points of failure in the therapy of cancer of the cervix: A reappraisal. *Am. J. Obstet. Gynecol.* **114**:755, 1972.

Helper, T. K., Dockerty, M. B., and Randall, L. M.: Primary adenocarcinoma of the cervix. *Am. J. Obstet. Gynecol.* **63**:800, 1952.

Henderson, P. H., and Buck, C. E.: Cervical leukoplakia. *Am. J. Obstet. Gynecol.* **82**:887, 1961.

Henriksen, E.: The lymphatic spread of carcinoma of the cervix and of the body of the uterus: A study of 420 necropsies. *Am. J. Obstet. Gynecol.* **58**:924, 1949.

Henriksen, E.: The dispersion of cancer of the cervix. *Radiology* **54**:812, 1950.

Henriksen, E.: Pyometra associated with malignant lesions of the cervix and the uterus. *Am. J. Obstet. Gynecol.* **72**:884, 1956.

Henriksen, E.: Distribution of metastases in Stage I carcinoma of the cervix. *Am. J. Obstet. ynecol.* **80**:919, 1960.

Hertig, A. T., and Gore, H.: *Tumors of the Female Sex Organs*, Part 2. In *Atlas of Tumor Pathology, Fasc. 33.* Armed Forced Institute of Pathology, Washington, D.C., 1960.

Heyman, J.: Radiological or operative treatment of cancer of uterus. *Acta Radiol.* **8**:363, 1927.

Hreshchyshyn, M. M., and Sheehan, F. R.: Lymphangiography in advanced gynecologic cancer. *Obstet. Gynecol.* **24**:525, 1964.

Hreshchyshyn, M. M., and Sheehan, F. R.: Collateral lymphatics in patients with gynecologic cancer. *Am. J. Obstet. Gynecol.* **91**:118, 1965.

Huffman, J. W.: Mesonephric remnants in the cervix. *Am. J. Obstet. Gynecol.* **56**:23, 1948.

Janeway, H. H.: Treatment of uterine cancer by radium. *Surg., Gynecol., Obstet.* **29**:242, 1919.

Johns, H. E.: *The Physics of Radiology.* Charles C Thomas, Springfield, Ill., 1961.

Johnson, L. D., Nickerson, R. J., Easterday, C. L., Stuart, R. S., and Hertig, A. T.: Epidemiologic evidence for the spectrum of change from dysplasia through carcinoma *in situ* to invasive cancer. *Cancer* **22**:901, 1968.

Jones, T. K., Levitt, S. H., and King, E. R.: Retreatment of persistent and recurrent carcinoma of the cervix with irradiation. *Radiology* **95**:167, 1970.

Jones, T. E., Newell, E. T., Jr., and Brubaker, R. E.: The use of alloy steel wire in the closure of abdominal wounds. *Surg., Gynecol., Obstet.* **72**:1056, 1941.

Kaplan, A. L., Hudgins, P. T., and Wall, J. A.: Postradiation pelvic fibrosis simulating recurrent carcinoma. *Am. J. Obstet. Gynecol.* **92**:117, 1965.

Keettel, W. C., Van Voorhis, L. W., and Latourette, H. B.: Management of recurrent carcinoma of the cervix. *Am. J. Obstet. Gynecol.* **102**:671, 1968.

Ketcheam, A. S., et al: Pelvic exenteration for carcinoma of the uterine cervix. *Cancer* **26**:513, 1970.

Kisclaw, M., Butcher, H. R., and Bricker, E. M.: Results of the radical surgical treatment of advanced pelvic cancer. *Ann. Surg.* **166**:428, 1967.

Kistner, R. W., Gorbach, A. C., and Smith, G. V.: Cervical cancer in pregnancy: Review of the literature with presentation of thirty additional cases. *Obstet. Gynecol.* **9**:554, 1957.

Kolstad, P., and Stafl, A.: *Atlas of Colposcopy.* University Park Press, Baltimore, Md., 1972.

Kottmeier, H. L.: Studies of dosage distribution in pelvis in radium treatment of carcinoma of uterine cervix according to Stockholm method. *J. Fac. Radiol.* **2**:312, 1951.

Kottmeier, H. L.: Ten-year end results, radiological treatment of carcinoma of the cervix. *Acta Obstet. Gynecol. Scand.* **41**:195, 1962.

Kottmeier, H. L.: Complications following radiation therapy in carcinoma of the cervix and their treatment. *Am. J. Obstet. Gynecol.* **88**:854, 1964.

Kottmeier, H. L.: Personal communication dated August 2, 1968, as quoted from Koss, L. G., Concept of genesis and development of carcinoma of the cervix. *Obstet. Gynecol. Surv.* **24**:851, 1969.

Krieger, J. S., and Embree, H. K.: Pelvic exenteration. *Cleveland Clin. Quart.* **36**:1, 1969.

Kurohara, S. S., Vongtama, V. Y., Webster, J. H., and George, F. W., III.: Post-irradiational recurrent epidermoid carcinoma of the uterine cervix. *Am. J. Roentgenol.* **111**:249, 1971.

Localio, S. A., and Friedman, M.: Surgical aspects of radiation enteritis. *Surg., Gynecol., Obstet.* **129**:1163, 1969.

Lapides, J.: Treatment of delayed intractable hemorrhagic cystitis following radiation and chemo-therapy. *J. Urol.* **104**:707, 1970.

Lewis, G. C., Raventos, A., and Hale, J.: Space dose relationships for points A and B in the radium therapy of cancer of the uterine cervix. *Am. J. Roentgenol.* **83**:432, 1960.

Liu, W., and Meigs, J. V.: Radical hysterectomy and pelvic lymphadenectomy. *Am. J. Obstet. Gynecol.* **69**:1, 1955.

Marchant, P. J.: Hemangioma of the cervix. *Obstet. Gynecol.* **17**:191, 1961.

Masterson, B. J., and Rutledge, F.: Irradiation ulcer of the urinary bladder. *Obstet. Gynecol.* **30**:23, 1967.

Masterson, J. G.: Analysis of untreated intraepithelial carcinoma of the cervix. In *Proceedings 3rd National Cancer Conference.* J. B. Lippincott, Philadelphia, 1957.

McGee, C. T., Cromer, D. W., and Greene, R. R.: Mesonephric carcinoma of the cervix: Differentiation from endocervical adenocarcinoma. *Am. J. Obstet. Gynecol.* **84**:358, 1962.

Meigs, J. V.: *Surgical Treatment of Cancer of Cervix.* Grune & Stratton, New York, 1954, p. 192.

Mikuta, J. J.: Invasive carcinoma of the cervix in pregnancy. *South Med. J.* **60**:843, 1967.

Mitra, S.: Cancer of the cervix: Prevalence, ethnology and treatment. *J. Obstet. Gynaec. India,* **7**:151, 1957.

Morton, D. G., and Dignam, W.: The cause of death in patients treated for cervical cancer. *Am. J. Obstet. Gynecol.* **64**:999, 1952.

Mountain, C. F.: Surgical management of pulmonary metastases. *Postgrad. Med.* **48**:128, 1970.

Navratil, E. and Kastner, H.: Unsere Erfahrungen mit 997 Amreichschen Operationen bei der Behandlung des invasiven Cervixkarcinoms. *Wien. Med. Wochenschr.* **116**:1012, 1966.

Newton, M.: Carcinoma of cervix: Use of matched pairs of cases to compare treatment by surgery or radiation. *Surg., Gynecol. Obstet.* **99**:29, 1954.

Ng, A. B., and Reagan, J. W.: Microinvasive carcinoma of the uterine cervix. *Am. J. Clin. Pathol.* **52**:511, 1969.

Nolan, J. F., Anson, J. H., and Steward, M.: A radium applicator for use in the treatment of cancer of the uterine cervix. *Am. J. Roentgenol., Radium Ther. Nucl. Med.* **79**:36, 1958.

Novak, E. R. and Woodruff, J. D.: *Gynecologic and Obstetric Pathology.* W. B. Saunders, Philadelphia, 1972.

Ortiz, R., Newton, M., and Longlois, P. L.: Colposcopic biopsy in the diagnosis of carcinoma of the cervix. *Obstet. Gynecol.* **34**:303, 1969.

Ortiz, R., and Odell, L. D.: Observations on the use of the colposcope for cervical neoplasia. *J. Reprod. Med.* **4**:97, 1970.

Ostergard, D. R., and Morton, D. G.: Multifocal carcinoma of the female genitals. *Am. J. Obstet. Gynecol.* **99**:1006, 1968.

Parker, R. T., Wilbanks, G. D., Yowell, R. K., and Carter, F. B.: Radical hysterectomy and pelvic lymphadenectomy with and without preoperative radiotherapy for cervical cancer. *Am. J. Obstet. Gynecol.* **99**:933, 1967

Parsons, L., and Friedell, G. J.: Radical surgical treatment of cancer of cervix. *Proc. Nat. Cancer Conf.* **5**:241, 1964.

Paunier, J. P., Delclos, L., and Fletcher, G. H.: Causes, time of death, and sites of failure in squamous cell carcinoma of the uterine cervix on intact uterus. *Radiology* **88**:555, 1967.

Perez, C. A., Bradfield, J. S., and Morgan, H. C.: Management of pathologic fractures. *Cancer* **29**:684, 1972.

Peterson, O.: Spontaneous course of cervical precancerous conditions. *Am. J. Obstet. Gynecol.* **72**:1063, 1956.

Radman, H. H.: Myoma of the cervix. *Am. J. Obstet. Gynecol.* **82**:361, 1961.

Rawls, W. E., Gardner, H. L., and Kaufman, R. L.: Antibodies to genital herpes virus in patients with carcinoma of the cervix. *Am. J. Obstet. Gynecol.* **107**:710, 1970.

Rawls, W. E., et al: Herpes virus Type 2: Association with carcinoma of the the cervix. *Science* **161**:1255, 1968.

Reagan, J. W.: Genesis of carcinoma of the uterine cervix. *Clin. Obstet. Gynecol.* **10**:883, 1967.

Richart, R. M.: Natural history of cervical intraepithelial neoplasia. *Clin. Obstet Gynecol.* **10**:748, 1967.

Richart, R. M., and Barron, B. A.: A follow-up study of patients with cervical dysplasia. *Am. J. Obstet. Gynecol.* **105**386, 1969.

Richart, R. M., and Vaillant, H. W.: Influence of cell collection techniques upon cytological diagnosis. *Cancer* **18**:1474, 1969.

Roddick, J. W., Jr., and Miller, D. H.: Factors affecting the management of recurrent cervical carcinoma. *Am. J. Obstet. Gynecol.* **101**:53, 1968.

Rutledge, F. N.: Combination irradiation and surgical therapy for carcinoma of the cervix. In *Cancer of the Uterus and Ovary*, Year Book Publishers, Chicago, 1969, p. 216.

Rutledge, F. N., and Burns, B. C., Jr.: Pelvic exenteration. *Am. J. Obstet. Gynecol.* **91**:692, 1965.

Rutledge, F. N., and Fletcher, G. H.: Transperitoneal pelvic lymphadenectomy following supervoltage irradiation for squamous cell carcinoma of the cervix. *Am. J. Obstet. Gynecol.* **76**:321, 1958.

Rutledge, F. N., Fletcher, G. H., and MacDonald, E. J.: Pelvic lymphadenectomy as an adjunct to radiation therapy in treatment for cancer of cervix. *Am. J. Roentgenol., Radium Ther. Nucl. Med.* **93**:607, 1965.

Rutledge, F. N., Gutierrez, A. G., and Fletcher, G. H.: Management of Stage I and II adenocarcinomas of the uterine cervix on intact uterus. *Am. J. Roentgenol., Radium Ther. Nucl. Med.* **102**:161, 1968.

Savlov, E. D., Nahhas, W. A., and May, A. G.: Iliac and femoral arteriosclerosis following pelvic irradiation for carcinoma of the ovary. *Obstet. Gynecol.* **34**:345, 1969.

Schier, J., Symmonds, R. E., and Dahlin, D. C.: Clinicopathologic aspects of actinic enteritis. *Surg., Gynecol., Obstet.* **119**:1019, 1964.

Schwarz, G.: Evaluation of Manchester system of treatment of carcinoma of cervix. *Am. J. Roentgenol., Radium Ther. Nucl. Med.* **105**:579, 1969.

Sherman, A. I.: *Cancer of the Female Reproductive Organs*. C.V. Mosby, St. Louis, 1963.

Smith, J. P., Golden, P. E, and Rutledge, F. N.: The surgical management of intestinal injuries following irradiation for carcinoma of the cervix. In *Cancer of the Uterus and Ovary*. Year Book Medical Publishers, Chicago, 1969, pg. 241.

Song, J.: *The Human Uterus: Morphogenesis and Embryological Basis for Cancer*. Charles C Thomas, Springfield, Ill. 1964.

Stallworthy, J.: Radical surgery following radiation treatment for cervical carcinoma. *Ann. Roy. Coll. Surg. Engl.* **34**:161, 1964.

Stern, E., and Dixon, W. J.: Cancer of the cervix: A biometric approach to etiology. *Cancer* **14**:153, 1961.

Stone, M. L., Weingold A. B., and Sall, S.: Cervical carcinoma in pregnancy. *Am. J. Obstet. Gynecol.* **93**:479, 1965.

Strockbine, M. F., Hancock, H. E., and Fletcher, G. H.: Complications in 831 patients with squamous cell carcinoma of the intact uterine cervix treated with 3000 rads or more whole pelvis irradiation. *Am. J. Roentgenol., Radium Ther. Nucl. Med.* **108**:293, 1970.

Suit, H., Wette, R., and Lindberg, F.: Analysis of tumor-recurrence times. *Radiology* **88**:311, 1967.

Symmonds, R. E., Pratt, J. H., and Welch, J. S.: Exenterative operations. *Am. J. Obstet. Gynecol.* **101**:66, 1968.

Taussig, F. J.: Iliac lymphadenectomy plus radiation in borderline cancer of cervix. *Am. J. Obstet. Gynecol.* **32**:777, 1936.

Taussig, F. J.: Iliac lymphadenectomy for Group II cancer of cervix. *Am. J. Obstet. Gynecol.* **45**:733, 1943.

Ter-Pogossian, M.: The physical aspects of radiation therapy of carcinoma of the cervix uteri. *Clin. Obstet. Gynecol.* **4**:466, 1961.

Townsend, D. E., and Ostergard, D. R.: Cryocauterization for preinvasive cervical neoplasia. *J. Reprod. Med.* **6**:171, 1971.

Townsend, D. E., Ostergard, D. R., and Lickrish, G. M.: Cryosurgery for benign disease of the uterine cervix. *J. Obstet. Gynaecol. Brit. Commonw.* **78**:667, 1971.

Townsend, D. E., Ostergard, D. R., Mishell, D. R., Jr., et al: Abnormal Papanicolaou smears: Evaluation by colposcopy, biopsies, and endocervical curettage. *Am. J. Obstet. Gynecol.* **108**:429, 1970.

Townsend, D. E., et al: Rational evaluation and treatment of the patient with preinvasive cervical neoplasia. Unpublished.

Twombly, G. H., and Taylor, H. C., Jr.: Treatment of cancer of cervix uteri: Comparison of radiation therapy and radical surgery. *Am. J. Roentgenol., Radium Ther. Nucl. Med.* **71**:501, 1954.

Ulfelder, H., Smith, C. J., and Costello, J. B.: Invasive carcinoma of the cervix during pregnancy. *Am. J. Obstet. Gynecol.* **98**:424, 1967.

Van Herik, M., Decker, D. G., Lee, R. A., and Symmonds, R. E.: Late recurrence in carcinoma of the cervix. *Am. J. Obstet Gynecol.* **108**:115, 1970.

Van Voorhis, L. W.: Carcinoma of the cervix. I. Therapeutic and patient factors affecting survival. *Am. J. Obstet. Gynecol.* **108**:105, 1970a.

Van Voorhis, L. W.: Carcinoma of the cervix. II. A critical evaluation of patient follow-up. *Am. J. Obstet. Gynecol.* **108**:115, 1970b.

Villasanta, U.: Complications of radiotherapy for carcinoma of the uterine cervix. *Am. J. Obstet. Gynecol.* **114**:717, 1972.

Wall, J. A., Collins, V. P., Hudgins, P. T., Kaplan, A. L., and Adams, R. M.: Carcinoma of the cervix. *Am. J. Obstet. Gynecol.* **96**:57, 1966.

Wertheim, E.: Radical abdominal operation in carcinoma of cervix uteri. *Surg., Gynecol., Obstet.* **4**:1, 1907.

Wertheim, E.: *Die Erweiterte Abdominale Operation bei Carcinoma Colli Uteri.* Urban & Schwarzenbert, Berlin, 1911.

Wheeles, C. R., Jr.: Small bowel bypass for complications related to pelvic malignancy. *Obstet. Gynecol.* **42**:661, 1973.

White, W. C., and Finn, F. W.: The late complications following irradiation of pelvic viscera. *Am. J. Obstet. Gynecol.* **62**:65, 1951.

Wied, G.: What is the place of colposcopy in modern gynecologic practice? *J. Reprod. Med.* **1**:17, 1968.

Wynder, E. L.: Epidemiology of carcinoma *in situ* of the cervix. *Obstet. Gynecol. Surv.* **24**:697, 1969.

CHAPTER THREE

Colposcopy

Colposcopy was developed in 1925 by Hans Hinselman of Hamburg, Germany. At that time it was believed that cervical cancer began as miniature nodules and that with increased magnification and illumination these small nodules should be detectable. Instead of miniature tumors Hinselman and his associates unexpectedly viewed a fascinating variety of both normal and abnormal tissue patterns. Being clinicians with little histopathological background and encumbered by the tumor nodule theory, they developed confusing concepts and a terminology that was cumbersome, lengthy, occasionally contradictory, and awkward for English translation.

Efforts were made to introduce colposcopy into the United States in the early 1930s as a means for early cervical cancer detection. Primarily because of the awkward terminology the method was generally ignored. With the introduction of cytology in the 1940s North American interest in colposcopy waned even further. In the 1950s and early 1960s attempts were again made in the English speaking countries to stimulate interest in this technique. Invariably, however, it was placed in competition with cytology for cervical cancer detection, and invariably it proved to be inferior. Cytology was more economical, considerably easier to learn, and had a lower false-negative rate. As a consequence, numerous critics of colposcopy appeared and at one point it was called the greatest gynecologic hoax of this or any other century.

More recently several significant developments have sparked a burgeoning interest in the technique in North America. First, the observed colposcopic changes have been placed on a solid scientific basis, which has been coupled with a logical and simplified terminology. Second, colposcopy is recommended primarily as a technique to provide the clinician with an additional dimension in the examination of the visible portion of the female genital tract (i.e., vulva, vagina, and cervix), therefore not placing it in competition with cytology but rather offering it as a complementary measure. Third, new reference materials, teaching aids, and instructional techniques have been developed. Last, and quite important, numerous articles have appeared in the English literature pointing out the value of colposcopy in avoiding diagnostic conization in the patient with an abnormal Papanicolaou test, i.e., a Pap test suggestive of dysplasia or worse (Class III or worse).

The colposcope is basically a stereoscopic "dissecting" microscope coupled with increased illumination. Various levels of magnification are available, the most practical being between 8 and 18x. A green filter is inserted between the light source and the tissue to accentuate the color tone differences between normal and abnormal patterns, as well as to enhance the vascular patterns. Interestingly, many instruments used in operating theaters and offices by ophthalmologists, neurosurgeons, and otolaryngologists are essentially "colposcopes."

Colposcopy is to be differentiated from colpomicroscopy, another method to carefully examine the cervix. Colpomicroscopy uses a magnification up to 200x, is more difficult to master, requires an expert knowledge of cytology, and takes a considerably longer time to complete. The examination of the visible portion of the female genital tract by colposcopy takes no more than a few minutes in the uncomplicated case. In patients with an abnormal Pap test, 15–20 minutes are usually required for a thorough evaluation.

One of the major concepts on which contemporary colposcopy is based is the transformation zone. A clear understanding of the transformation zone is vital not only to colposcopy but also in comprehending the origin and development of cervical neoplasia. The transformation zone is defined as the area of the cervix (or cervix and vagina) that was initially covered by columnar epithelium which, through a process called metaplasia, has been replaced in whole or in part by squamous epithelium.

It has been generally believed that the cervix is normally covered by squamous epithelium and that the presence of endocervical columnar epithelium on the ectocervix is an abnormal location for this tissue. Recent studies in Australia and the United States, however, have established the fact that columnar tissue initially exists on the ectocervix in at least 70% of females and extends onto the vagina in an additional 5% of the female population. Moreover, the location of columnar epithelium on the ectocervix is determined early in embryologic development.

Metaplasia (i.e., transition from columnar to squamous epithelium) probably occurs throughout an individual's lifetime; however, it has been suggested that this normal physiologic transition is most active at three phases: fetal stage, adolescence, and the first pregnancy. The process is enhanced by an acid environment and is no doubt influenced by steroids such as estrogen and progesterone. Embryologically the fallopian tubes, uterus, cervix, and vagina are derived from the paired mullerian ducts. Initially the vagina is lined by a simple columnar epithelium, but early in fetal life a stratified cuboidal epithelium, which eventually differentiates into squamous epithelium, begins to displace this müllerian derived columnar tissue. Virtually all of the columnar epithelium in the vagina and a variable portion of the ectocervical columnar tissue are replaced in the balance of female fetuses. The location of columnar tissue on the ectocervix and in a few cases in the vagina is therefore not the result of outward growth from the cervix as once believed. The replacement of the columnar tissue apparently stops around the fifth gestational month. After the initial replacement of müllerian columnar epithelium by the urogenital sinus cuboidal epithelium is completed, any further replacement of the columnar tissue by squamous tissue is accomplished by the process referred to as metaplasia. Metaplasia in the fetus takes place in the latter half of pregnancy and is probably due to the influence of maternal steroids. After delivery, metaplasia slows because of a drop in steroids and the neutral secretions of the vagina. With the onset of menstruation, the vagina becomes more acid after the establishment of a bacterial population. When the columnar ectocervical tissue is exposed to the acid environment, the transformation process is once again activated.

The metaplastic squamous epithelium originated both as a peripheral ingrowth from the squamous epithelium laid down early in fetal life and from multipotential cells that are usually found subjacent to the columnar epithelium. The multipotential cells differentiate into immature squamous epithelium when exposed to an acid environment. The squamous cells then displace the overlying columnar epithelium and develop into multiple foci or islands. The islands broaden, coalesce, and eventually join the peripheral contribution from the original squamous epithelium. Gland openings develop that permit the egress of mucus from the deeper secreting columnar cells. In some instances the gland openings become occluded and nabothian cysts form. The complete transformation from columnar to squamous epithelium probably requires many years. Patients who are on oral contraceptives seem to have a slower transformation, probably because of the buffering effect from increased production of mucus in response to the steroids contained in the pills. With advancing age, the transformation zone matures, nabothian cysts and gland openings disappear, and the constantly changing squamocolumnar junction gradually migrates up the endocervical canal. The upward migration is relatively slow because of the anatomical location of the canal and neutral pH of the environment.

In the reproductive years, the transformation zone is characterized by areas of columnar epithelium interspersed with areas of metaplastic squamous epithelium, gland openings, and nabothian cysts. With advancing age, the transformation zone becomes less apparent and only the very fine vascular structure will reveal its location. Occasionally the metaplastic squamous epithelium appears slightly whiter than the original squamous epithelium. This is due to an increased number of relatively large nuclei in the intermediate and parabasal cell layers. In some instances, the immature metaplastic epithelium lacks glycogen and only partially stains with iodine.

In most women a normal tranformation zone develops and cytology is likewise normal. However, in a few instances, due to an unknown cause or causes, a DNA change occurs in the immature metaplastic squamous epithelium and potentially malignant cells develop. As a consequence an abnormal transformation zone evolves. It is in the abnormal transformation zone that patterns characteristic of the earliest forms of cervical neoplasia are invariably found.

3-1 ABNORMAL TRANSFORMATION ZONE

A transformation zone is classified as abnormal when one or more of the following patterns are viewed: white epithelium, mosaic structure, punctation, leukoplakia, and abnormal vascular pattern. Although each pattern may exist as a separate and distinct entity, in most cases several patterns will be present simultaneously. The basic component of all patterns is white epithelium, which is due to an increased number of nuclei which may have an increase in DNA. When light from the colposcope illuminates an area with increased nuclear concentration, it does not completely penetrate the area and is reflected through the lens of the instrument. As a consequence these areas appear white. The optical density and, therefore, the degree of whiteness vary directly with the nuclear concentration. Normal epithelium is pinkish white, whereas dysplasia and carcinoma *in situ*, which have greater nuclear density, are significantly whiter. In some instances the white epithelium will develop into a pattern referred to as mosaic or punctation. Mosaic structure and punctation are due to the retention and/or crowding out of the individual villus capillaries of the columnar epithelium. Leukoplakia is a raised white plaque that is visible with the naked eye before the application of acetic acid. Acetic acid is a mucolytic agent that assists in the removal of mucus and also has a dehydrating effect, causing a relative increase in the nuclear-cytoplasmic ratio.

Invariably one border of white epithelium, mosaic structure or punctation is made up by the active or physiologic squamocolumnar junction. On the other hand, leukoplakia is seldom present at the physiolgic squamocolumnar junction; however, it is invariably within the transformation zone. Atypical vessels have patterns that are highly irregular and have been termed "commas," "spaghetties," "corkscrews," or "earthworms." They are to be differentiated from the regular branching of normal vessels frequently seen over large nabothian cysts. Atypical vessels are most important since they may herald the site of early invasive carcinoma. Examples of the various patterns in the abnormal transformation zone are seen in Figs. 3-1 to 3-5.

With experience it is possible to grade the colposcopic abnormalities and to make an extremely accurate prediction as to the histologic diagnosis. Factors considered in grading include the vascular structures (i.e., regular or irregular), surface contour, (i.e., flat, depressed, raised, and/or irregular), color and opacity, or degree of whiteness, and line of demarcation from apparently normal epithelium. The green filter enhances the color tone differences and the vascular changes; the latter are best viewed before acetic acid application. Acetic acid is very important in enhancing the color tone differences. Immature metaplastic squamous epithelium may also appear white because of the relatively increased number of immature cells with large nuclei. It is possible to differentiate it from mildly dysplastic epithelium in that the border between metaplastic and normal epithelium is highly irregular, whereas the border between normal and potential dysplastic tissue is usually sharp.

Most of the abnormal patterns will be unifocal, although in some instances multifocal appearances are seen. Invariably, multifocal disease is confined to the ectocervix and transformation zone. We have not seen a case of disease high in the canal and low on the ectocervix without an intervening bridge of abnormal epithelium.

3-2 COLPOSCOPICALLY OVERT CARCINOMA

There are instances in which the naked eye can detect no suggestive evidence of invasive carcinoma. However, when these patients are examined with colposcopy, features consistent with invasive cancer, that is, raised irregular surface contour, thick epithelium, and markedly atypical vascular pattern, are most apparent. In these cases the colposcope is particularly valuable in pinpointing the exact area for sampling for early diagnosis and prompt initiation of therapy.

3-3 SATISFACTORY OR UNSATISFACTORY EXAMINATION

Critical to every colposcopic evalutaion of the cervix is the ablity to view the entire limits of the active or physiologic squamocolumnar junction. If the entire limits of this most important landmark cannot be seen, the examination must be judged unsatisfactory and the possibility of invasive cancer in a patient with an abnormal Pap test cannot be excluded. However, if invasive cancer has been recognized and confirmed by a biopsy on the visible portion of the cervix, obviously the patient has had an appropriate evaluation.

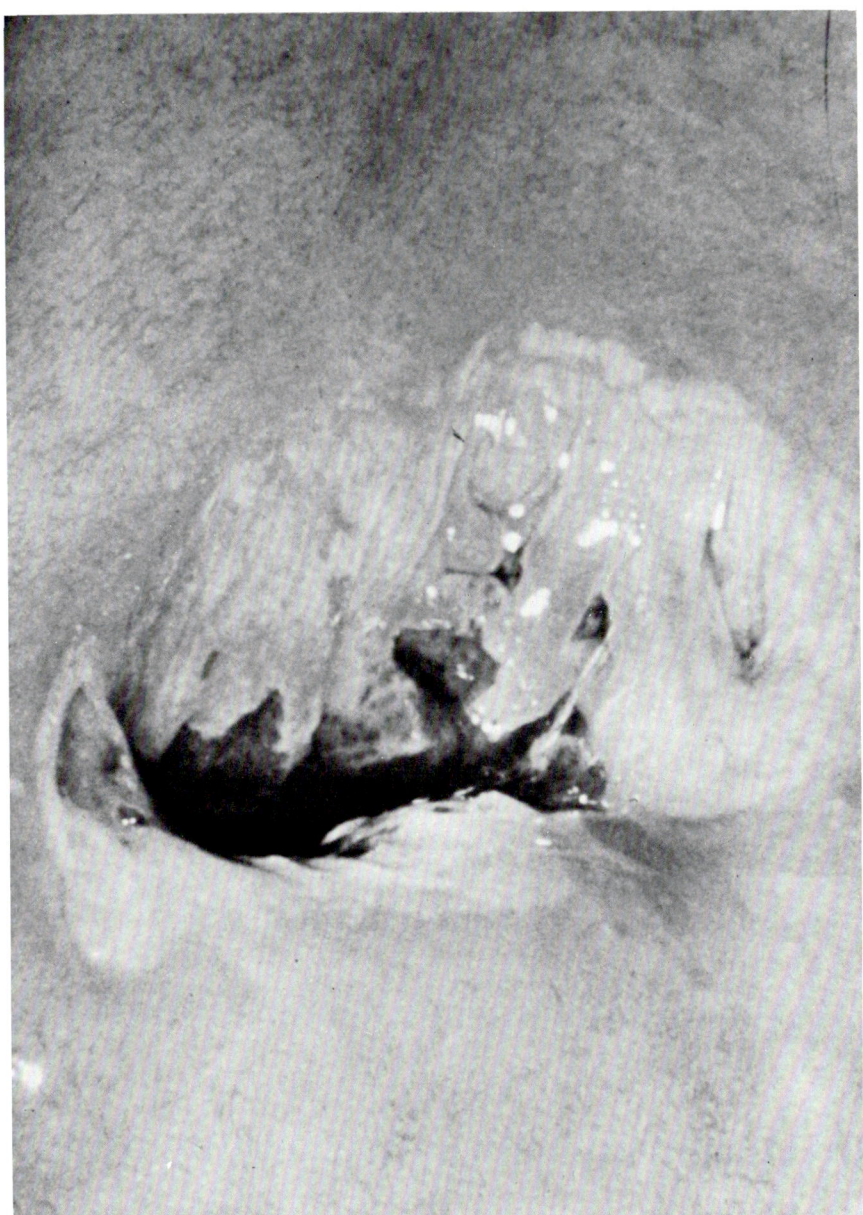

Fig. 3-1 Colpo-photograph of 19 year add nulliparous female whose Pap test was suggestive of moderate dysplasia. An abnormal transformation zone characterized by white epithelium is present. Directed biopsy showed moderate dysplasia. Entire limits of physiologic squamocolumnar junction is seen; therefore diagnostic conization is unnecessary.

In cases were cervical intraepithelial neoplasia is present and the entire junction cannot be seen, the examination must be considered unsatisfactory and the patient must be given a vigorous endocervical curettage. If invasive cancer is not found in this test or by other office biopsies in the presence of CIN, a diagnostic conization must be performed.

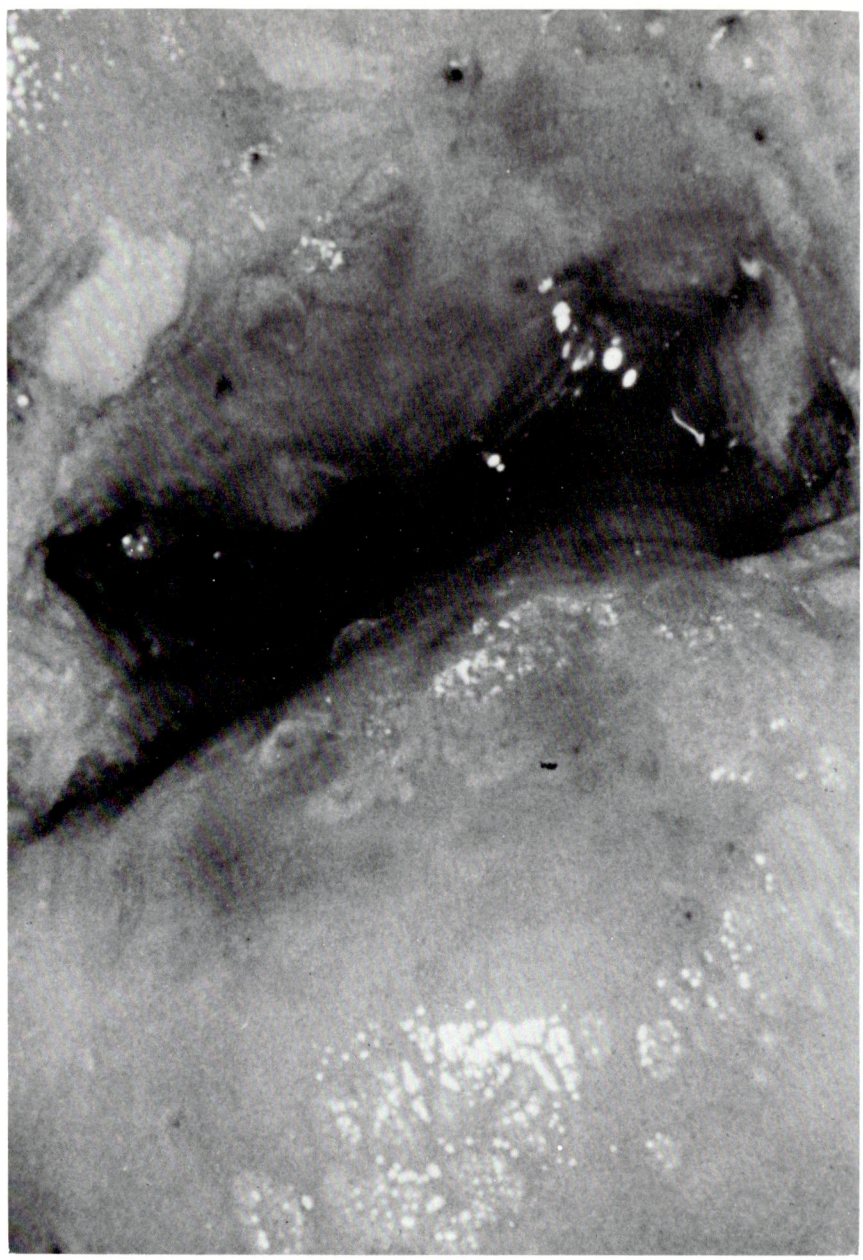

Fig. 3-2 Colpo-photograph of 27 year old gravida 2 para 2 whose Pap test was consistent with mild to moderate dysplasia. Leukoplakia present at 11 o'clock in the transformation zone but not at the squamocolumnar junction. Patient had white epithelium extending into the canal, and upper limits of the lesion could not be seen. Endocervical curettage revealed moderate dysplasia, and diagnostic conziation was necessary for complete evaluation of endocervical canal. The small area of leukoplakia was visible to the naked eye before the application of acetic acid. 16X.

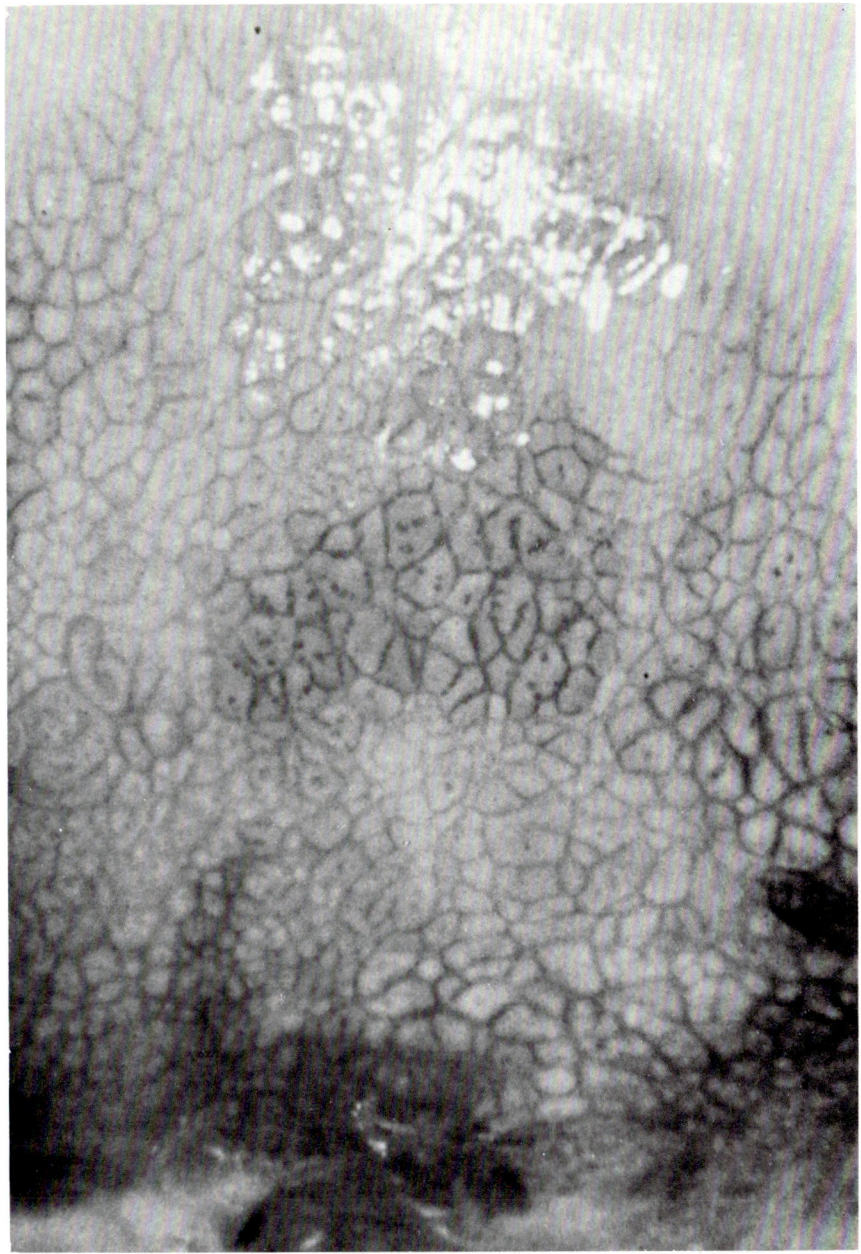

Fig. 3-3 Atypical transformation zone characterized by mosaic structure with an occasional area of punctation. The mosaic structure is regular, and the punctation has a moderate increase in intercapillary distance. Directed biopsy showed carcinoma *in situ*. Entire limits of this lesion could be seen; therefore diagnostic conization was unnecessary.

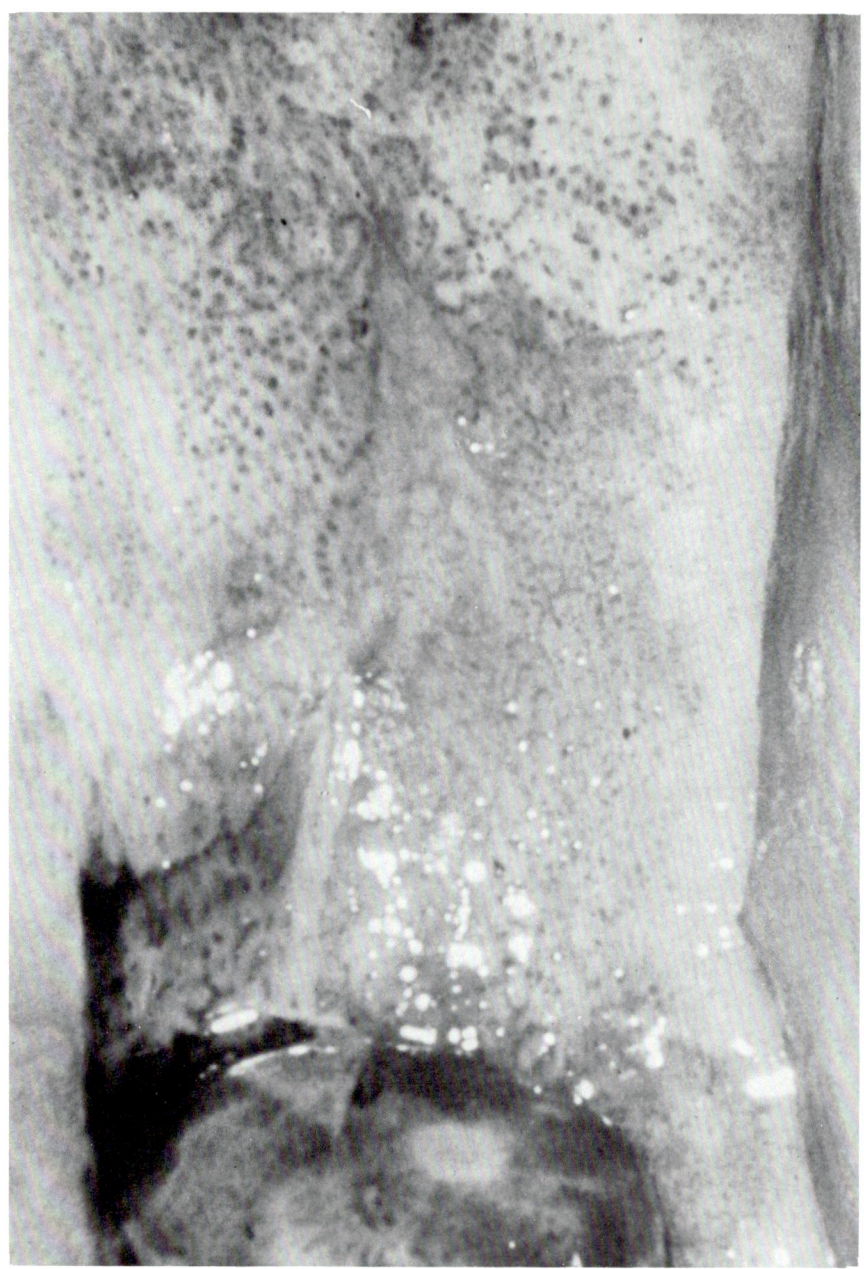

Fig. 3-4 Atypical transformation zone characterized by punctation. Large polyp occluding the external os present at the bottom of the colpo-photograph. Directed biopsy revealed carcinoma *in situ*, but entire limits of lesion could not be viewed and conization was necessary since endocervical curettage showed only carcinoma *in situ*. Conization revealed a carcinoma *in situ*. 16X.

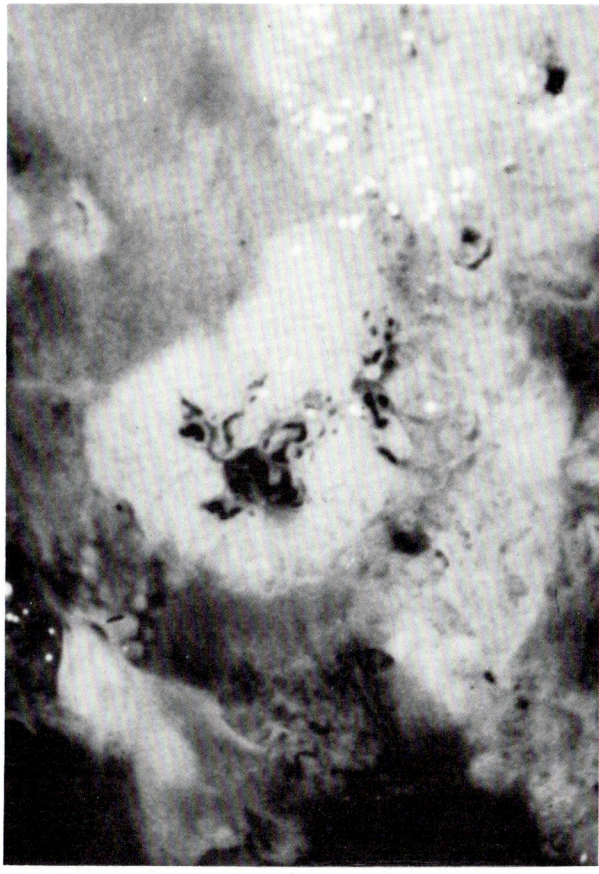

Fig. 3-5 Atypical transformation zone characterized by heavy white epithelium with a focus of atypical vascular structure within the center of this epithelium. Directed biopsy of the atypical vascular pattern revealed microinvasive carcinoma. Conization was necessary to assess the lesion completely since the microinvasive cancer was present and the lesion extended well into the canal. An endocervical curettage revealed severe dysplasia. 16X.

3-4 OTHER COLPOSCOPIC FINDINGS

The single largest subdivision of colposcopic findings consists of those that are of minor significance. Most frequently encountered include condylomas, papillomas, cervical polyps, true erosions (which are usually traumatic because of speculum insertion), vaginocervicitis, and atrophic epithelium. The most important of the miscellaneous patterns are condylomas and papillomas (Fig. 3-6) since they give rise to abnormal Pap tests. These lesions are more frequently seen during pregnancy and are usually recognized because of their striking surface contours and vascular structures. Most are associated with

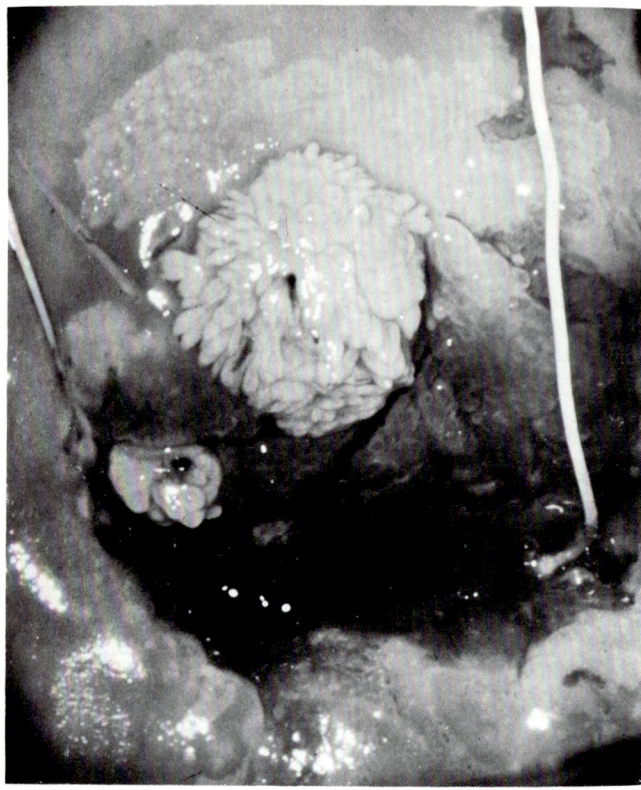

Fig. 3-6 Typical condyloma accuminata present at 12 o'clock and a smaller satellite lesion at 11 o'clock. Patient had a Pap test suggestive of mild to moderate dysplasia. White epithelium present on the anterior lip with a very irregular border consistent with squamous metaplasia. Entire limits of the lesion could be seen. Directed biopsy of the lesion at 12 o'clock revealed condyloma, and directed biopsy of the white epithelium revealed active metaplasia. IUD string present passing out of the os at 4 and at 10 o'clock. 16X.

vulvar and vaginal components and are invariably multifocal. Although one may believe that he is viewing a papilloma or condyloma, it is mandatory that such lesions always be sampled because in a few instances a keratinizing invasive cancer has mistakenly been diagnosed as a condyloma.

With the recognition of the above colposcopic patterns, it is possible to categorize these changes on the basis of a simplified and logical terminology (see Table 3-1).

3-5 APPLICATIONS OF COLPOSCOPY

Abnormal Papanicolaou Test

The single greatest value of colposcopy is for the patient who has an abnormal Pap test, be she pregnant, nonpregnant, or postradiation. The evaluation of the patient with an abnormal Pap test was covered thoroughly in Chapter 2. In pregnancy, colposcopy

TABLE 3-1   COLPOSCOPIC TERMINOLOGY

Normal colposcopic findings
1. Original squamous epithelium
2. Columnar epithelium
3. Transformation zone

Abnormal colposcopic findings
1. Atypical transformation zone
   White epithelium
   Punctation
   Mosaic structure
   Leukoplakia
   Abnormal blood vessels
2. Suspect frank invasive cancer

Unsatisfactory colposcopic findings

Other colposcopic findings
   Vagino-cervicitis
   True erosion
   Atrophic epithelium
   Condyloma, papilloma

permits a rapid, accurate assessment and conization is seldom needed. In patients who have abnormal Pap tests after radiotherapy, it is frequently easy to locate the cause of the abnormal result by colposcopy, thereby eliminating the need for hospitalization and extensive diagnostic steps, including surgery. In other cases, a very early recurrence may be detected, thereby permitting a more expiditous route for further therapy.

Benign Cervical Changes

Physicians often are faced with a patient who has a red, "angry" appearing cervix. In these cases colposcopic examination will permit an accurate evaluation of the abnormality, thereby assuring both the physician and the patient that a more serious problem is not present. The red, somewhat hypertrophied, granular appearance of the cervix in these patients is invariably due to the single-cell columnar epithelium overlying the highly vascular stroma. This appearance is sometimes exaggerated in women taking birth control pills. It is normal for columnar epithelium to be located on the ectocervix, and therapy is not necessary unless there are associated symptoms such as vaginal discharge. Patients with cervical polyps can also be assessed by colposcopy. In most cases the base of the polyp can be viewed.

Vulva

Vulvar disease is amenable to colposcopic evaluation, although the patterns are not as striking as those on the cervix. Intraepithelial vulvar lesions are frequently mulifocal, and with the colposcope it is possible to note how many lesions are present. In some cases there will be only a single focus, thereby precluding the need for radical excision. When keratinized lesions are present, however, colposcopy is of less value. Keratinized lesions must be totally excised because of inability to assess the vascular pattern.

The most frequent pattern encountered on the vulva is white epithelium, which may have a keratinized surface. Mosaic structure and punctation are infrequently seen since the lack of columnar epithelium precludes the formation of these patterns. Infectious disease such as herpes and syphilis present no particular diagnostic features, although small vesicles of herpes progenitalis can be detected early, permitting a prompt initiation of therapy and possibly aborting the full blown disease. Condylomas and papillomas are quite assessable by colposcopy and in the very young individual colposcopic examination will exclude the presence of a more serious problem, avoiding hospitalization and anesthesia for evaluation.

Vagina

Benign and malignant vaginal lesions can be evaluated by colposcopy. Granulation tissue at the apex of the vagina is an all too frequent occurrence after hysterctomy. It is not always possible to assess this lesion accurately, and as a consequence granulation tissue must always be biopsied since it has atypical vascular features. Intraepithelial vaginal lesions have a tendency to be multifocal and are ideally suited for colposcopic evaluation. When evaluating vaginal intraepithelial lesions it is important that Lugol's solution be used to assist in the location of tiny foci that may be hidden in the vaginal folds. The prominent patterns in the vagina are white epithelium and punctation. If there has been columnar tissue in the vagina, as does occur in a small minority of patients and is particularly prominent in diethylstilbestrol exposed offspring, all the features seen on the cervix, such as mosaic structure, punctation, leukoplakia, and atypical vessels, may be present.

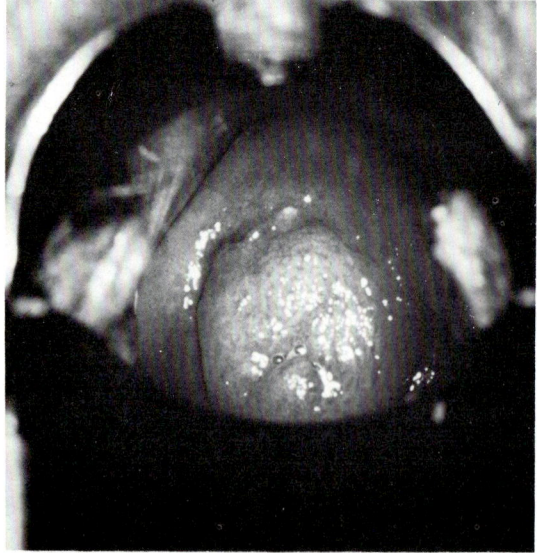

Fig. 3-7 Gross photograph of a 19 year old DES exposed female with a classic cervical collar. Patient had an erythematous appearing cervix which extended onto the collar. 16X.

Diethylstilbestrol Exposed Offspring

The recent finding of clear cell adenocarcinoma as well as other anomalies in DES exposed offspring provides the colposcopist with a fertile field for investigation. With the naked eye, it is almost impossible to know the extent of changes in the vagina and cervix in the DES exposed individual. With the colposcope, it is possible to assess the changes precisely and to preclude the necessity of multiple punch biopses, which are invariably required when only a naked eye examination is carried out. Although clear cell adenocarcinoma is relatively rare in DES exposed offspring, squamous cell lesions are beginning to be seen with alarming frequency. Since these abnormalities are occurring in very young individuals, a colposcopic evaluation becomes mandatory in any DES exposed offspring who has an abnormal Pap test. The total impact that DES will have on female offspring remains to be determined, and only well designed prospective studies with long-term follow-up will identify the significant changes that should be evaluated.

In DES exposed offspring, one invariably sees a vast transformation zone, which usually covers the entire ectocervix and extends onto the vagina, occasionally down to the

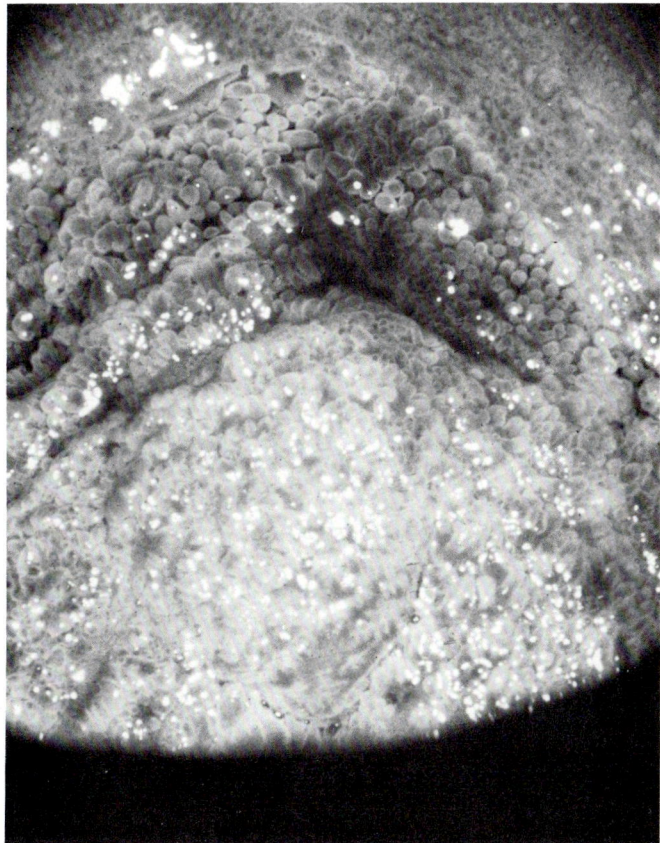

Fig. 3-8   Colpo-photograph of the same patient as in Fig. 3-7. Grapelike appearance of columnar tissue present. Above the area of columnar tissue is active squamous metaplasia. Patient also had areas of adenosis in the vagina and an extensive transformation zone in the vagina. 16X.

introitus. The metaplastic squamous epithelium of the vagina usually appears white, forming mosaic and punctation patterns. Atypical vessels are rare. As the metaplastic squamous epithelium matures, the white appearance tends to lessen. However, considerable time is required for the tissue to become mature enough to accept Lugol's iodine. Adenosis, cervical hoods, ridges, and cock's combs that are viewed grossly can be promptly and soberly examined colposcopically, permitting a positive and tranquil assurance to the patient and her parents that no truly serious abnormality exists. Examples of gross and colposcopic changes encountered in DES exposed offspring are shown in Figs. 3-7 to 3-10.

Research and Education

It is possible with colposcopy to provide the medical student, intern, and resident with a more meaningful appreciation of "benign" as well as premalignant disease of the cervix. It is particularly satisfying to point out the areas where cervical neoplasia is most likely to occur, so that the Pap sampling is more accurate, thereby lowering the false-negative rate. In patients from whom specific areas of tissue are needed for research, one can precisely

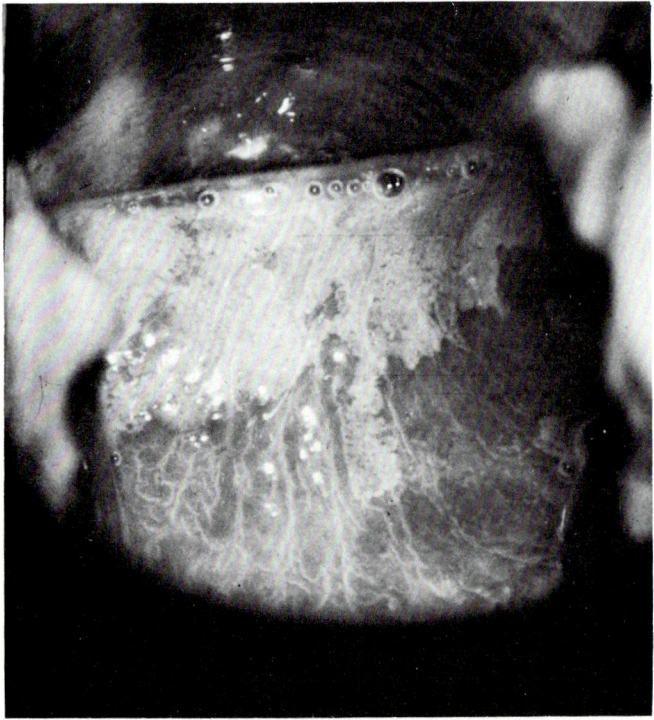

Fig. 3-9   Colpo-photograph of midvagina in a 12 year old female who was exposed to DES during the first trimester. Entire vagina was lined by velvety appearing columnar epithelium. Immature metaplastic squamous epithelium is present with an irregular border on the anterior portion of the photograph and the vertical ridges of columnar epithelium seen in the lower half. 16X.

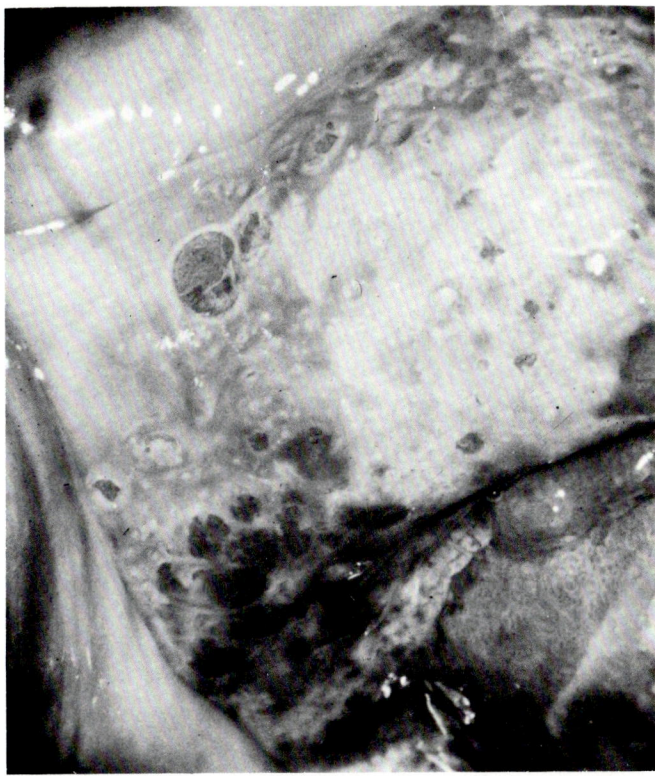

Fig. 3-10   Colpo-photograph of upper third of vagina of a 23 year old female exposed to DES during the first trimester. Normal squamous epithelium seen in the upper extreme left hand border of the photograph. White metaplastic epithelium present in the right mid portion of the photograph. Gland openings are throughout the vagina, and large islands of persistent columnar tissue are present. In the extreme lower right hand corner of the photograph is a portion of a cervical hood which·is covered entirely by columnar epithelium. 16X.

sample both normal and abnormal tissue without significantly disturbing the cervical architecture or surface epithelium.

Infertility

In selected cases colposcopic inspection of the infertile patient is helpful in determining the cause of postcoital bleeding and has been of assistance in collecting cervical mucus. Although the technique has not been of significant value in enhancing the possiblity of fertility, it certainly provides a more thorough assessment of the cervix in the infertile individual.

REFERENCES

Beller, F. K., and Khatamee, M.: Evaluation of punch biopsy of cervix under direct colposcopic observation (target punch biopsy). *Obstet. Gynecol.* 28:622, 1966.
Coppleson, M., Pixley, E., and Reid, B.: *Colposcopy*. Charles C Thomas, Springfield, Ill. 1971.

Coppleson, M., and Reid, B.: *Preclinical Carcinoma of the Cervix Uteri*. Pergamon Press, New York, 1967.

Donohue, L., and Meriwether, D.: Colposcopy as a diagnostic tool in the investigation of cervical neoplasia. *Am. J. Obstet. Gynecol.* 113:107, 1972.

Gondos, B., Townsend, D. E., and Ostergard, D. R.: Cytologic diagnosis of squamous dysplasia and carcinoma of the cervix. *Am. J. Obstet. Gynecol.* 110:107, 1971.

Hinselman, H.: Verbesserung de Inspektionsmoglichkeiten von Vulva, Vagina und Portio. *Münch. Med. Wochenshr.* 73:1733, 1925. Cited by Coppleson.

Hollyock, V. E., and Chanen, W.: The use of the colposcope in the selection of patients for cervical cone biopsy. *Am. J. Obstet. Gynecol.* 114:185, 1972.

Kostad, P. and Stafl, A.: *Atlas of Colposcopy*. University Park Press, Baltimore, Md. 1972.

Krumholz, B. A., and Knapp, R. C.: Colposcopic selection of biopsy sites. *Obstet. Gynecol.* 39:22, 1972.

Lang, W. R., and Rakoff, A. E.: Colposcopy and cytology: Comparitive values in the diagnosis of cervical atypism and malignancy. *Obstet. Gynecol.* 8:312, 1956.

Limburg, Hans; Comparison between cytology and colposcopy in the diagnosis of early cervical carcinoma. *Am. J. Obstet. Gynecol.* 75:1298, 1958.

Navratil, E., Burghardt, E., Bajardi, F., and Nash, W.: Simultaneous colposcopy and cytology used in screening for carcinoma of the cervix. *Am. J. Obstet. Gynecol.* 75:1292, 1958.

Ortiz, R., Newton, M., and Langlois, P. L.: Colposcopic biopsy in the diagnosis of carcinoma of the cervix. *Obstet. Gynecol.* 34:303, 1969.

Ries, E.: Erosion, leukoplakia and the colposcope in relation to carcinoma of the cervix. *Am. J. Obstet. Gynecol.* 23:393, 1932.

Salzer, R. B: Colposcopy: An aid in the detection of early cancer and precancerous conditions of the cervix. *Obstet. Gynecol.* 13:451, 1959.

Scott, J. W., and Vence, C. A.: Colposcopy, cytology and biopsy in the office diagnosis of uterine malignancy. *Cancer Cytol. J.* 5, No. 1, 1963.

Stafl, A., and Mattingly, R. F.: Colposcopic diagnosis of cervical neoplasia. *Obstet. Gynecol.* 41:168, 1973.

Townsend, D. E., Ostergard, D. R., Mishell, D. R., Jr., and Hirose, F. M.: Abnormal papanicolaou smears: Evaluation by colposcopy, biopsies, and endocervical curettage. *Am. J. Obstet. Gynecol.* 108:429, 1970.

Tredway, D. R., Townsend, D. E., Hovland, D. N., and Upton, R. T.: Colposcopy and cryosurgery in cervical intra-epithelial neoplasia. *Am. J. Obstet. Gynecol.* 114:1020, 1972.

CHAPTER FOUR

Cancer
of the Corpus

4-1 HYPERPLASIAS AND CARCINOMA *IN SITU* OF THE ENDOMETRIUM

A number of patients in the menopausal and reproductive eras develop various grades of endometrial hyperplasia. Unfortunately, this entity is particularly common in patients with a disturbed pituitary ovarian axis and anovulatory cycles (polycystic ovarian disease or Stein-Leventhal-like syndrome). These young women are often childless, and preservation of the uterus is very desirous.

To properly manage these patients one must first be aware of the malignant potential of these endometrial hyperplasias. Much has been written during the past 30 to 40 years about endometrial hyperplasia as a precursor of corpus cancer, but most studies were based on retrospective examination of previous endometrial biopsies from patients with endometrial carcinoma, or they dealt with older patients. Chamlain and Taylor (1970) did an especially interesting study of 97 young women with endometrial hyperplasia. In 24 of 97 (25%) of these patients the endometrial hyperplasia was associated with sclerocystic ovaries consistent with the so-called Stein-Leventhal syndrome. Fertility in the entire group of patients was low: only 27% in spite of desire and effort, conceived in the years after endometrial hyperplasia was diagnosed, and only 12% carried their pregnancies to term. In 14 of these women, the lesion progressed to adenocarcinoma 1-14 years after the initial diagnosis of endometrial hyperplasia, in spite of the fact that 41% of the patients underwent hysterectomy at some interval after the diagnosis was made.

This particular study points up two important factors in regard to endometrial hyperplasia. First, these patients are poor candidates, without induction of ovulation, for future childbearing and generally have very low fertility. Second, there is a significant chance of progression of the lesion from a noninvasive to an invasive state.

It is known that prolonged periods of anovulation occur most often during the postmenarchial and premenopausal periods in the human female. In the premenopausal female anovulation is the result of inability of the aging ovary to respond to sequential gonadotropin stimulation. In the reproductive female the causes may be multiple, involving abnormal function of the pituitary, thyroid, adrenal glands, or ovaries. Prolonged periods of unopposed estrogens with stimulation of the endometrium may produce cystic and adenomatous hyperplasia and, in certain patients, carcinoma *in situ*. The reason for a variation in response is unknown.

Patients with certain types of adenomatous endometrial hyperplasia are more likely to develop carcinoma than those with more benign lesions of the endometrium. The general figure of 5-12% of patients with atypical adenomatous hyperplasia (carcinoma *in situ*) is the risk for invasive cancer quoted for this group. The process is often relatively slow, and progression from hyperplasia to carcinoma may take 5 or more years. It should be remembered, however, that various hyperplastic patterns may be found in the nonmalignant endometrium of patients with endometrial carcinoma. Careful sampling of the endometrial cavity is a prerequisite to consideration of conservative therapy. The next question is whether this progression is reversible at a specific point. In this connection it would appear that progestins can be effective. Not only have potent progestational agents been shown to cause marked changes in endometrial hyperplasia and carcinoma *in situ*, but also they have a marked morphologic and histochemical effect on invasive carcinoma of the endometrium, both in the intrauterine site and in the metastatic foci. In addition, in selected patients with atypical endometrial patterns associated with the Stein-Leventhal syndrome, wedge resection has been followed by ovulation, secretion of progesterones, and reversion of hyperplastic processes. Indeed, recently many, such as Kistner et al (1966), have suggested the use of Clomid to induce ovulation as a treatment for endometrial hyperplasia.

Although an association between endometrial hyperplasia and subsequent carcinoma has been observed by many authors, the relationship of estrogen to this sequence is unclear. The available data from human material would suggest the following:

1. There is little, if any, evidence that estrogenic substances are carcinogenic in the premenopausal woman.
2. Only meager evidence is available to indicate that cystic ("Swiss cheese") hyperplasia is causally related to endometrial carcinoma.
3. In predisposed individuals, the unopposed action of estrogenic substances for considerable periods of time will result in endometrial hyperplasia, anaplasia, carcinoma *in situ*, and, eventually, carcinoma.

The therapeutic regimens suggested for the management of atypical endometrial hyperplasia and carcinoma *in situ*, are as follows:

Postpubescence—treat with estrogen-progestin artificial cycles for 6 months, and then attempt to secure ovulation.

Patients within the childbearing period—treat with estrogen-progestin artificial cycles for 3 months, followed by sampling of the endometrium to ensure reversion to a benign pattern, and then attempt to secure ovulation with the use of cortisone, clomiphene, or wedge resection of the ovaries. If the patient is not interested in childbearing at the present time, use the estrogen-progestin artificial cycles continuously until reversion to a benign pattern, and discontinue only when the patient is desirous of pregnancy.

Premenopausal women who, for some reason are interested in preserving their childbearing capacities—treat with estrogen-progestin artificial cycles until the age of

50-55, with a backup of hysterectomy in uncontrolled cases. Otherwise hysterectomy is the treatment of choice in this age group.

Postmenopausal women—hysterectomy, of course, is recommended. Some of these women, however, are quite elderly and are not operative candidates, and in these instances high doses of Depo-Provera (400 mg IM every 2 weeks) or Megace (40 mg daily) for at least a year are used. The endometrial cavity can be sampled by endometrial biopsy and Gravlee jet wash.

In summary, it appears that prolonged stimulation of the endometrium by endogenous or exogenous estrogen results in the development of endometrial hyperplasia. Intermittent secretory differentiation of the endometrial glands, by either progesterone or synthetic progestins, prevents the development of hyperplasia. Retrospective studies of patients having endometrial cancer suggest a progression of abnormal endometrial glandular patterns from cystic to adenomatous hyperplasia, and then to atypical hyperplasia or carcinoma *in situ*. Hysterectomy specimens indicate that carcinoma *in situ* and invasive carcinoma of the endometrium frequently occur simultaneously and suggest that carcinoma may arise in or from the atypical endometrial glands. Prospective studies in the human female have shown that approximately 10% of patients having atypical endometrial hyperplasia will eventually develop invasive cancer if untreated. Although the precise factors that convert premalignant to malignant epithelium are unknown, recent investigations indicate that the cells and glands which subsequently become malignant demonstrate abnormal DNA distribution and aneuploidy.

Both progesterone and synthetic progestins have been shown to be capable of producing reversion of adenomatous and atypical adenomatous hyperplasia to an atrophic pattern. In women desirous of pregnancy this may also be effected by induction of ovulation. During the premenopausal years, the administration of a synthetic estrogen-progestin combination, as found in combined oral contraceptives, produces reversion of adenomatous hyperplasia. In this age group, atypical adenomatous hyperplasia has been converted into atrophic endometrium by the parenteral administration of synthetic progesterones. Although the progestational agents are able to produce striking changes in the morphology of the endometrial glands, they should not be regarded as a panacea, and in no way should they be construed by the clinician as a substitute for the usual diagnostic procedures and appropriate therapy. We recommend that these patients be subjected to hysterectomy at the completion of the childbearing period.

4-2 INVASIVE CANCERS OF THE ENDOMETRIUM

Cancers of the endometrium have become of increasing interest because of a rise in their incidence, which is probably due to the increase in the number of women who reach the age group in which cancer of the corpus uteri is most likely to occur. In addition, one must keep in mind, the continuing debate concerning the background of cancer of the endometrium, especially in regard to the role of estrogens as possible carcinogens. The malignancies that most commonly occur in the endometrium are the following:

    I. Preinvasive (carincoma *in situ*)
 II. Invasive
      A. Adenocarcinoma
          1. Adenocanthoma
          2. Adenosquamous carcinoma

B. Squamous carcinoma
C. Sarcoma
   1. carcinosarcoma
   2. stromal sarcoma
   3. mixed mesodermal tumors

Adenocarcinoma

The term carcinoma of the endometrium is selected for lesions that arise in the endometrial epithelium. Adenocarcinoma of the endometrium constitutes about 90% of all endometrial neoplasms. These lesions are sometimes divided into carcinoma of the corpus (Stage I) and carcinoma corporis et colli (Stage II). Extension of the process into the cervix constitutes a change in staging and often in treatment.

Epidemiology

Carcinoma of the corpus is most common in the sixth and seventh decades of life. Seventy five per cent of corpus cancer occurs after the age of 50, and only 4% before the age of 40. Hertig (1949) has reported the youngest case authenticated, which was in a 16 year old girl. In contrast to cervical carcinoma, which is more common in the fourth and fifth decades of life, corporeal carcinoma classically is a disease that afflicts nulliparous, obese, diabetec, and hypertensive postmenopausal women. Cancer of the corpus uteri is one of the lesions prevalent in "cancer families"; a history of cancer in the immediate family background has been found in 12-28% of cases. As mentioned previously, a high percentage of patients who develop this disease before the menopause have a history of anovulatory menstrual cycles consistent with Stein-Leventhal-like syndrome.

Microscopic Pattern

In some endometrial carcinomas, the reproduction of the endometrial glands is so complete that the tissue is quite similar to benign endometrium. The cancer may be described as a well-differentiated carcinoma (Fig. 4-1) or as severe atypical adenomatous hyperplasia. At the other extreme, there may be only groups of cells or fragments of glands suggestive of benign structures; this is described as poorly differentiated carcinoma of the corpus. Well-differentiated lesions are designated as Grade 1, and poorly differentiated lesions as Grade 3. Table 4-1 gives the distribution of lesions by grade in Stage I disease.

Occasionally the microscopic pattern will defy differentiation from sarcoma of the endometrium, and the tumor may be classified as anaplastic carcinoma of the endometrium. It would appear from several studies that the prognosis for the patient varies inversely with the degree of differentiation; well-differentiated tumors appear to do much better than anaplastic corpus cancer. This is undoubtedly related to the facts that undifferentiated lesions have a higher incidence of node involvement (Table 4-2) and that the rate of recurrence increases with grade (Table 4-3). The incidence of spread beyond the uterus and cervix in Grade 3 lesions has been reported as 45%, as opposed to 11% in Grade 1 lesions (Table 4-4). All of these parameters are, of course, reflected in the fact that survival with 5 year cure rates in patients with Grade 3 lesions is roughly 50% of that for Grade 1 lesions (Table 4-5).

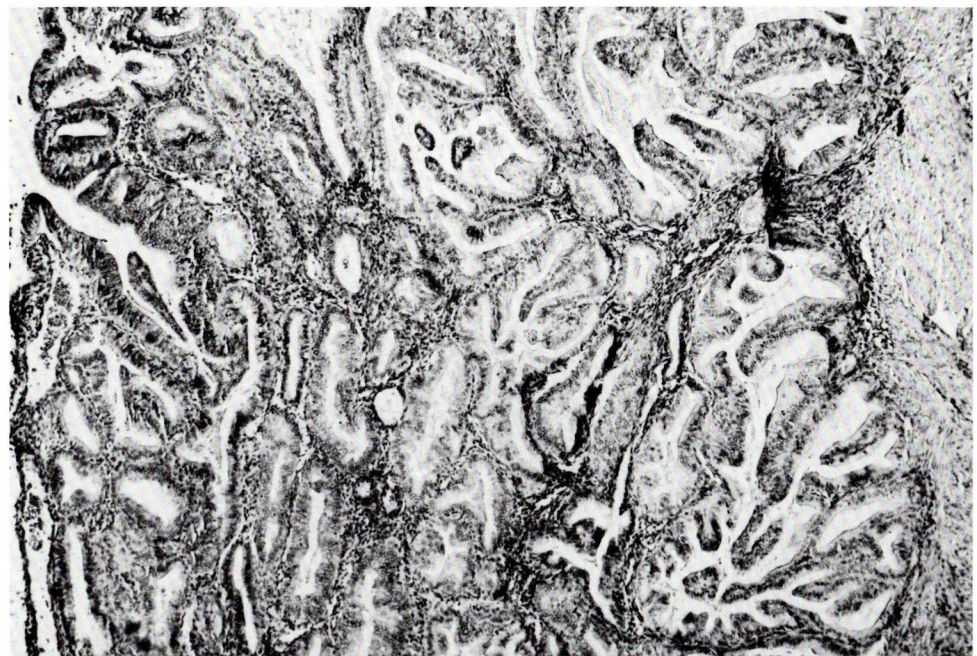

Fig. 4-1 Well-differentiated (Grade I) adenocarcinoma of the endometrium.

Lines of Spread (Fig. 4-2)

1. *Spread to the Lymph Nodes.* Although there is some lack of agreement among authors, the incidence of lymphatic involvement in Stage I and Stage II endometrial carcinoma appears to be appreciable. In a review article by Morrow, DiSaia, and Townsend (1973), 369 patients with Stage I carcinoma of the endometrium treated by radical hysterectomy and pelvic lymphadenectomy were analyzed for the incidence of positive pelvic nodes. It was found that 10.6% of the patients with Stage I disease, as opposed to 36.5% with Stage II disease, had positive pelvic nodes (Table 4-6). As noted above, the incidence of positive nodes increases appreciably in patients with Grade 3 lesions. Deep myometrial invasion also was associated with a 31% incidence of positive

TABLE 4-1 ENDOMETRIAL ADENOCARCINOMA: STAGE I LESIONS

Grade	Percent of Total
1	42.5
2	34.4
3	23.1

Based on 1284 cases reported by Gusberg et al (1960); Roman et al (1967): Wade et al (1967); Cheon (1969); Lewis et al (1970).

TABLE 4-2 ENDOMETRIAL ADENOCARCINOMA: RELATIONSHIP OF NODE METASTASIS TO GRADE

Grade	Positive Nodes (%)
1	7.6
2	13.0
3	28.6
All cases	14.0

Based on 178 cases reported by Lees (1969) and Lewis et al (1970).

TABLE 4-3 ENDOMETRIAL
ADENOCARCINOMA: INFLUENCE OF
GRADE ON RECURRENCE

Grade	Recurrence (%)
1	8
2	20
3	44

From Finn (1950).

TABLE 4-4 ENDOMETRIAL
ADENOCARCINOMA: SPREAD
BEYOND UTERUS AND
CERVIX BY GRADE

Grade	Per Cent of Total
1	10.6
2	12.1
3	45.0

From Wade et al (1967) and Cheon (1969).

TABLE 4-5 ENDOMETRIAL
ADENOCARCINOMA: INFLUENCE OF
GRADE ON SURVIVAL

Grade	5 Year Survival (%)
1	81.7
2	75
3	43.3

From Wade et al (1967); Cheon (1969);
Nahhas et al (1971)

nodes, as compared with a 3% incidence in patients with minimal myometrial invasion (Table 4-7).

In essence, the operative series reviewed indicated that the involvement of pelvic nodes is not much less common in endometrial than in cervical cancer. Since treatment of the pelvic nodes is always a consideration in cervical cancer, it would seem appropriate to give corporeal lesions the same attention. This is especially relevant when one considers that 40% of the patients with positive nodes survived for 5 years (Table 4-8), destroying the myth that patients are not salvageable once endometrial carcinoma disseminates beyond the uterus. Theoretically, corporeal cancer can disseminate via the utero-ovarian ligaments to the infundibulopelvic ligaments and avoid the deeper pelvic lymphatics. However, pelvic node involvement is not uncommon, especially when the cervix and/or isthmus of the uterus is involved.

2. *Spread to the Myometrium.* Gusberg et al (1960) have shown that tumors with a high degree of differentiation have a lower incidence of deep myometrial involvement than poorly differentiated tumors (Table 4-9). However, myometrial invasion can occur in a significant number of patients with well-differentiated lesions (Fig. 4-3); therefore, careful inspection of the uterus after hysterectomy is necessary. Unfortunately, prior irradiation therapy can alter the histologic proof of deep myometrial invasion. Table 4-10 shows the incidence of myometrial invasion in two groups of patients; one group was treated with surgery alone, and the other with surgery following preoperative irradiation therapy. It is obvious that the incidence of deep myometrial invasion was reduced by two thirds in the irradiated group and suggests strongly that the tumor shrinkage produced by the radiation gives a distorted pathological specimen. This may be somewhat hazardous since the incidence of positive nodes increases considerably with the presence of deep

SPREAD OF ADENOCARCINOMA
OF THE CORPUS UTERI

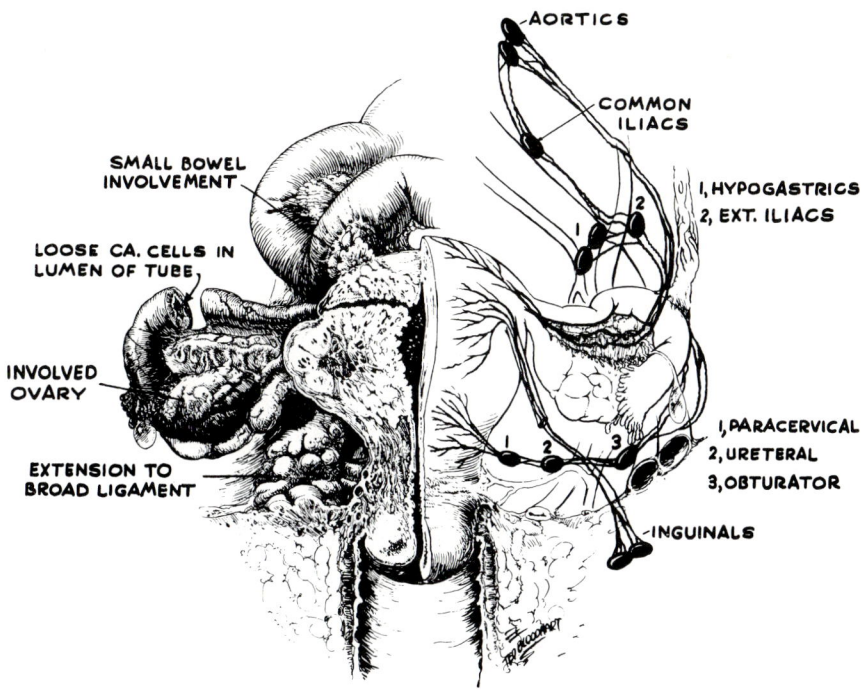

Fig. 4-2 Lines of spread of adenocarcinoma of the endometrium. (Courtesy of E. Henriksen, M.D., Clinical Professor of Ob/Gyn, University of Southern California School of Medicine, Adenocarcinoma of the corpus uteri: A clinicopathological study, *Surg., Obstet. Gynecol.* **58**:331,1950.)

myometrial invasion. This fact presents one of the strong arguments for hysterectomy before radiation therapy in Stage I lesions without undifferentiated histology or cervical involvement.

The depth of myometrial invasion also correlates closely with the incidence of recurrence. Twenty-seven per cent of patients with deep myometrial invasion are subject to recurrent disease, as opposed to 9% with minimal or superficial invasion (Table 4-11).

TABLE 4-6 ENDOMETRIAL
ADENOCARCINOMA: INCIDENCE OF
PELVIC NODE METASTASIS

	Stage I	Stage II
Total cases	369	85
Nodes positive	39	31
Per cent of total	10.6%	36.5%

From Liu and Meigs (1955); Lefevre (1956); Schwartz and Brunschwig (1957); Roberts (1961); Hawksworth (1964); Rickford (1968); Lees (1969); Lewis et al (1970).

TABLE 4-7   ENDOMETRIAL ADENOCARCINOMA:
INCIDENCE OF POSITIVE PELVIC
NODES VS MYOMETRIAL INVASION

Myometrial Invasion	Number of Cases	Number with Nodes Positive	Per cent of Total
None	22	0	0
Slight	71	2	2.8
Moderate	52	9	17.3
Advanced	62	19	30.7
All cases	207	30	14.5

From Javert (1952) and Lewis et al (1970).

This, of course, influences survival, and the 5 year survival figures (Table 4-12) reflect the poor prognosis for patients with deep myometrial invasion.

3. *Involvement of the Isthmus and Cervix*. Extension of the cancer to the isthmus and cervix must be carefully considered since it mandates a more extensive type of treatment. As seen in Table 4-6, the incidence of positive pelvic nodes in Stage II endometrial carcinoma is quite significant. Once the cervix is involved in the disease process, the mode of dissemination is quite similar to that in cervical cancer.

4. *Spread to the Vagina*. Vaginal metastases are rare when a patient is first seen and are usually indicative of disseminated disease. However, a 5-10% incidence of vaginal cuff recurrence after hysterectomy has been reported by many investigators. Cuff recurrence is most common in patients who have not received pre- or postoperative irradiation therapy. The recurrence rate in patients who have received adjunctive irradiation varies between 2-5%; thus vaginal recurrence can be dramatically reduced with concomitant use of radiotherapy. Although further studies are necessary, it would appear that a patient with a well-differentiated lesion not deeply invading the myometrium or involving the cervix or isthmus does not need adjunctive radiotherapy to avoid cuff occurrence.

5. *Spread to Pelvic Structures*. Spread to the broad ligaments, fallopian tubes, and ovaries is common. For this reason the surgical attack on this disease always includes a total abdominal hysterectomy with bilateral salpingo-oophorectomy. The frequency of these metastases is too great to allow preservation of the ovaries, even when the patient is not of menopausal age. In addition, evidence suggests that many of these tumors may be estrogen dependent, providing another justification for removal of the ovaries even in a premenopausal patient.

TABLE 4-8   ENDOMETRIAL
ADENOCARCINOMA: SURVIVAL
WITH PELVIC NODE
METASTASIS

Total cases	25
Number living for 5 years	10
Survival rate (%)	40

From Schwartz and Brunschwig (1957);
Lewis et al (1970); Dobbie et al (1965).

**TABLE 4-9   ENDOMETRIAL ADENOCARCINOMA:
RELATIONSHIP OF GRADE TO INVASION**

Grade	None	Superficial (percent of total)	Deep
1	56	28	16
2	48	25	27
3	36	14	50

Adapted from Gusberg et al (1960) and Cheon (1969).

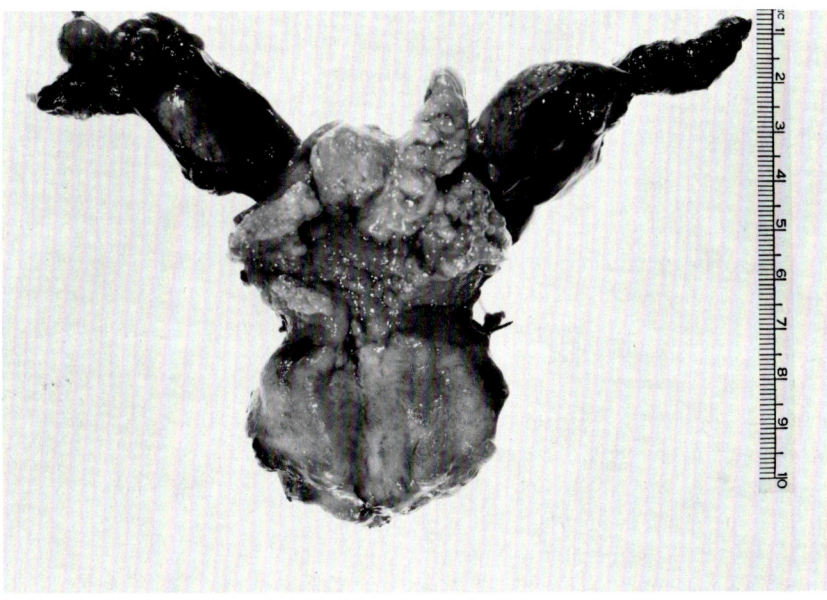

Fig. 4-3 Gross specimen (uterus has been opened) of a patient with a well-differentiated Stage I adenocarcinoma of the endometrium, illustrating deep myometrial invasion. Patient also had positive pelvic nodes.

**TABLE 4-10   ENDOMETRIAL ADENOCARCINOMA: PERCENT
DISTRIBUTION OF MYOMETRIAL INVASION—
SURGERY VS RADIATION AND SURGERY**

Myometrial Invasion	No Preoperative X-ray Therapy %	Preoperative X-ray Therapy %
No tumor	7	46
Endometrium only	28	24
Myometrium < one third	40	22
Myometrium > one third	25	8

From Lewis et al (1974).

TABLE 4-11   ENDOMETRIAL CARCINOMA:
INFLUENCE OF INVASION ON RECURRENCE

Myometrial Invasion	Number of Cases	Recurrence (%)
None	111	9.0
Superficial	59	8.5
Deep	29	27.0

From Finn (1950).

6. *Distant Metastases*. The distribution of distant metastases is often different from the pattern of spread from cancer of the cervix. Generalized implantation metastasis on the abdominal serosa is more prevalent in endometrial than in cervical cancers because the former type penetrates the wall of the uterus and seeds the abdominal cavity. Cul-de-sac implants, masses in the omentum, and ascites are common in advanced disease. The cancer may travel via the ovarian vascular drainage pathway and metastasize to the para-aortic nodes. Inguinal node, supraclavicular node and lung metastases are also seen.

Staging

Clinical staging of adenocarcinoma of the endometrium remains more indefinite than that of cervical carcinoma because the limits of the cancer spread cannot be determined as easily. In spite of these limitations a clinical staging has been devised that has practical value. Such staging considers the size of the uterus, palpable evidence of cancer extending beyond the serosal surface of the uterus, and spread to the cervix, as shown by gross lesion or microscopic confirmation by biopsy after fractional curettage. On the basis of this information, four stages are described as follows:

Stage I   The carcinoma is confined to the corpus.
  Stage Ia   The length of the uterine cavity is 8 cm or less.
  Stage Ib   The length of the uterine cavity is more than 8 cm.
  Stage I cases should be subgrouped with regard to the histologic type of adeno-
          carcinoma as follows:

        G1   Highly differentiated adenomatous carcinomas.
        G2   Differentiated adenomatous carcinomas with partly solid areas.
        G3   Predominantly solid or entirely undifferentiated carcinomas.

TABLE 4-12   ENDOMETRIAL
ADENOCARCINOMA, STAGE I:
INFLUENCE OF INVASION
ON SURVIVAL

Invasion	5 Year Survival (%)
None	98
Superficial	90
Deep (> one third)	68

From Lindgren (1957); Keller et al (1974); Welander et al (1972).

Stage II   The carcinoma involves corpus and cervix.
Stage III The carcinoma extends outside the corpus but not outside the true pelvis (it
           may involve the vaginal wall or the parametrium but not the bladder or the
           rectum).
Stage IV   The carcinoma involves the bladder or rectum or extends outside the pelvis.

The distribution of endometrial carcinoma by stage is seen in Table 4-13. Stage I is
obviously of considerable importance, since the incidence appears to be rising along with
the general incidence of cancer.

Diagnosis

Persistent unusual perimenopausal bleeding or any postmenopausal bleeding is the most
common symptom of this malignancy. These patients should be subjected to endometrial
biopsy and liberal use of dilatation and curettage. The Papanicolaou smear is unreliable in
detecting this particular malignancy; the most optimistic figures report only 50% pick-up.
Suction biopsy is reliable in about 80% of cases of cancer of the corpus in most series. An
enlarged uterus in a postmenopausal woman with postmenopausal bleeding should be
regarded as indicative of carcinoma of the endometrium until proved otherwise. Other
symptoms and signs of this malignancy, such as pain, are late manifestations of the
disease and are therefore associated with a very poor prognosis.

Treatment

Hysterectomy is still the mainstay and generally accepted basis for the management of
endometrial carcinoma. The value of adjunctive radiation therapy lies in the improvement
of survival rates and the lowering of local recurrence rates. Accumulated evidence has
established four practical points of therapeutic importance:

1. The field at risk with endometrial carcinoma is similar to that with carcinoma of
the cervix, although the percentage distribution of metastasis may be different.
2. For Stage I tumors a 5 year cure rate over 80% can be obtained by total abdominal
hysterectomy with bilateral salpingo-oophorectomy combined with pre-or postoperative
radiation.

TABLE 4-13 ENDOMETRIAL
CARCINOMA: STAGE
DISTRIBUTION

Stage	Per Cent of Total
I	76.5
II	8.5
III	10.4
IV	4.7

Based on 2432 cases re-
ported by Boronow (1969);
Kottmeier (1969); Wade et
al (1967); Sall et al (1970);
Shah and Green (1972); Welander et al (1972).

3.   The risk of pelvic node metastasis is minimal when the primary tumor is superficial, but is 30-40% with deep myometrial penetration or with involvement of the cervix or isthmus.

4.   Poor differentiation and anaplasia of the primary tumor increase the danger of dissemination both within the field of risk and beyond the pelvis.

In regard to treatment, the *well-differentiated lesion* in a uterus of normal size may be treated with hysterectomy and bilateral salpingo-oophorectomy alone. Excellent results in a small series of selected patients utilizing this treatment technique have been reported by Keller et al (1974). However, the uterus should be carefully inspected for myometrial invasion. Should myometrial invasion be present to a significant degree (greater than one third of depth) or unsuspected involvement of the cervix or isthmus be revealed, the operative procedure should be followed with whole pelvis irradiation and possibly the installation of vaginal ovoids.

Moderately or *poorly differentiated lesions* of the endometrium in a uterus of normal size can be treated with preoperative radiation in the form of two radium insertions (Fig. 4-4), followed in 6 weeks with total abdominal hysterectomy and bilateral salpingo-oophorectomy. An alternative and possibly preferable treatment plan for the moderately differentiated lesion calls for initial exploration with total abdominal hysterectomy and bilateral salpingo-oophorectomy, followed by careful pathologic study of the specimen and tailored postoperative irradiation based on the histologic findings. Whole pelvis irradiation is given when the criteria for nodal treatment are found, and vaginal cuff radium alone when they are not.

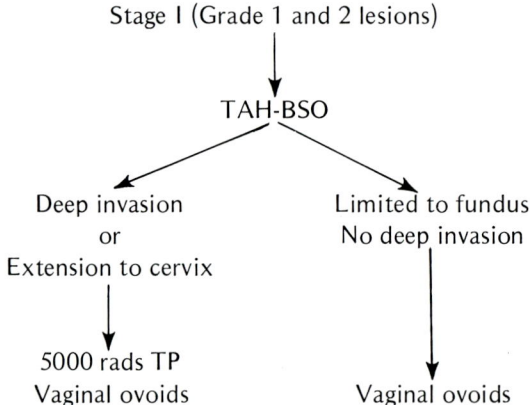

Stage I (Grade 1 and 2 lesions)

TAH-BSO

Deep invasion
or
Extension to cervix

Limited to fundus
No deep invasion

5000 rads TP
Vaginal ovoids

Vaginal ovoids

Lesions with a poorly differentiated carcinoma by histology and/or *involvement of the cervix* should be treated with 4000 rads whole pelvis preoperatively, along with one radium insertion (Figs. 4-5 and 4-6) 1-6 weeks before total abdominal hysterectomy and bilateral salpingo-oophorectomy. In addition, some authorities recommend total pelvic (TP) irradiation for the enlarged uterus (Stage Ib) on the basis that it represents bulky disease; often, however, the uterus is enlarged by fibroids, not tumor, the volume of disease is not large, and minimal invasion of the myometrium is present. The issue of the best therapy for Stage Ib is equivocal, and until further studies are available the treatment plan must be left to the judgment of the physician.

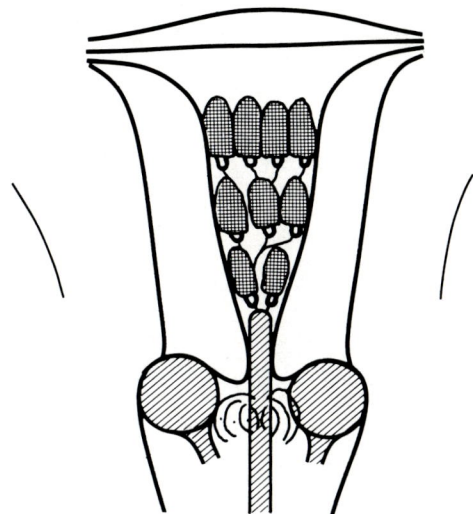

Fig. 4-4 Heyman packing of uterus with nine capsules, short tandem, and two ovoids.

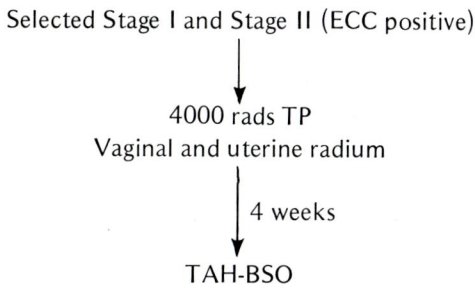

Selected Stage I and Stage II (ECC positive)

↓

4000 rads TP
Vaginal and uterine radium

↓ 4 weeks

TAH-BSO

Tables 4-14 and 4-15 provide detailed radiation treatment plans based on the M.D. Anderson Hospital experience. Cumulative 5 year survival rates for endometrial carcinoma are listed in Table 4-16.

Management of Recurrent or Disseminated Carcinoma
of the Endometrium

Recurrences in the lower third of the vagina can be treated with interstitial irradiation in the form of radium needles. Superficial recurrences located higher in the lateral wall can be treated with a vaginal cylinder, also containing radium. Whole pelvis irradiation is typically used for the apical cuff recurrence common in this disease. Well-differentiated lesions respond well to whole pelvis irradiation, but poorly differentiated lesions appear to show less improvement.

Progestins have been used in the treatment of disseminated adenocarcinoma of the endometrium. Most reports show a response rate of between 35 and 50% of patients, with distant metastases being more sensitive than pelvic recurrences. Several dramatic reports of complete disappearance of pulmonary metastasis can be found in the literature. The

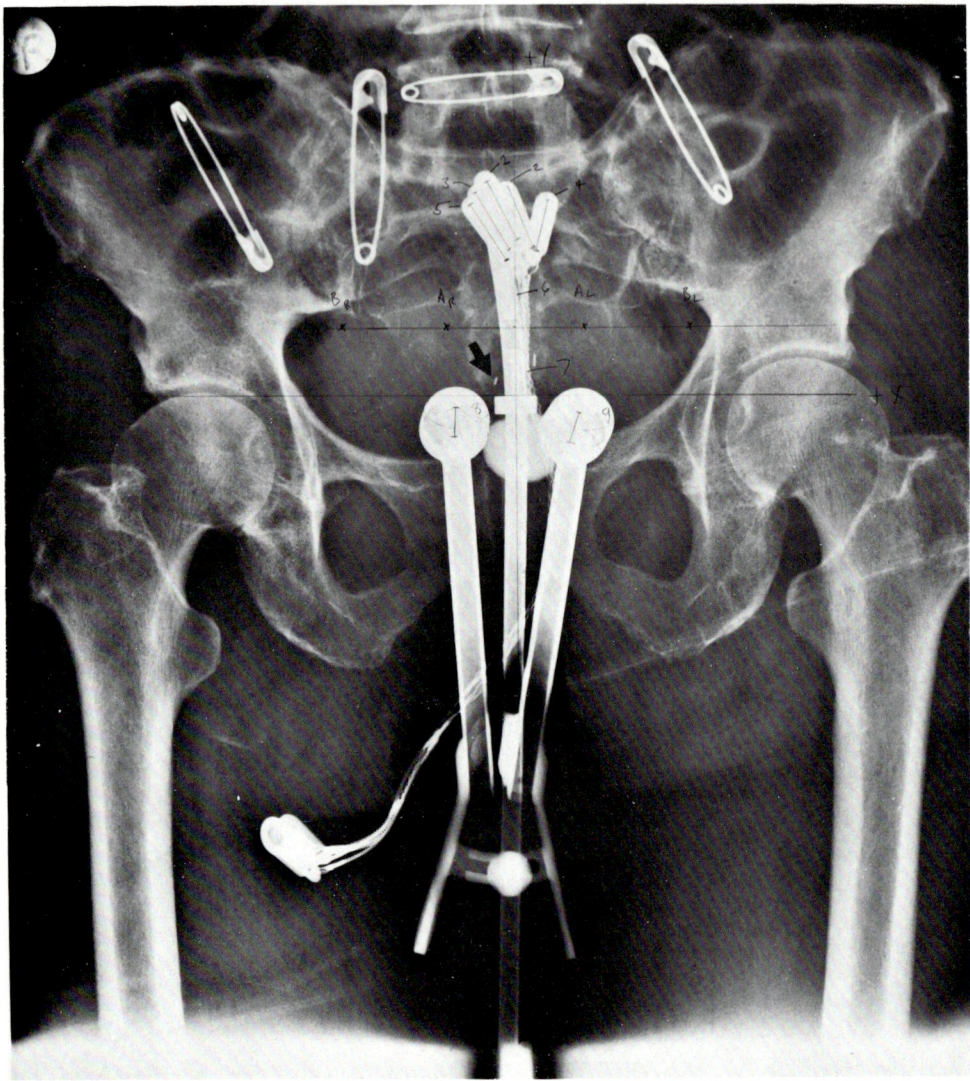

Fig. 4-5 Anterior-posterior view of the pelvis, illustrating six Heyman capsules, a short cervical tandem, and vaginal ovoids in place. Silver seeds (arrows) are embedded 0.5 cm into the cervix.

survival rate of responders appears to be considerably better than that of nonresponders in almost every series reported. Dosages of 500-1000 mg of Depo-Provera (medroxyprogesterone acetate) weekly have been considered therapeutic. Delalutin (hydroxyprogesterone caproate) has been used in doses of 500-1000 mg IM twice weekly. Recently an oral synthetic progestin, Megace (megestrol acetate), at a dose of 40-80 mg b.i.d., has proved to be effective as an alternative to Depo-Provera.

Other Cancers of the Corpus

Adenoacanthoma is managed as if the squamous elements were not present and the malignancy were composed entirely of the adenomatous elements. Adenosquamous

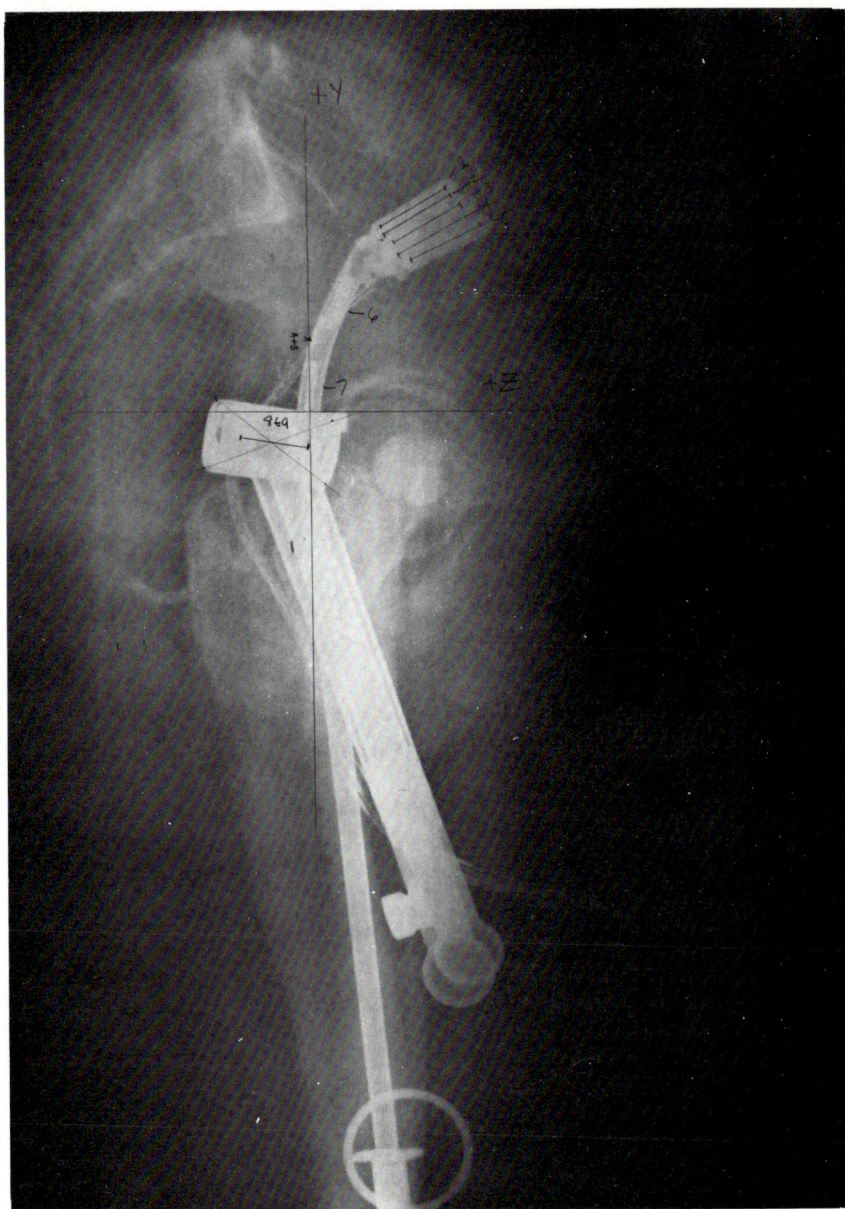

Fig. 4-6 Lateral view of the pelvis of the patient shown in Fig. 4-5.

carcinoma of the endometrium has demonstrated high virulence in many studies and may best be considered in a category with undifferentiated lesions.

Sarcomas may arise from the endometrial stroma or the myometrium (Table 4-17) and often present as a polypoid mass protruding through the cervix. The most common lesions are the carcinosarcoma and mixed mesodermal tumors of the endometrium (Fig. 4-7) Leiomyosarcomas are less common and frequently are diagnosed only when the uterus is examined after hysterectomy. Again the mainstay of treatment is total abdominal hysterectomy with bilateral salpingo-oophorectomy. Although these sarco-

TABLE 4-14 ENDOMETRIAL ADENOCARCINOMA, STAGE I: TREATMENT POLICIES AND TECHNIQUES

CLINICAL SITUATION	WHOLE PELVIS IRRADIATION	RADIUM UTERINE CAVITY	RADIUM VAGINA	COMMENTS
Small uterus, well differentiated tumor	TAH, BSO	—Adjunctive radiation if warranted by pathological findings		
Preoperative irradiation followed by simple hysterectomy				
1. Small uterine cavity	—	Tandem (e.g., 20-15-10) (3000-3500 mg-hr) x 1	Surface dose 7000 rads (ovoids or protruding source)	Hysterectomy immediately after last radium insertion; check carefully for myometrial invasion
2. Slightly or moderately enlarged uterus, well differentiated tumor	—	Heyman packing or tandem x 2 (2500 mg-hr each) two-three weeks apart	Surface dose 8000 rads 2 applications [ovoid(s)] or Surface dose 7000 rads 1 application [ovoid (s)]	
3. Large uterus and/or anaplastic tumor	4000 rads/ 4 weeks	Heyman packing (2500 mg-hr) x 1	Surface dose 4000 rads 1 application (ovoid or protruding source)	Hysterectomy to follow in 4-6 weeks
4. Perforation before or during treatment	4000 rads/ 4 weeks		Individualize	Consider hysterectomy without radium first

TABLE 4-14 (cont.)

Technically operable but surgery contraindicated				
1. Small or normal size uterine cavity, well differentiated tumor	—	If tandem used, 2 applications (72 and 72 hr) (5000-6000 mg-hr)	Surface dose 7000 rads 1 application [ovoid(s)] or Surface dose 8000 rads 2 applications [ovoid(s)]	Physicians should be fully congnizant that deletion of hysterectomy lowers the probability of cure by 20%
2. Slightly or moderately enlarged uterus, well differentiated tumor	—	Increased Heyman Packing or tandem to 3000 mg-hr × 2 two-three weeks apart		
3. Large uterus and/or anaplastic tumor	4000 rads/ 4 weeks	3500-4000 mg-hr 2 applications with Heyman packing or tandem 2 or 3 weeks apart	Surface dose 4000 rads	
Technically inoperable	4000 rads/4 weeks to 6000 rads/6 weeks	May add 1 radium packing if geometry permits	Surface dose 2500-4000 rads, depending upon external dose	These patients may benefit from concommitant use of progestins
Postoperative irradiation				
1. Nodes to be treated	5000 rads/6 weeks		Vaginal ovoids surface dose 3000 rads	Treatment of nodes is necessary if there is significant myometrial invasion, involvement of the isthmus or cervix, or spread outside the uterus
2. Nodes not treated	—		Vaginal ovoids surface dose 6000-7000 rads	

Modified from Fletcher (1973).

TABLE 4-15 ADENOCARCINOMA OF THE CORPUS AND CERVIX, STAGE II: TREATMENT POLICIES AND TECHNIQUES

CLINICAL SITUATION	WHOLE PELVIS IRRADIATION	UTERUS	VAGINA	PARAMETRIA	COMMENTS
Preoperative irradiation					
1. Normal size uterus, well differentiated tumor; no extension beyond uterus or cervix	—	Tandem and ovoids 4000 mg-hr X 2 two weeks apart		3000-4000 rads	Hysterectomy to follow in 4-6 weeks
2. Slightly or moderately enlarged uterus, well differentiated tumor; no extension beyond uterus or cervix	4000 rads	2500 mg-hr tandem or Heyman packing	Vaginal surface dose (ovoids) 4000 rads	No additional	Hysterectomy to follow in 4-6 weeks
3. Normal size uterus, anaplastic tumor	4000 rads	Tandem and ovoids 4000 mg-hr; vaginal surface dose 4000 rads		No additional	Hysterectomy to follow in 4-6 weeks
Technically operable but surgery contraindicated					
1. Normal size uterus, well differentiated tumor; no extension beyond uterus or cervix	—	Tandem and ovoids X 2 two weeks apart 5000 mg-hr each; vaginal surface dose 7000-8000 rads		3000-4000 rads	

TABLE 4-15 (cont.)

2. Slightly or moderately enlarged uterus, well differentiated tumor; no extension beyond uterus or cervix	4000 rads	2 insertions 2000 mg-hr each Heyman packing or tandem	Ovoids X 2 vaginal surface dose 4000-5000 rads
3. Normal size uterus, ana-plastic tumor	4000 rads	Tandem and ovoids 3000 mg-hr 2 weeks apart	Vaginal surface dose 4000-5000 rads (ovoids)
Technically inoperable	4000 rads/4 weeks to 6000 rads/6 weeks	May add 1 radium packing if geometry permits	Surface dose 2500-4000 rads, depending on ex-ternal dose	These patients may benefit from concomitant use of progestins

Modified from Fletcher, (1973).

129

TABLE 4-16
ENDOMETRIAL ADENOCARCINOMA:
5 YEAR (UNCORRECTED)
SURVIVAL RÅTES

Stage	Survival (%)
I	76.2
II	51.0
III	25.6
IV	8.8
All cases	68.3

Based on 2432 cases reported
by Boronow (1969); Kott-
meier (1969); Wade et al
(1967); Sall et al (1970) Shah
and Green (1972); Welander et
al (1972).

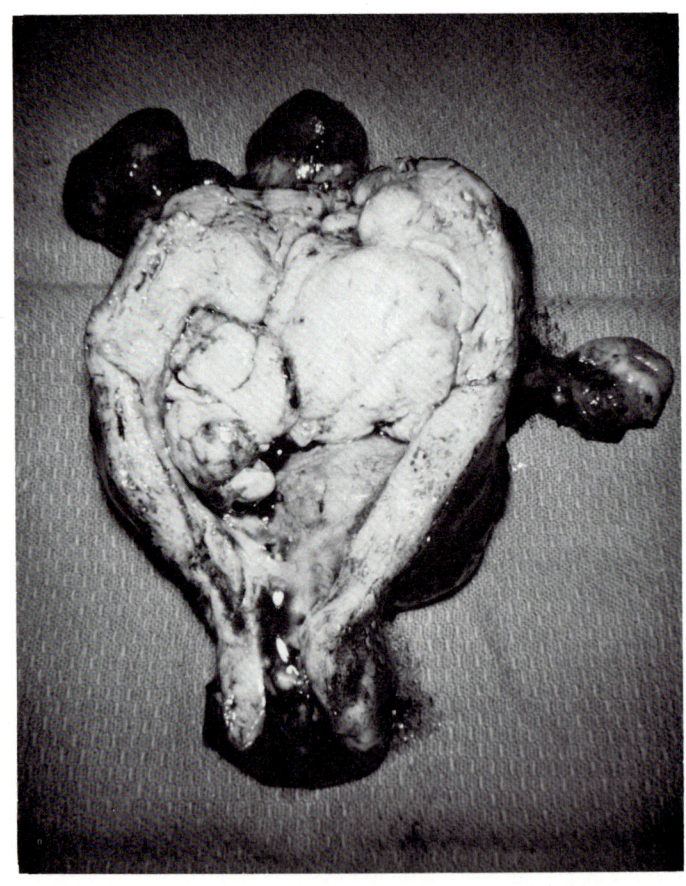

Fig. 4-7 Endometrial cavity is distended by a bulky mixed mesodermal sarcoma; myometrial invasion is evident.

TABLE 4-17 OBER CLASSIFICATION OF UTERINE SARCOMAS

Type	Homologous	Heterologous
Pure	Stromal sarcoma (endolymphatic stromal myosis)	Rhabdomyosarcoma
	Leiomyosarcoma	Chondrosarcoma
	Angiosarcoma	Osteosarcoma
	Fibrosarcoma	Liposarcoma
Mixed	Carcinosarcoma	Mixed müllerian tumors (mixed mesodermal tumor)

matous lesions of the endometrium have variable radiosensitivity, they are usually treated when possible with preoperative whole pelvis irradiation, consisting of 4000-5000 rads through parallel opposed fields, and intrauterine and vaginal radium before hysterectomy. Evidence from a limited number of studies implies that this combination of irradiation therapy and surgery produces the best survival rate for these devastating malignancies.

Other evidence suggests that central and pelvic recurrence is so frequent in these cancers that more consideration should be given to a radical surgical attack, including radical hysterectomy with node dissection. The common occurrence of distant metastases in endometrial sarcomas has discouraged a surgical approach, but it is likely that more efficient pelvic control would reduce this incidence and contribute to higher survival. More extensive study of this hypothesis is necessary. At our institution, patients with

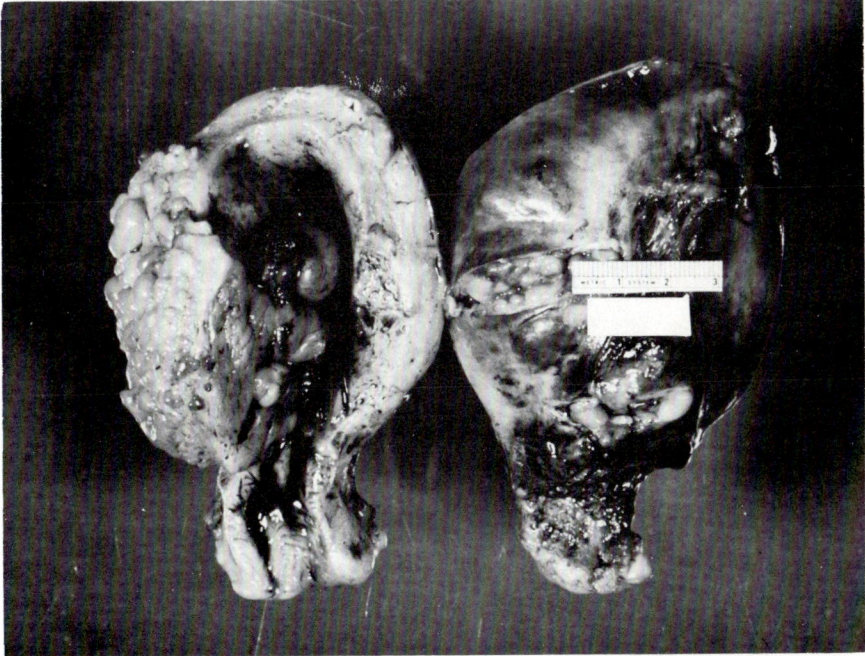

Fig. 4-8 Gross specimen of a uterus with endolymphatic stromal myosis, showing deep invasion of the myometrium and extension into the parametrium on the right. Patient had negative pelvic nodes.

poorly differentiated endometrial sarcomas receive multiple drug chemotherapy for at least 12 months in addition to conservative surgery and radiotherapy or radical surgery. This is done in an effort to destroy occult mestastases that are already out of the treatment field at the time of primary treatment. Survival rates of 20-40% have been reported for lesions limited to the uterus, the prognosis for stromal sarcoma being somewhat better than that for mixed mesodermal tumors. This is especially true for stromal sarcomas when the number of mitotic figures per 10 high power fields is less than 10; survival in these cases approaches 100% with appropriate therapy. These low grade endometrial sarcomas of the stromal variety may be appropriately treated with radical hysterectomy and pelvic lymphadenectomy, since their radiosensitivity is often poor and their spread pattern is usually of the local pelvic type. This is particularly true of the

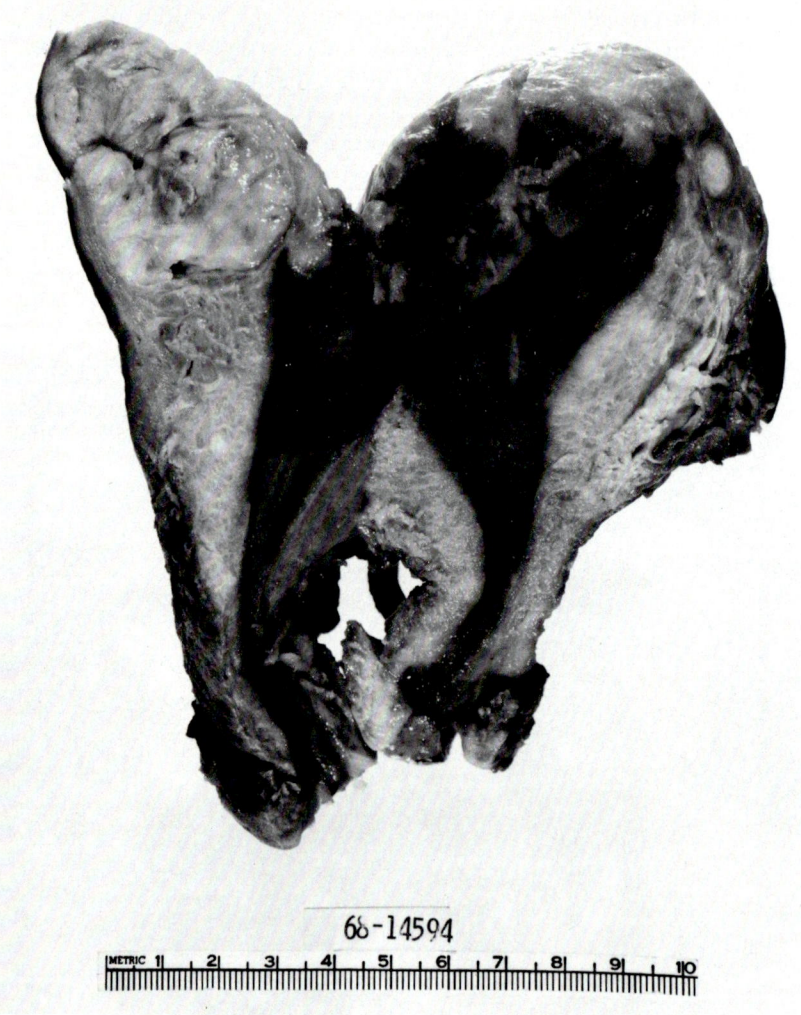

Fig. 4-9 Leiomyosarcoma in the right cornu of the uterus. The patient was operated on for menorrhagia and "fibroid" uterus.

lowest grade stromal sarcoma, endolymphatic stromal myosis (Fig. 4-8), which consistently invades by local extension through the myometrium out into the parametrial tissues.

The exact incidence of leiomyosarcoma of the uterus (Fig. 4-9) is not known, but it is indeed low. Its particular interest lies in its possible relationship to leiomyomas of the uterine myometrium. Thorton and Carter (1951) reported 14 cases of myometrial sarcoma along with 2459 cases of leiomyoma, and only 6 cases (0.24%) definitely arose in "fibromyoma." Gusberg et al (1960) reported 32 cases arising in myoma, along with 17,353 patients with fibromyoma of the uterus from the same institution in the same time period, for an incidence of 0.18%. These lesions occur primarily in the fifth and sixth decades of life, with a definite number appearing after the menopause. Postmenopausal bleeding, fever, lower abdominal pain, and a rapid increase in uterine size may all be symptoms of this disease. The majority of cases are diagnosed postoperatively after removal of a myomatous uterus. Total hysterectomy is the treatment of choice. The results with irradiation treatment have been generally quite poor, and the role of chemotherapy is untested. The survival rate for patients with no myometrial invasion (cellular myoma or "leiomyosarcoma *in situ*") is quite good (80-90%), whereas those with evidence of invasion invariably succumb to the disease.

REFERENCES

Alford, C. D., Betson, J. R., Jr., and DiSanti, N.: Wertheim hysterectomy and pelvic lymphaden-ectomy for carcinoma of the uterine corpus. *Am. J. Obstet. Gynecol.* **83**:1306, 1962.

Anderson, J., and Stephens, S.: Survival in carcinoma of the endometrium following pelvic node dissection. *Dan. Med. Bull.* **11**:160, 1964.

Austin, J. H., and MacMahon, B.: Indicators of prognosis in carcinoma of the corpus uteri. *Surg. Gynecol. Obstet.* **128**:1247, 1969.

Bickenbach, W., Lochmüller, H., Dirlich, G., et al: Factor analysis of endometrial carcinoma in relation to treatment. *Obstet. Gynecol.* **29**:632, 1967.

Boronow, R. C.: Carcinoma of the Corpus: Treatment at M.D. Anderson Hospital. In *Cancer of the Uterus and Ovary*, Year Book Medical Publishers, Chicago, 1969a.

Boronow, R. C.: Therapeutic considerations in endometrial cancer. *J. Miss. State Med. Assoc.* **10**:451, 1969b.

Bourne, A. W., and Williams, L. N.: Cancer of the uterine body. In *Recent advances in Obstetrics and Gynecology*, 10th Ed. Little, Brown, Boston, 1962.

Carmichael, J. A., and Bean, H. A.: Carcinoma of the endometrium in Saskatchewan. *Am. J. Obstet. Gynecol.* **97**:294, 1967.

Chamlain, D. L., and Taylor, H. B.: Endometrial hyperplasia in young women. *Obstet. Gynecol.* **36**:619, 1970.

Cheon, H. K.: Prognosis of endometrial carcinoma. *Obstet. Gynecol.* **34**:680, 1969.

Classification and staging of malignant tumors in the female pelvis. *Acta Obstet. Gynecol. Scand.* **50**:1, 1971.

DiSaia, P. J., Castro, J. R., and Rutledge, F. N.: Mixed mesodermal sarcoma of the uterus. *Am. J. Roentgenol. Radium Ther. Nucl. Med.* **117**:632, 1973.

Dobbie, B. M. W., Taylor, C. W., and Waterhouse, J. A. H.: A study of carcinoma of the endometrium. *J. Obstet. Gynaecol. Brit. Commonw.* **72**:659, 1965.

Finn, W. F.: Time, site and treatment of recurrences of endometrial carcinoma. *Am. J. Obstet. Gynecol.* **60**:773, 1950.

Fletcher, G. H., Ed.: *Textbook of Radiotherapy*. Lea & Febiger, Philadelphia, 1973.

Graham, J. B.: Treatment of choice in cancer of the uterine corpus. *N. Engl. J. Med.* **254**:1112, 1956.

Graham, J.: The value of preoperative or postoperative treatment by radium for carcinoma of the uterine body. *Surg. Gynecol. Obstet.* **132**:855, 1971.

Gusberg, S. B., et al: Selection of treatment for corpus cancer. *Am. J. Obstet. Gynecol.* **80**:374, 1960.

Hawksworth, W.: The treatment of carcinoma of the body of the uterus. *Proc. Roy. Soc. Med.* **57**:467, 1964.

Hertig, A. T., Sommers, S. C., and Bengloff, H.: Genesis of endometrial carcinoma. *Cancer* **2**:957, 1949.

Hirabayashi, K., and Graham, J.: Clinical classification of carcinoma of the uterine body. *Surg. Gynecol. Obstet.* **126**:75, 1968.

Javert, C. T.: The spread of benign and malignant endometrium in the lymphatic system with a note on coexisting vascular involvement. *Am. J. Obstet. Gynecol.* **64**:780, 1952.

Kistner, R. W., Lewis, J. L., and Steiner, C. T.: Effects of clomiphene citrate on endometrial hyperplasia in the premenopausal female. *Cancer* **19**:115, 1966.

Keller, D., Kempson, R. L., Levine, G., and McLennan, C.: Management of the patient with early endometrial carcinoma. *Cancer* **33**:1108, 1974.

Kottmeier, H. L.: Individualization of therapy in carcinoma of the corpus. In *Cancer of the Uterus and Ovary*, Year Book Medical Publishers, Chicago, 1969, pp. 102-108.

Krieger, P. D., and Gusberg, S. B.: Endolymphatic stromal myosis—a Grade 1 endometrial sarcoma. *Gynecol. Oncol.* **1**:299, 1973.

Kurohara, S. S., George, F. W., III, and Vongtama, V.: Method of staging system construction. *Acta Radiol.* **11**:65, 1972.

Lampe, I.: Endometrial carcinoma. *Am. J. Roentol., Radium Ther. Nucl. Med.* **90**:1011, 1963.

Lees, D. H.: An evaluation of the treatment of carcinoma of the body of the uterus. *J. Obstet. Gynaecol. Brit. Commonw.* **76**:615, 1969.

Lefevre, H.: Node dissection in cancer of the endometrium. *Surg. Gynecol. Obstet.* **102**:649, 1956.

Lewis, B. V., Stallworthy, J. A., and Cowdell, R.: Adenocarcinoma of the body of the uterus. *J. Obstet. Gynaecol Brit. Commonw.* **77**:343, 1970.

Lewis, G. C., Jr., Slack, N. H., Mortel, H., and Brass, I. D. J.: Adjuvant progestogen therapy in the primary definitive treatment of endometrial cancer. *Gynecol. Oncol.* **2**:368, 1974.

Lindgren, L.: The prognosis of carcinoma of the endometrium in its different stages treated by surgery combined with post-operative radiotherapy. *Acta Obstet. Gynecol. Scand.* **36**:426, 1957.

Liu, W. and Meigs, J. V.: Radical hysterectomy and pelvic lymphadenectomy. *Am. J. Obstet. Gynecol.* **69**:1, 1955.

McLennan, C. E.: The argument against pre-operative radium for endometrial cancer. *Trans. Pacif. Coast Obstet. Gynecol. Soc.* **25**:122, 1957.

Morrow, C. P., DiSaia, P. J. and Townsend, D. T.: Current management of endometrial carcinoma. *Obstet. Gynecol.* **42**:399, 1973.

Moss. W. T., and Grand, W. W.: *Therapeutic Radiology*, 4th ed, C. V. Mosby, St. Louis, 1974.

Nahhas, W. A., Lund, C. J., and Rudolph, J. H.: Carcinoma of the corpus uteri. *Obstet. Gynecol.* **38**:564, 1971.

Ng, A., and Reagan, J.: Incidence and prognosis of endometrial carcinoma by histological grade and extent. *Obstet. Gynecol.* **35**:437, 1970.

Nilsen, P. A. and Koller, O.: Carcinoma of the endometrium in Norway. 1957-1960, with special reference to treatment results. *Am. J. Obstet. Gynecol.* **105**:1099, 1969.

Nolan, J. F., and Harrison, L. A.: Carcinoma of the endometrium: An evaluation of pre-operative radiation therapy. *Obstet. Gynecol.* **17**:601, 1961.

Ober, W. B. and Jason, R. S.: Sarcoma of the endometrial stroma. *Am. Med. Assoc. Arch. Pathol.* **56**:301, 1953.

Parsons, L., and Cesare, F.: Wertheim hysterectomy in the treatment of endometrial carcinoma. *Surg. Gynecol. Obstet.* **108**:582, 1959.

Peterson, E. P.: Endometrial carcinoma in young women. *Obstet. Gynecol.* **31**:702, 1968.

Reddi, P. R., Nussbaum, H., Wollin, M., and Kagan, A. R.: Treatment of uterine cancer with special reference to radium system. *Obstet. Gynecol.* **43**:238, 1974.

Rickford, R. B. K.: Involvement of the pelvic lymph nodes in carcinoma of the endometrium. *J. Obstet. Gynaecol Brit. Commw.* **75**:580, 1968.

Roberts, D. W. T.: Carcinoma of the body of the uterus at Chelsea Hospital for Women, 1943-1953. *J. Obstet. Gynaecol. Brit. Commonw.* **68**:132, 1961.

Roman, T. N., Beck, R. R., and Latour, J. P. A.: Correlation of histologic grading with 5-year survival rates in endometrial carcinoma. *Am. J. Obstet. Gynecol.* **97**:117, 1967.

Sall, S., Sonnenblick, B., and Stone, M. L.: Factors affecting survival of patients with endometrial carcinoma. *Am. J. Obstet. Gynecol.* **107**:116, 1970.

Schwartz, A. E., and Brunschwig, A.: Radical pan-hysterectomy and pelvic node excision for carcinoma of the corpus uteri. *Surg. Gynecol. Obstet.* **105**:675, 1957.

Shah, C. A., and Green, T. H.: Evaluation of current management of endometrial carcinoma. *Obstet. Gynecol.* **39**:500, 1972.

Stallworthy, J. A.: Surgery of endometrial cancer in the Bonney tradition. *Ann. Roy. Coll. Surg. Engl.* **48**:293, 1971.

Steele, S. J., Scott, J. M., and Stephens, T. W.: Endometrial stromal sarcoma. *Brit. J. Surg.* **55**:943, 1968.

Thornton, W. W., and Carter, J. P.: Sarcoma of the uterus: A clinical study. *Am. J. Obstet. Gynecol.* **62**:294, 1951.

Wade, M. E., et al: Adenocarcinoma of the endometrium. *Am. J. Obstet. Gynecol.* **99**:869, 1967.

Wagner, D., Richart, R. M., and Terner, J. Y.: Deoxyribonucleic acid content of presumed precursors of endometrial carcinoma. *Cancer* **20**:2067, 1967.

Welander, C., Griem, M. L., and Newton, M.: Staging and treatment of endometrial carcinoma. *J. Repod. Med.* **8**:41, 1972.

CHAPTER 5

Tumors of the Ovary

5-1 NONNEOPLASTIC CYSTS AND HYPERPLASIAS

Nonneoplastic (functional) cysts, derived from the graafian follicle, and ovarian hyperplasias are the most common clinically detectable enlargements of the ovary occurring during the reproductive years (Table 5-1). They are of importance primarily because they cannot be distinguished readily on clinical grounds from true neoplasms.

Functional Cysts

Follicular cysts are usually asymptomatic. They may be accompanied by minor degrees of unilateral pelvic pain, however, and occasionally dyspareunia is experienced. Some patients report menstrual irregularities. Spontaneous rupture may occur, accompanied by bleeding that is rarely serious. Follicular cysts infrequently undergo torsion and infarction, producing a surgical emergency.

TABLE 5-1
NONNEOPLASTIC
CYSTS AND
HYPERPLASIAS OF THE OVARY

1. Functional cysts
   A. Follicle cysts
   B. Corpus luteum cysts
2. Theca-lutein cysts
3. Pregnancy luteoma
4. Sclerocystic ovaries
5. Endometriotic cysts

Corpus luteum cysts are less common than follicular cysts and are more likely to be associated with symptoms. Often the menstrual period is delayed, and vaginal spotting occurs. If pain and intra-abdominal bleeding develop and the cystic mass is palpable, the clinical picture may simulate precisely an ectopic pregnancy.

Functional cysts are characterized by their dimensions. They seldom exceed 10 cm in diameter, are unilateral, and are freely mobile. During the reproductive years an adnexal mass of this description can be presumed to be a functional cyst rather than a true neoplasm. Their rather transitory existence is of prime importance in distinguishing them from true neoplasms. Tradition and clinical experience have taught that functional cysts usually persist for only a few days or weeks, and reexamination during a different phase of the menstrual cycle has been common practice. Many gynecologists prescribe combination oral contraceptive pills to accelerate the involution of functional cysts on the presumption that these cysts are gonadotropin dependent. The inhibitory effect of the contraceptive steroids on the release of pituitary gonadotropins should abbreviate the life span of these cysts, hastening their identification as functional or nonneoplastic. Failure of the enlargement to regress during the period of observation mandates operative removal.

Spanos (1973) studied 286 cases of clinically apparent functional cysts in women. Steroid contraceptives were prescribed, and the women reexamined in 6 weeks. In 72% of the individuals the mass disappeared during this observation interval. Of the 81 patients whose mass persisted, none was found to have a functional cyst at laparotomy (Table 5-2). The fact that five of the removed tumors were malignant underscores the importance of avoiding unnecessary delay in operative investigation.

Theca-Lutein Cysts

Multiple follicle cysts with luteinization of the thecal cells are referred to as theca-lutein cysts and are believed to result from high levels of human chorionic gonadotropin (hCG)

TABLE 5-2 ADNEXAL "CYSTS"
PERSISTENT IN 286 PATIENTS
BETWEEN THE AGES OF 16 AND 48
YEARS TREATED WITH ESTROGEN AND
PROGESTERONE FOR 6 WEEKS

Diagnosis	Number of Patients	
Nonneoplastic cysts		35
Functional	0	
Endometriotic	28	
Paraovarian	4	
Hydrosalpinx	3	
Neoplasms		46
Dermoid	9	
Epithelial, benign	32	
Epithelial, malignant	4	
Dysgerminoma	1	
Total		81

From Spanos (1973).

or an increased sensitivity of theca cells to hCG. Typically theca-lutein cysts are found in association with hydatidiform mole (one third to one half of the cases) and choriocarcinoma, but occasionally they occur in pregnant patients with Rh sensitization, multiple gestation, toxemia, or diabetes, and (rarely) in a normal single pregnancy. Administration of gonadotropins or clomiphene to induce ovulation may produce theca-lutein cysts and multiple corpora lutea ("overstimulation syndrome"). Theca-lutein cysts are characteristically bilateral and may achieve a size greater than 25 cm in diameter. Theca-lutein cysts do not usually require special treatment as regression occurs subsequent to the lowering of gonadotropin levels. Return to normal size, however, often lags behind the decline in gonadotropin levels.

Pregnancy Luteoma

Pregnancy luteoma is a nodular hyperplasia of ovarian lutein cells. It occurs exclusively during pregnancy, predominantly in multiparous Negro women. Nearly all cases have been discovered incidentally at the time of cesarean section or postpartum tubal ligation. Maternal and fetal virilism have been reported in association with pregnancy luteoma. Pregnancy luteomas range in size from 6 to 16 cm, are frequently bilateral, and are invariably multinodular. Spontaneous regression occurs postpartum, but the hyperplasia may recur with subsequent pregnancies. When doubt exists regarding the nature of the lesion, pathologic examination should be made before excising the ovary.

Sclerocystic Ovaries

Bilateral ovarian enlargement may be found in young women with the Stein-Leventhal syndrome of infertility, oligomenorrhea, and menstrual irregularities. The ovaries may be 2-3 times normal size. The etiology of the ovarian enlargement usually is apparent clinically because of the characteristic history and physical features of this syndrome.

Endometriosis

About 5% of patients with endometriosis will have a clinically detectable adnexal mass. This endometriotic cyst or "endometrioma" presumably results from cyclic hemorrhage into a focus of ovarian endometriosis. Accumulation of blood within the cavity results in the classical "chocolate" cyst. These cysts are thin walled and minor degrees of leakage often occurs, producing intermittent pain and inducing adhesion formation to surrounding structures. Physical examination may reveal other findings consistent with endometriosis, including uterosacral nodularity, retroversion of the uterus, and cul-de-sac tenderness. Management of the patient with an adnexal mass and endometriosis must be directed toward the adnexal mass. If uterosacral nodularity is present, prompt surgical exploration is even more urgent since the nodules may represent implants from ovarian carcinoma.

5-2 TRUE OVARIAN NEOPLASMS—GENERAL CONSIDERATIONS

An enlarged ovary constitutes one of the most frequent and potentially serious conditions in gynecology. The etiologic possibilities range from the harmless follicular cyst to some of the most ruthless malignancies in human oncology. The clinician is charged with the responsibility of determining the exact nature of an ovarian enlargement and the threat it poses to the patient's life and reproductive function. Recognition of the malignant potential of an ovarian tumor is of paramount importance since the patient's life often depends on appropriate therapy.

Every woman at birth has a 5 to 7% risk of developing an ovarian neoplasm sometime during her life. No other organ has the capacity to produce such a wide variety of tumors with respect to both histologic structure and biologic behavior. The clinical manifestations are protean and constitute one of the most remarkable features of these neoplasms. Ovarian tumors may be associated with the production of estrogenic, androgenic, progestational, and adrenal steroid hormones, as well as the clinical manifestations reflecting the physiologic function of these agents. The elaboration of the polypeptide chorionic gonadotropin may mimic early pregnancy or induce pseudopuberty. A hyperthyroid state can result from functioning teratomatous thyroid tissue, and such paraendocrine disorders as hypercalcemia and hypoglycemia have been reported. Autoimmune hemolytic anemia rarely is caused by the common dermoid cyst. Ascites and hydrothorax suggestive of advanced malignancy can be manifestations of the generally harmless ovarian fibroma, and peritoneal implants occasionally develop from benign epithelial tumors and benign teratomas. Although an ovarian neoplasm is often silent or productive of only minor symptoms, it may present as a surgical emergency secondary to infarction, rupture, or hemorrhage. Thus ovarian tumors are able to produce a wide spectrum of disease states requiring individualization of management based on sound pathologic diagnosis and accurate knowledge of the natural history of the individual neoplasm.

Symptoms

The diverse ovarian tumors generally manifest themselves in a similar manner. As enlargement occurs, there is progressive compression of the surrounding pelvic structures, producing such commonplace symptoms as urinary frequency, constipation, pelvic discomfort, and a feeling of heaviness. Dyspareunia is reported in some instances. When the diameter of the mass exceeds 12—15 cm in the adult, it begins to rise out of the pelvis, which can no longer accommodate it. At this stage of development the patient is likely to notice abdominal enlargement, which she may attribute to weight gain. During the late reproductive years the coincidental occurrence of menopausal amenorrhea and abdominal swelling may be misinterpreted as a pregnancy. Pain of various degrees is one of the most common presenting symptoms of ovarian tumors, whether neoplastic or functional. Rapid enlargement producing capsular stretching, twisting of the tumor on its vascular pedicle, intracystic hemorrhage, and rupture are all mechanisms by which the pain may originate. Occasionally such an event initiates severe pain and the clinical features of a surgical emergency. In childhood and the early reproductive years, torsion of an ovarian tumor frequently simulates acute appendicitis. Menstrual irregularity, often associated with functional cysts, is an uncommon symptom of benign neoplasms of the ovary.

Malignant ovarian tumors seldom are discovered in asymptomatic patients, a fact attributable to their rapid growth. Abdominal pain and abdominal swelling are consistently the two most frequent complaints reported. In the presence of ascites or mestatases to the upper abdomen, gastrointestinal symptoms such as bloating, heartburn, nausea, anorexia, and abdominal discomfort are often experienced. It is understandable that the patient frequently seeks advice from an internist because these symptoms are suggestive of cholecystitis, peptic ulcer, and other gastrointestinal disturbances. When ascites is clinically apparent, a tentative diagnosis of liver disease is often entertained. Abnormal vaginal bleeding is more commonly a symptom of ovarian cancer than of benign ovarian neoplasia. In the reproductive years the bleeding abnormality may take the form of absent, irregular, or excessive menses. Some women before reporting for medical care will have noticeable weight loss because of chronic anorexia and nausea.

The relative frequencies of the various presenting complaints in ovarian cancer are given in Table 5-3. Since the individual with ovarian carcinoma has no unique appearance or characteristic symptoms that distinguish her from the numerous patients with the ordinary problems encountered in everyday office practice, the physician must excercise constant vigilance.

Physical Findings

An adequate pelvic examination is the key to the diagnosis of ovarian neoplasms. Prerequisites include an empty bladder and rectum with relaxed pelvic and abdominal muscles. Even under optimal conditions a small ovarian mass may not be detected, particularly in the obese patient. As a rule the lower genital tract is normal in the patient with an ovarian tumor, but the cervix and vagina may be displaced by extrinsic pressure. Although an adnexal mass may be palpable on vagino-abdominal bimanual examination, of greater value and an indispensable step in the evaluation of the female pelvis is rectovaginal bimanual examination of the pelvic organs. This maneuver permits an assessment of the posterior uterine surface, uterosacral ligaments, the pouch of Douglas, and the parametria. Small ovarian tumors, cul-de-sac nodularity, and neoplastic disease involving the rectovaginal septum, that might otherwise not be appreciated on physical examination may be detected in this manner. The uterus is often distinctly separate from an adnexal mass, but at times such discrimination is impossible. Although dermoids and

TABLE 5-3 PRESENTING SYMPTOMS OF
PATIENTS WITH OVARIAN CANCER

Symptom	Per cent
Abdominal swelling	70
Abdominal discomfort	50
Gastrointestinal	20
Urinary	15
Abnormal bleeding	15
Weight loss	15
Asymptomatic	?

endometriotic cysts tend to occupy the anterior cul-de-sac, most ovarian tumors lie posterior to the uterus or have ascended into the abdomen.

It is not possible on physical examination alone to identify with certainty whether an ovarian mass is benign or malignant; but if the mass is unilateral, cystic, mobile, and less than 10 cm in diameter, a benign diagonsis is favored, whereas solid, bilateral, fixed, larger masses are more likely to be malignant. Paradoxically, a huge cystic tumor filling the abdomen is usually benign. Although the presence of ascites is a strong indication of a malignant tumor, it is not pathognomonic (see the discussion of Meigs's syndrome, p. 187). The delineation of a large ovarian mass on abdominal examination is frequently a simple matter, particularly in a thin subject with a solid or semisolid tumor (Figs. 5-1 and 5-2), but differentiation of ascites from a large ovarian cyst may be exceedingly difficult. A fluid wave can be elicited in either condition. However, the tympanitic note of the small intestine should be central in a supine patient with ascites and lateral when the distension is secondary to a tumor. Furthermore, ascites will balloon an umbilical hernia, but a neoplastic mass within the abdomen will not.

It is imperative that the physical examination not be limited to the pelvis in the patient with a gynecologic tumor. The lymph node bearing areas must be carefully palpated. Both the supraclavicular and inguinal nodes are frequent sites of metastases from ovarian cancer, and even the axillary nodes may be clinically involved. The breast and rectum are more common sites of primary cancer in women than any of the genital organs, and they should always be examined. Other features to be looked for include pleural effusions and leg edema. The physical examination of a patient with an ovarian mass should also include a search for the stigmata of abnormal hormone production.

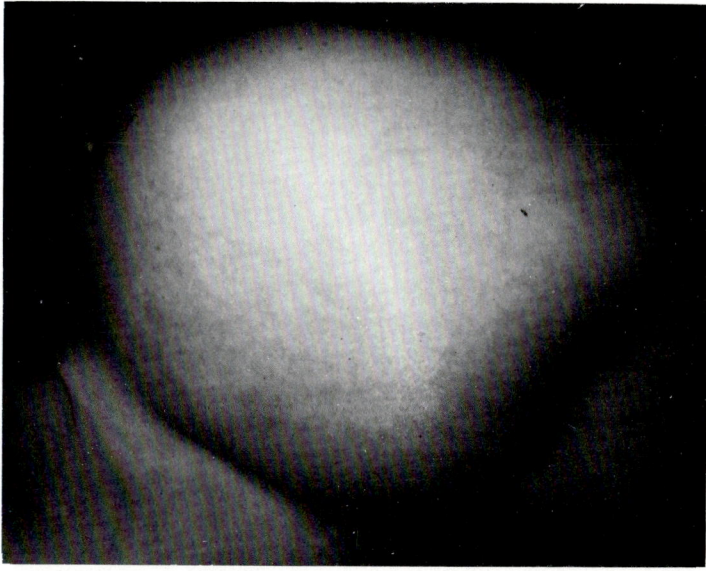

Fig. 5-1 Marked protuberance of the abdomen in a 64 year old female. The enlargement occurred gradually over several months and was accompanied by minor abdominal discomfort. The umbilicus is at the top center of the picture, and the upper thigh and mons pubis to the left. The apparent "flaring" of the flank is due to subcutaneous adipose tissue and not ascites. A large, solid tumor was easily outlined on abdominal palpation.

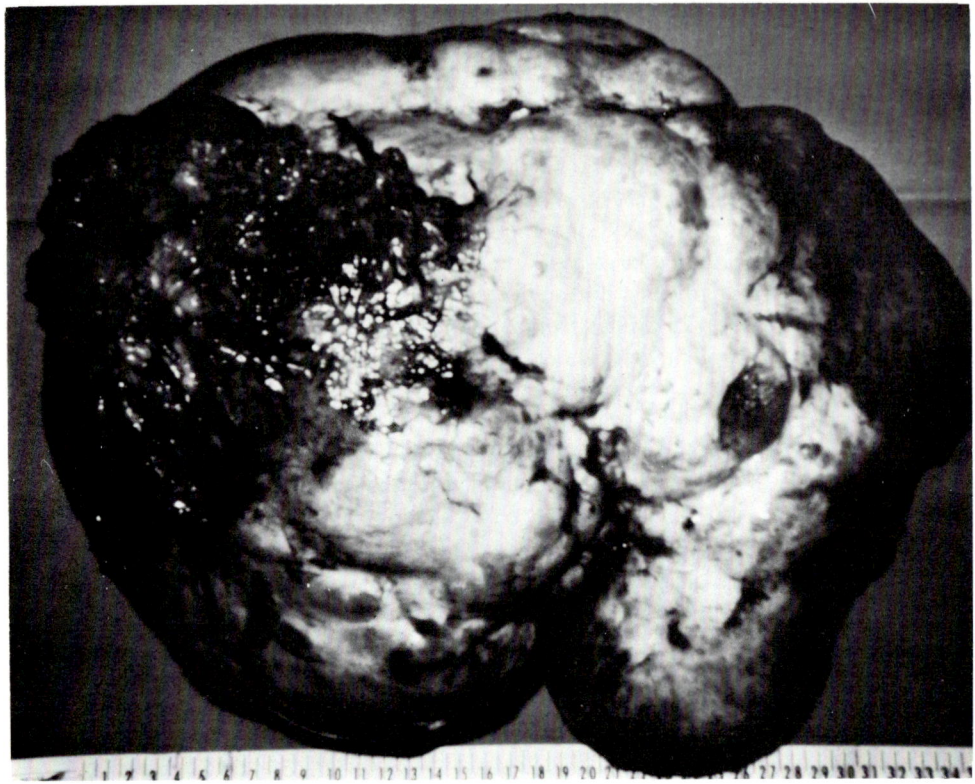

Fig. 5-2 Huge ovarian neoplasm removed from the patient in Fig. 5-1. On cut section the tumor was predominantly solid with areas of cystic degeneration, hemorrhage, and necrosis. Microscopically mixed endometrioid and clear cell carcinoma were found arising in a fibroadenoma.

Preoperative Evaluation

The diagnosis and management of ovarian neoplasia, benign or malignant, are ultimately dependent on surgical exploration. The preoperative work-up should be tailored to the physical findings, the patient's symptomatology, and her general medical condition. Table 5-4 presents some of the numerous conditions that may masquerade as ovarian tumors and must therefore be borne in mind during the preoperative assessment of the patient with a pelvic mass. A plain film of the abdomen frequently provides clues to the nature of such a mass. About one half of ovarian dermoid cysts can be positively identified in this manner because of three characteristic radiographic features: (1) calcifications due to tooth and bone formation (Fig. 5-3), (2) a radiolucent shadow cast by the lipidic fluid filling the cyst, and (3) the "capsule sign," a rim of radiodensity circumscribing the cyst (Fig. 5-4). Papillary serous tumors, benign or malignant, may contain sufficient calcifications, psammoma bodies, to be visible radiographically. Metastases from malignant serous tumors with psammoma bodies similarly may be visualized (Fig. 5-5).

Intravenous urography is of great importance in the preoperative assessment of the patient with a pelvic mass. It will provide the surgeon with valuable information about renal function, urinary tract anomalies, and ureteral obstruction. The last of these is of special importance when retroperitoneal dissection is necessary. The chest x-ray is

**TABLE 5-4 NONOVARIAN CAUSES
OF AN APPARENT ADNEXAL MASS**

1. Neoplastic
    Uterine and ligamentous myomata
    Tubal carcinoma
    Carcinoma of sigmoid, cecum, appendix
    Retroperitoneal neoplasm
2. Nonneoplastic
    Tube-ovarian abscess
    Diverticulitis
    Appendiceal abscess
    Matted bowel and omentum
    Peritoneal cyst
    Stool in sigmoid
    Pelvic kidney
    Full bladder
    Urachal cyst
    Anterior sacral meningocoele
    Pregnancy (intrauterine, tubal, abdominal)

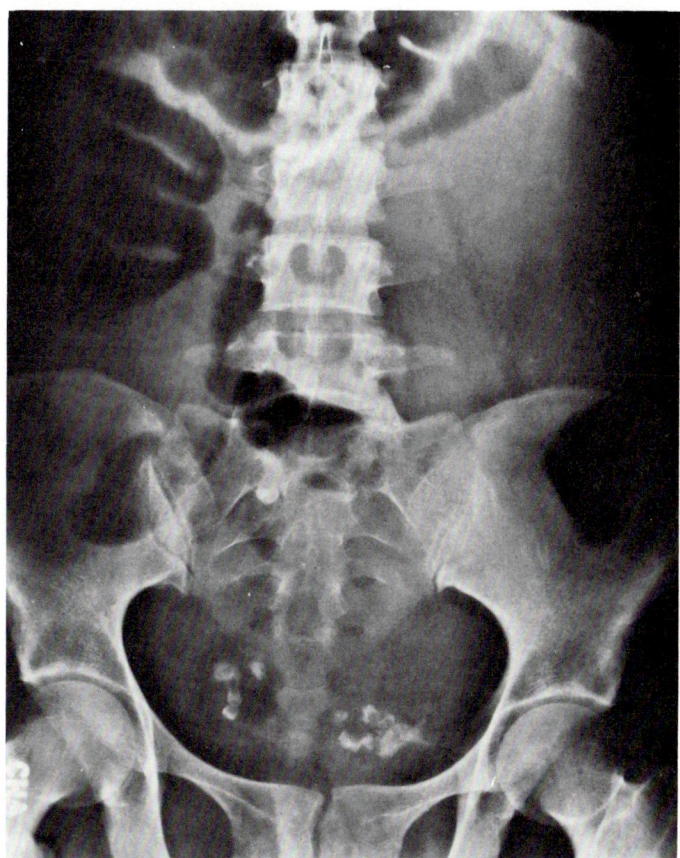

Fig. 5-3 Anterior-posterior radiograph of the abdomen and pelvis. The two sets of calcifications in the pelvis represent teeth in bilateral ovarian dermoids. The teeth on the patient's right occupy a radiolucent shadow cast by the lipid fluid in the cyst. (From C.P. Morrow and W.R. Hart.: The Ovaries, in *Gynecology and Obstetrics: The Health Care of Women*, Seymour Romney et al, Eds., McGraw-Hill, New York, in press.)

143

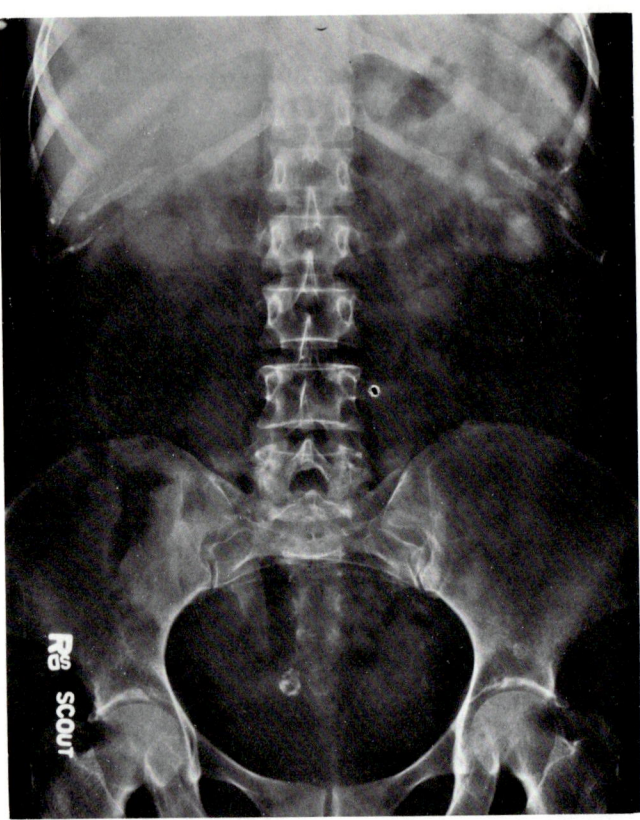

Fig. 5-4 Anterior-posterior radiograph of the abdomen and pelvis. A circular rim of radiodensity in the patient's right lumbar region identifies the dermoid cyst. The mottled calcification in the pelvis proved to be a uterine myoma. (From C.P. Morrow and W.R. Hart.: The Ovaries, in *Gynecology and Obstetrics: The Health Care of Women*, Seymour Romney et al., Eds., McGraw-Hill Book, New York, in press.)

indispensable. It not only provides important information about the status of the heart and lungs but also detects clinically silent metastases and pleural effusions. In the patient with symptoms referable to the colon or with a fixed or irregular pelvic mass, a large bowel contrast study is indicated. Inflammatory and neoplastic disease of the colon can be easily confused with ovarian malignancy. Although upper gastrointestinal symptoms in a patient with an adnexal mass may suggest ovarian cancer with abdominal metastases, the symptoms may actually be unrelated to the pelvic mass and hence radiographic studies of the gallbladder and stomach are necessary. It also should be remembered that gastric cancer can metastasize to the ovaries, especially in a premenopausal woman. Liver function studies are essential in the evaluation of a patient with ascites, but paracentesis or cul-de-sac aspiration for cytology is seldom warranted if a pelvic mass is present.

   Cervical cytology is of limited practical value in the work-up of a pelvic mass but should be performed to evaluate the cervix for neoplasia. An endometrial biopsy will exclude corpus carcinoma and is indicated particularly in the patient with a history of abnormal bleeding or an enlarged uterus. The value of ultrasound and laparoscopy in the investigation of a pelvic mass has not been established. Laparoscopy, culdoscopy, and pelvic pneumonography can be useful in defining ovarian enlargement that is suspected

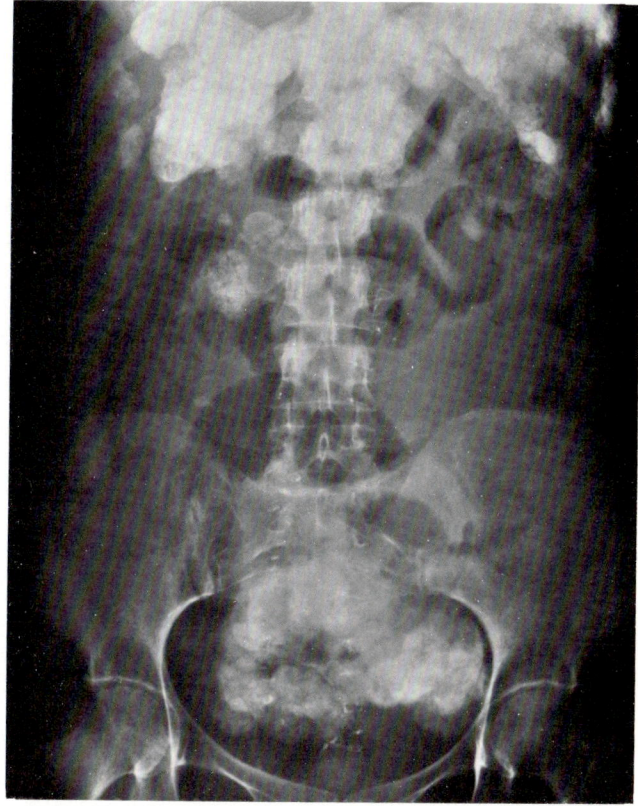

Fig. 5-5 Anterior-posterior radiograph of the abdomen and pelvis. Extensive pelvic and abdominal calcifications due to psammoma bodies in a papillary serous carcinoma of the ovary. (From C.P. Morrow and W.R. Hart.: The Ovaries, in *Gynecology and Obstetrics: The Health Care of Women*, Seymour Romney et al, Eds., McGraw-Hill, New York, in press.)

but uncertain on pelvic examination. Lymphangiography, venography, arteriography, and gallium scintigraphy have all been used to study pelvic masses, but none has an established role in this clinical problem.

Operative Management

Any patient suspected of having an ovarian neoplasm, malignant or benign, should be subjected to laparotomy as soon as the diagnostic studies are completed. Only individuals whose general condition is too poor to tolerate surgery should be excluded. In these cases a presumptive diagnosis of benign or malignant disease must be made on the basis of physical examination, laboratory aids, and peritoneal cytology. The abdominal incision selected must be adapted to the type of operative procedures that the surgeon envisions, considering the different diagnostic possibilities. A longitudinal midline incision permits the greatest flexibility but will not always be necessary. There is a natural reluctance, especially in young women, to extend an incision to facilitate the intact removal of a cystic ovarian tumor. Although such a tumor is likely to be benign, the critical issue is whether rupture of a malignant cyst might be harmful to the patient. To assume that spillage of fluid from a malignant cyst is innocuous seems insupportable since exfoliated malignant cells are often present in the fluid of malignant cysts. To incur the risk of contaminating the peritoneal cavity with cancer cells by unnecessarily decompressing or otherwise rupturing an ovarian cyst at surgery is contrary to the most fundamental principles of cancer surgery. These principles must not be abandoned on the basis of empirical clinical data. Although some reports in the literature have shown no deleterious influence on prognosis when rupture of a malignant cyst occurs, none has involved sufficient cases to take into account the differences in stage, grade, cell type, and treatment.

Frequently at the time of surgery the preservation or sacrifice of the reproductive and endocrine functions of the genital tract depends on recognition of the malignant potential of the ovarian neoplasm. Although in most cases absolute identification must await histopathologic studies, several gross features that suggest malignancy may be observed at surgery (Table 5-5). None of these findings per se is diagnostic of malignancy, but hemorrhagic ascitic fluid, excrescences on the cortical surface of the tumor, and peritoneal implants (Fig. 5-6) are rarely found with benign neoplasms. Additional information can be obtained by sectioning the neoplasm after it has been removed. Areas of hemorrhage and necrosis, numerous intracystic papillary growths, friable tissue, and a cystic and solid composition are suggestive of malignancy (Figs. 5-7 and 5-8). By contrast, when a tumor is composed of one or more smooth walled cysts free of papillary excrescences and having no solid areas, it is in all likelihood benign. The finding of hair, teeth, and sebaceous material identifies the tumor as a cystic teratoma, which, with few exceptions, is benign (Fig. 5-9).

In a child or young woman of reproductive age, for whom conservative surgical management is a major consideration, microscopic examination of the tumor by frozen section analysis should be obtained to guide the surgeon in his selection of therapy whenever doubt exists about the nature of the neoplasm. If the diagnosis of malignancy is uncertain, or if the neoplasm is malignant but confined to one ovary (Stage Ia), peritoneal washings, omental biopsy, and wedge biopsy of the uninvolved ovary should be performed in conjunction with unilateral salpingo-oophorectomy. A careful, systematic search for evidence of extraovarian disease is, of course, mandatory before conservative surgical therapy can be selected as the form of treatment.

TABLE 5-5   FREQUENT GROSS FEATURES
OF BENIGN AND MALIGNANT OVARIAN TUMORS

Benign	Malignant
Unilateral	Bilateral
Capsule intact	Capsule ruptured
Freely mobile	Adherent to adjacent organs
Smooth surface	Excrescences on surface
No ascitic fluid	Ascites, especially hemorrhagic
Smooth peritoneal surfaces	Peritoneal implants
Entire tumor viable	Areas of hemorrhage and necrosis
Cystic	Solid or semisolid
Smooth cyst lining	Intracystic papillations
Uniform appearance	Variegated

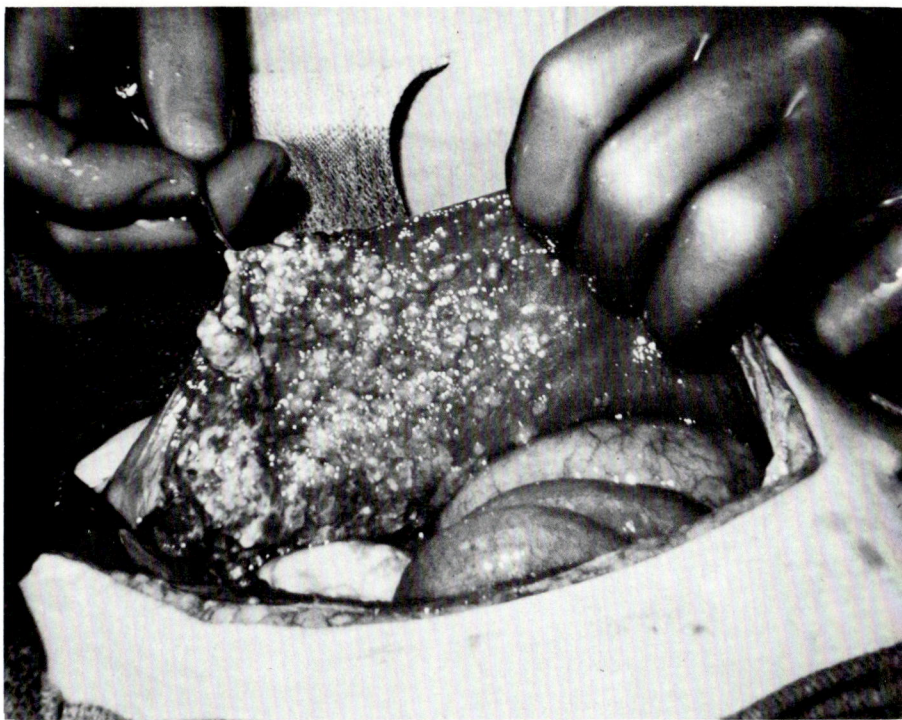

Fig. 5-6 Studding of the anterior parietal peritoneum from serous carcinoma of the ovary. Distended loops of small bowel are in the right foreground.

Classification of Ovarian Tumors

In view of the prodigious variety of ovarian neoplasms it is not surprising that numerous systems of classification have been devised, none of which is without shortcomings. Currently the most popular and practical scheme of classification is based on the histogenesis of the ovary. In this system the primary ovarian neoplasms are divided into four major groups according to their origin from the celomic (surface or germinal) epithelium, primitive germ cells, specialized gonadal stroma, or nonspecific mesenchyme (Table 5-6). When ovarian tumors are grouped into this histogenetic schema, it is generally observed that 60–70% of all ovarian neoplasms are derived from the celomic epithelium, while 15–20% are of germ cell origin. The ovarian stroma groups, specialized and nonspecific, each account for 5–10% of ovarian tumors (Table 5-7). About 5% of ovarian tumors are secondary or metastatic in origin, if only clinically significant ovarian metastases are included.

5-3 NEOPLASMS DERIVED FROM CELOMIC EPITHELIUM

Ovarian neoplasms of celomic epithelial origin constitute the largest subgroup in the histogenetic classification scheme. These tumors are believed to arise from the ovarian surface (germinal) epithelium, which is of paramesonephric derivation. Most neoplasms in

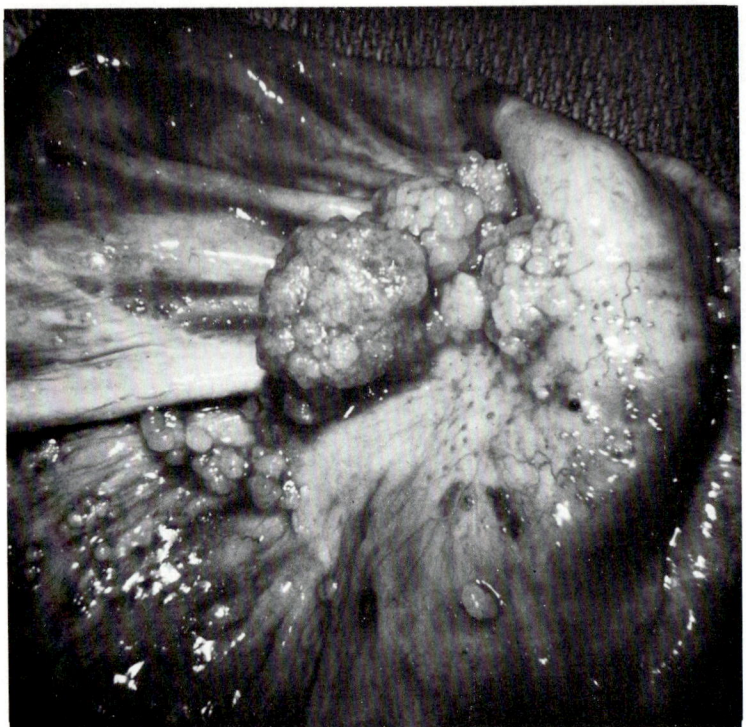

Fig. 5-7 Unilocular serous ovarian neoplasm. Condylomatous intracystic growths are suggestive of malignancy. This case proved to be a papillary serous tumor of borderline malignant potential.

this group contain epithelium histologically similar to that lining the endocervix, endometrium, or endosalpinx and are designated as mucinous, endometrioid, or serous tumors, respectively. Mixtures of these cell types are not uncommon, and such tumors are categorized according to the dominant cell type. Less common varieties of ovarian neoplasms derived from the celomic epithelium include the clear cell (mesonephroid) carcinoma, the Brenner tumor, and the rare carcinosarcoma and mixed mesodermal tumor. Most epithelial neoplasms can be further classified according to histologic and cytologic features as benign, borderline, or malignant. The degree of histologic differentiation may vary widely within the same neoplasm, and each tumor must be classified according to the least differentiated region. Occasionally the stromal component of an epithelial tumor predominates, and the neoplasm is then referred to as a cystadenofibroma.

Benign Epithelial Neoplasms

Serous Cystadenomas

Serous cystadenomas account for approximately 25% of all benign ovarian neoplasms. They occur predominantly during the reproductive years and are rare before puberty. The incidence of bilaterality is reported to be 15%. Serous cystadenomas have a smooth outer surface (Fig. 5-10). The simple serous cysts have a smooth lining and are unilocular.

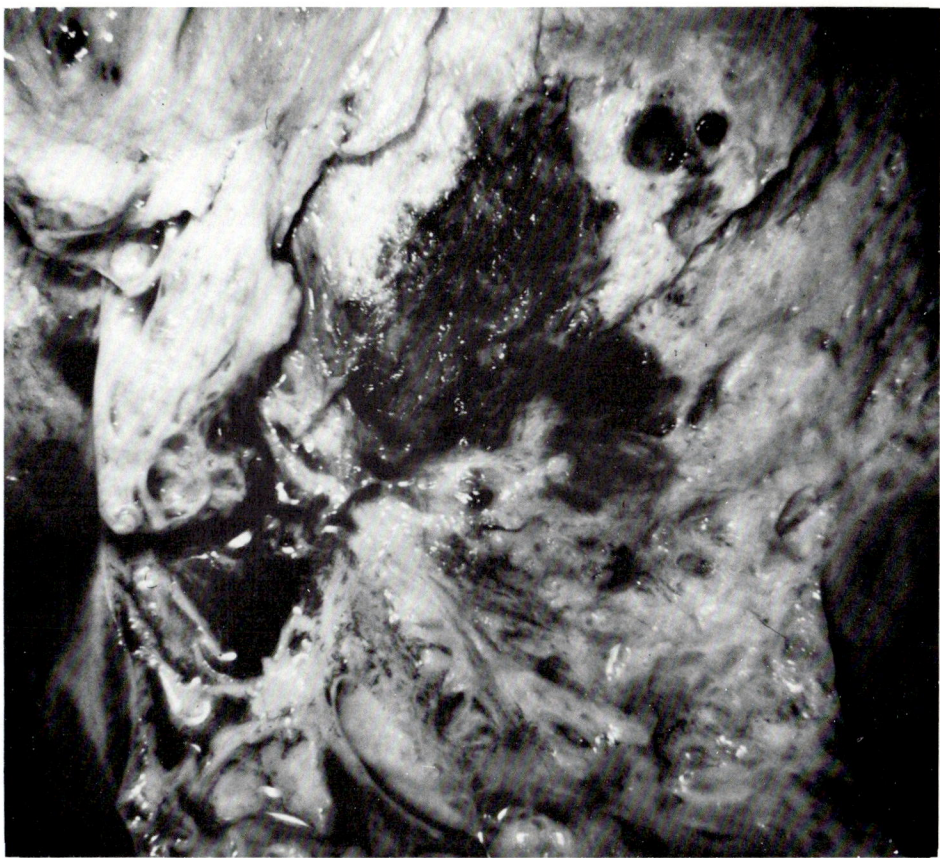

Fig. 5-8 Cut section of an ovarian neoplasm, demonstrating solid and cystic composition with an area of hemorrhage and necrosis, both very suggestive of malignancy. (Same case as in Figs. 5-1 and 5-2.)

Papillary serous cystadenomas are characterized by warty growths protruding into the lumen of the tumor. They are frequently multilocular. Papillary tumors are more likely to be bilateral. About one fourth of papillary serous tumors contain microscopic calcospherites, psammoma bodies, which may be extensive enough to be detected by pelvic radiographs. Spontaneous rupture of a papillary serous cystadenoma may rarely result in peritoneal implants.

Mucinous Cystadenoma

Benign mucinous cystadenomas occur with less frequency than the serous variety and are less often bilateral. These neoplasms are generally multilocular and are lined by simple mucus secreting columnar epithelium reminiscent of endocervical epithelium. The occasional coexistence of mucinous epithelium with endometrioid or serous epithelium supports an origin from surface celomic epithelium; however, some mucinous cystadenomas have an epithelial lining containing goblet cells, argentaffin cells, and occasionally Paneth's cells, suggesting a teratomatous origin. Dermoid cysts have been found in association with mucinous cystadenomas in about 5% of cases. The majority of

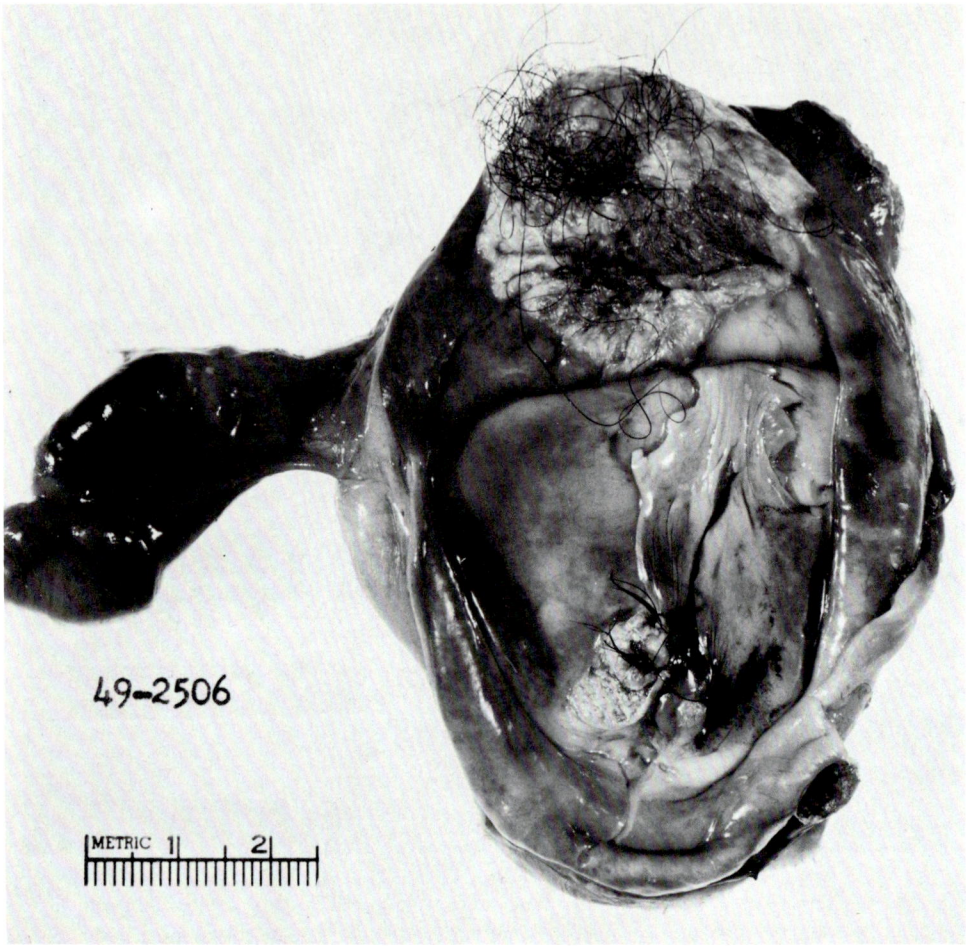

Fig. 5-9 Benign cystic teratoma of the ovary (dermoid cyst). The unilocular cyst has been opened, and the sebaceous contents removed. Although not as abundant as in many dermoids, the hair so characteristic of these neoplasms is quite evident.

the so-called giant tumors of the ovary are of the mucinous variety (Fig. 5-11), and in general benign serous cystadenomas tend to be smaller than mucinous tumors. Mucinous cystadenomas may develop papillary excrescences protruding from the cyst lining. Rupture may result in implantation of the tumor on the peritoneum and in a profuse outpouring of mucinous material. However, the occurrence of pseudomyxoma peritonei is far more commonly associated with rupture of a malignant or borderline malignant mucinous neoplasm.

Benign Endometrioid and Mesonephroid Tumors

Few authorities accept the ovarian endometrioma as a true neoplasm. If these lesions are excluded, endometrioid cysts are an extremely rare form of benign ovarian tumor, as is the mesonephroid variety. Occasionally endometrioid and mesonephroid epithelium may be found in cystadenofibromas.

TABLE 5-6   HISTOGENETIC
CLASSIFICATION OF OVARIAN NEOPLASMS

1. Neoplasms derived from celomic epithelium
    Serous tumor
    Mucinous tumor
    Endometrioid tumor
    Mesonephroid (clear cell) tumor
    Brenner tumor
    Undifferentiated carcinoma
    Carcinosarcoma and mixed mesodermal tumor
2. Neoplasms derived from germ cells
    Teratoma
        a. Mature teratoma
            Solid adult teratoma
            Dermoid cyst
            Struma ovarii
            Malignant neoplasms secondarily arising from
            mature cystic teratoma
        b. Immature teratoma (partially differentiated
            teratoma)
    Dysgerminoma
    Embryonal carcinoma (endodermal sinus tumor)
    Choriocarcinoma
    Gonadoblastoma
3. Neoplasms derived from specialized gonadal stroma
    Granulosa-theca tumors
        a. Granulosa tumor
        b. Thecoma
    Sertoli-Leydig tumors
        a. Arrhenoblastoma
        b. Sertoli tumor
    Gynandroblastoma
    Lipid cell tumors
4. Neoplasms derived from nonspecific mesenchyme
    Fibroma, hemangioma, leiomyoma, lipoma, etc.
    Lymphoma
    Sarcoma

Brenner Tumor

Brenner described a tumor composed of nests of transitional-like epithelial cells
embedded in an abundant fibrous stroma. He believed the tumor to be related to the
granulosa tumors and designated it as "oophoroma folliculare." This tumor accounts for
1% of all ovarian tumors; over half occur in the postmenopausal age group. Bilaterality is
uncommon, and only rarely are Brenner tumors malignant. Five to ten per cent of
Brenner tumors occur in conjunction with mucinous cystadenomas and dermoid cysts.
Many of the reported Brenner tumors were discovered only incidentally on microscopic
examination of the ovary. The typical histologic features are shown in Fig. 5-12.

Management of Benign Epithelial Tumors

Surgical removal is adequate therapy for any benign ovarian neoplasm, but factors other
than excision of the tumor enter into the plan of therapy. In postmenopausal women the

TABLE 5-7   RELATIVE FREQUENCY OF PRIMARY OVARIAN NEOPLASMS ACCORDING TO HISTOGENETIC CATEGORY

Histogenetic Category	Per Cent
1. Celomic epithelium	70
2. Germ cell	20
3. Specialized gonadal stroma	5
4. Nonspecific mesenchyme	5

uterus, tubes, and ovaries are considered to be expendable from both a physiologic and a psychologic perspective. Since the ovary and uterus (inclusive of the cervix) are relatively common sites for cancer, it has become established practice to remove these organs when pelvic surgery is required after the menopause. During the reproductive years preservation of the childbearing and hormonal functions of the reproductive tract is of major importance in the treatment of benign ovarian tumors, and consequently conservative surgery is the rule. The risk of preserving the contralateral ovary has been studied by Randall et al (1972), who followed 213 women after unilateral oophorectomy for a benign serous or mucinous cystadenoma. This group did not seem to show any increase or decrease in the risk of developing a benign or malignant ovarian tumor, as compared with the general population.

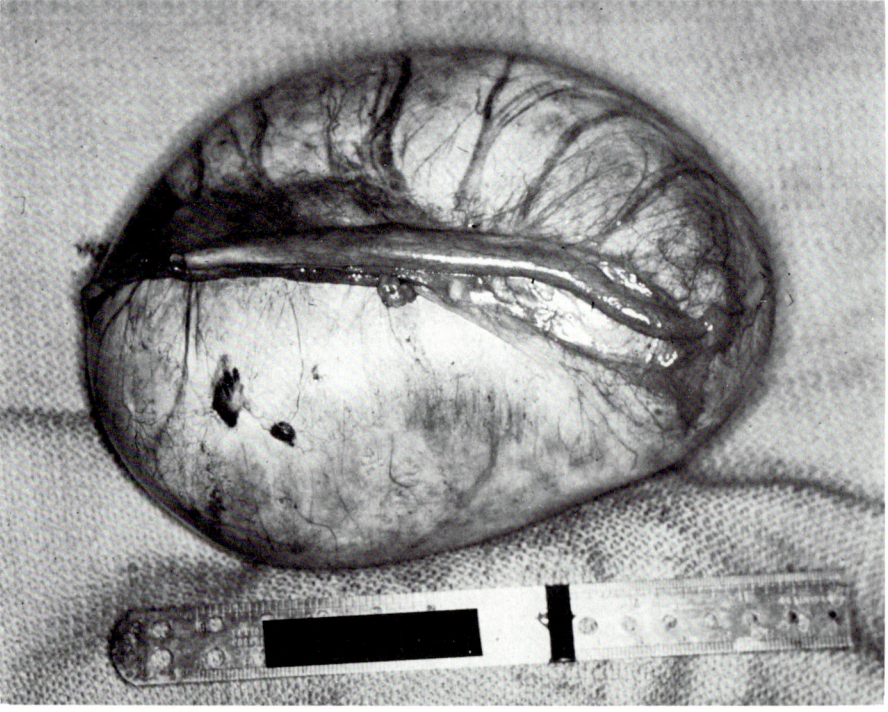

Fig. 5-10 Gross appearance of a simple serous cystadenoma. The neoplasm was composed of a unilocular, smooth walled cyst entirely free of papillary growths on the outer and inner surfaces. The fallopian tube crosses the outer surface of the cyst.

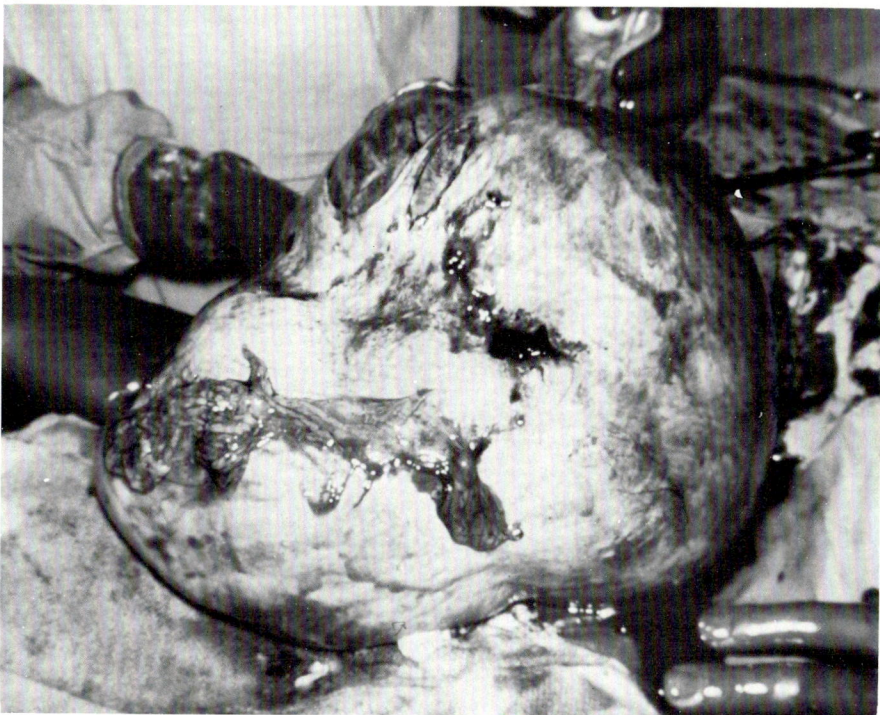

Fig. 5-11 Large mucinous cystadenoma. Cut section disclosed typical multilocular composition. The locules were lined by an entirely smooth epithelium, and no solid areas were found. Slightly viscous mucoid fluid filled the locules.

Enucleation of a benign appearing unilateral cystic ovarian neoplasm is frequently recommended to conserve ovarian tissue. This maneuver is especially applicable to the young patient with bilateral benign cysts or with only a single ovary. In Randall's study, 4 of 42 patients with an enucleated benign cystadenoma subsequently developed a second neoplasm in the same ovary. None of the four neoplasms was malignant, and none was of the same cell type as the original lesion. Surgical incision of the uninvolved ovary has been recommended to uncover an occult neoplasm. There is no doubt that an otherwise inapparent tumor can be discovered in this manner, but neither the rate of discovery nor the morbidity to the bivalved ovary has been determined.

Borderline Malignant Epithelial Tumors

For many years the existence of a group of epithelial ovarian tumors that have histologic and biologic features occupying a position between those of the clearly benign and frankly malignant ovarian epithelial neoplasms (Taylor, 1929) has been recognized. The International Federation of Gynecology and Obstetrics (FIGO) accorded these tumors official status in its 1961 classification of epithelial ovarian tumors and designated them as cystadenomas of low potential malignancy (Table 5-8). These borderline malignancies, which account for approximately 15% of all epithelial ovarian cancers, are often referred to as proliferative cystadenomas. Histologically the general epithelial structures are

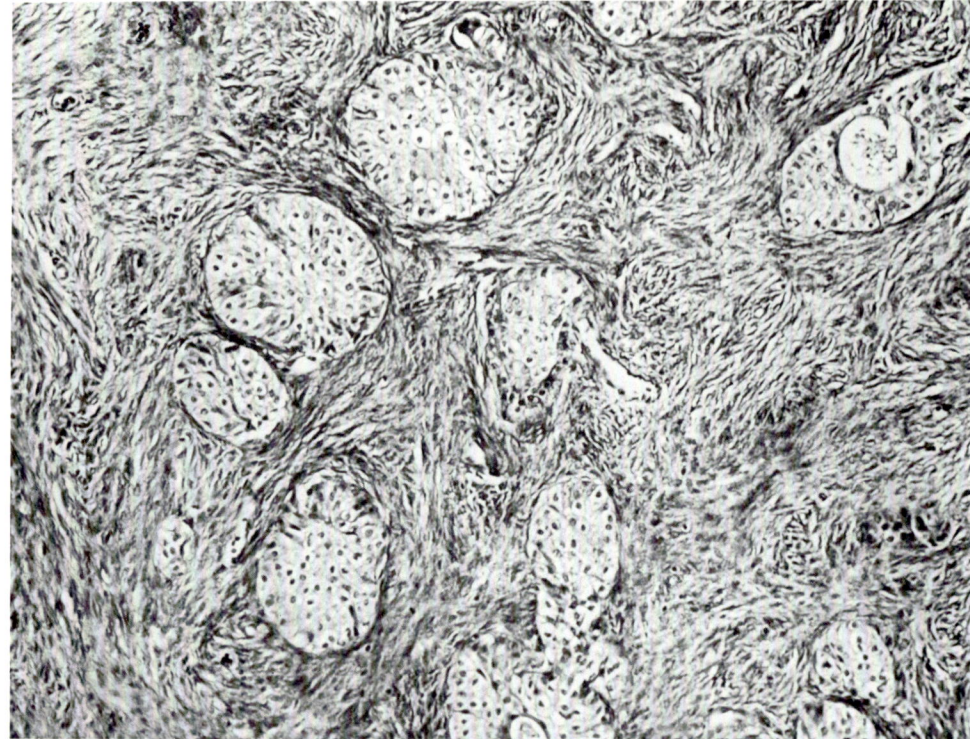

Fig. 5-12 Brenner tumor of the ovary. Anastomosing cords of transitional-like epthelium embedded in an abundant fibrous stroma. The epithelial "islands" tend to form central cavities which may be lined by mucinous epithelium. Malignant forms are rarely encountered. ×80.

maintained as in benign tumors, but the epithelial cells show proliferative activity, nuclear abnormalities, and abnormal mitoses. There is no evidence of infiltrative destructive growth in the stroma of these borderline neoplasms (Fig. 5-13a, 5-13b, 5-13c). Implantation metastases may occur on the peritoneal surface, and spontaneous regression after excision of the primary tumor has been reported.

Aure et al (1971a) reported 10 year life-table survival rates of approximately 95% for both serous and mucinous cystadenomas, Stage I, of low potential malignancy. However, symptomatic recurrences and death developed as long as 20 years posttherapy in some patients (Fig. 5-14). Hart and Norris (1973) recorded a series of borderline mucinous tumors confined to one or both ovaries at the time of diagnosis with a corrected 10 year

**TABLE 5-8   FIGO HISTOLOGIC
CLASSIFICATION OF THE
COMMON PRIMARY EPITHELIAL
TUMORS OF THE OVARY**

A. Benign cystadenomas.
B. Cystadenomas with proliferative activity of the epithelial cells and nuclear abnormalities but with no infiltrative destructive growth (low potential malignancy).
C. Cystadenocarcinomas.

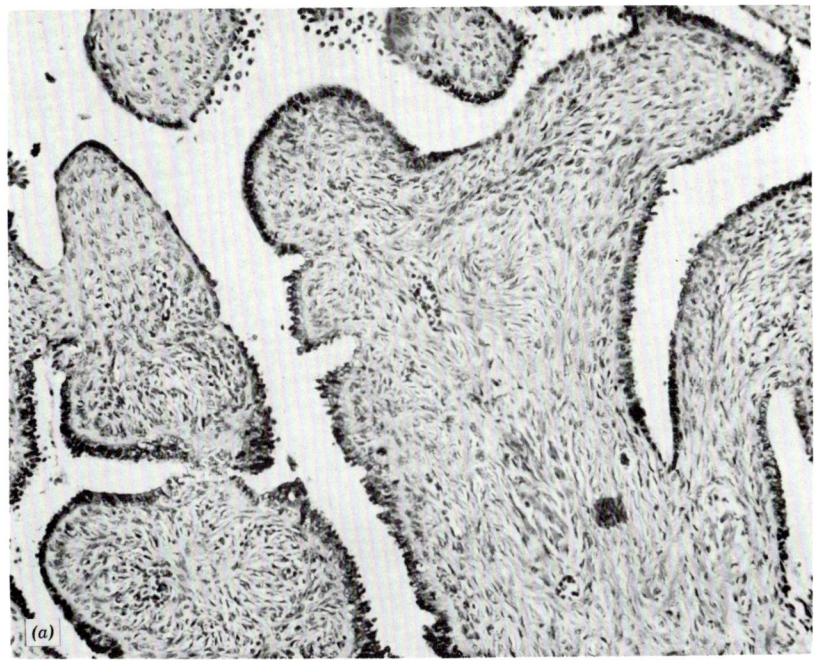

Fig. 5-13a Benign serous cystadenoma. The papillary growths are composed of a broad connective tissue core covered by a simple tubal type epithelium free of nuclear aberrations.

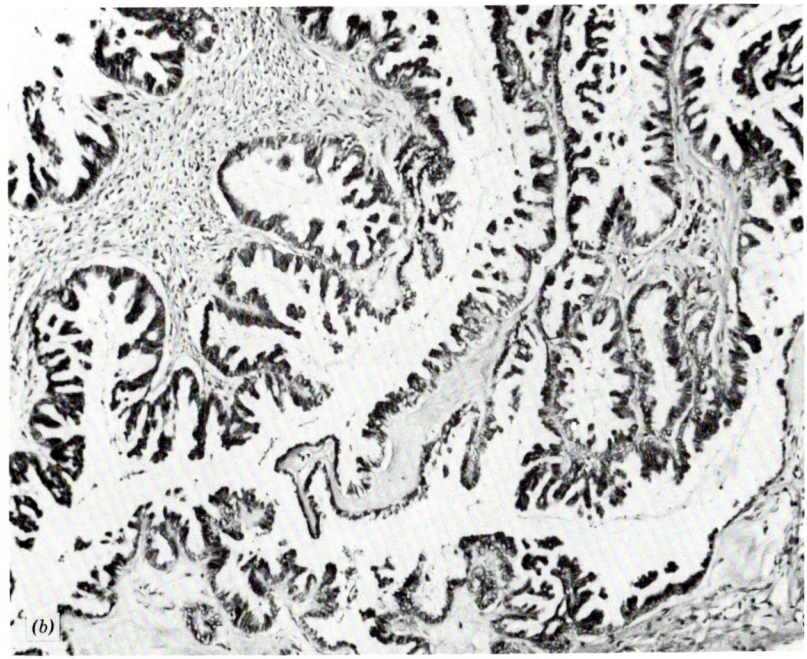

Fig. 5-13b Low potential malignancy serous tumor. The papillary growths are more extensive with secondary and tertiary branching. The epithelial proliferation results in a piling up of cells. The individual cells have the cytologic features of malignancy, but there is no evidence of infiltrative, destructive growth.

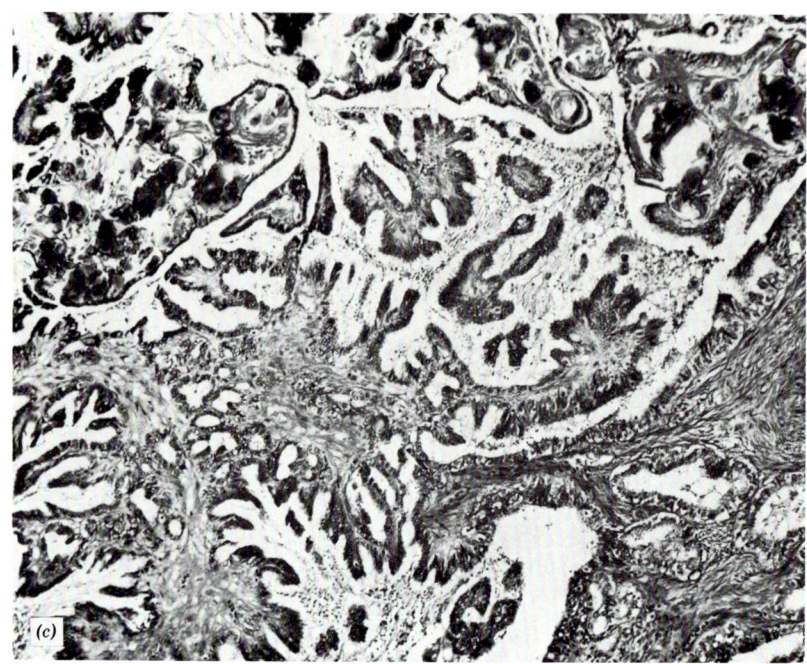

Fig. 5-13*c* Serous carcinoma. The epithelium is anaplastic and the orderly papillary branching lost. There is invasion of the stroma, unequivocal evidence of malignancy. Numerous psammoma bodies can be seen at the top of the picture.

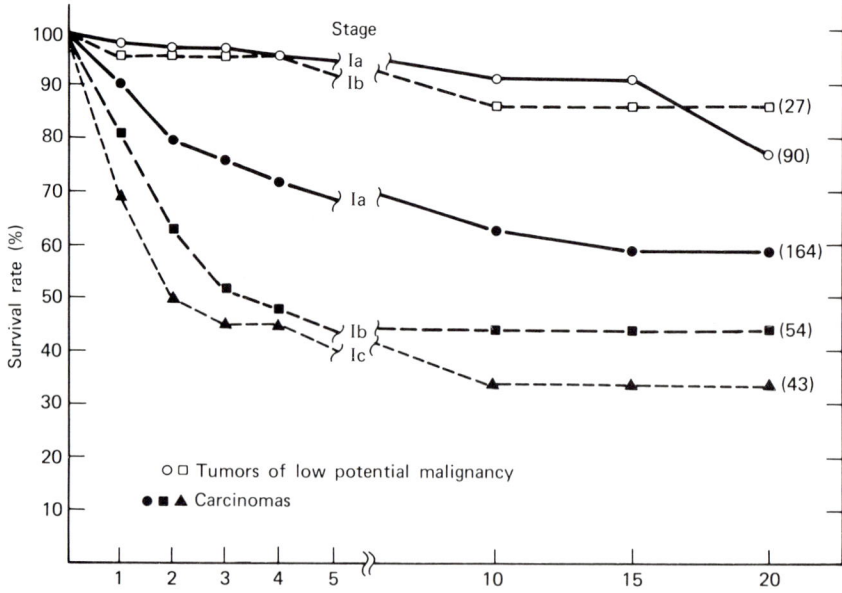

Fig. 5-14 Comparison of survival rates for FIGO Stages Ia, Ib, and Ic ovarian carcinoma (numbers of patients in parentheses). The better prognosis for tumors of low malignant potential is evident. (Reprinted with permission from J.C. Aure, K. Hoeg, and P. Kolstad, Clinical and histologic studies of ovarian carcinoma: Long-term followup of 990 cases, *Obstet. Gynecol.* 37:1, 1971.)

actuarial survival rate of 96%. Obviously the borderline tumors carry an excellent prognosis and need to be separated from the "true" carcinomas if meaningful data regarding prognosis and therapy are to be obtained.

Malignant Epithelial Neoplasms

Malignant tumors of the ovary derived from celomic epithelium account for 85% of all ovarian cancers. They demonstrate a broad variation in biologic behavior that correlates rather well with the degree of histologic differentiation. The cell type of the epithelial component can usually be identified as serous, mucinous, endometrioid, mesonephroid, or a mixture of these. Approximately 15% of cases are too poorly differentiated to characterize the cell type. The prognosis for this group is especially bleak.

Serous Carcinoma

Serous carcinoma accounts for 50% of all epithelial malignancies and is the most common ovarian cancer in the adult female (Table 5-9). The tumor is usually partly cystic and partly solid with areas of extensive papillary growths. As in the benign and borderline forms, psammoma bodies are encountered in approximately 30% of serous carcinomas. Bilateral involvement occurs in about one third of the cases (Fig. 5-15) and is more common in the advanced stages of the disease. The neoplasm tends to grow rapidly with

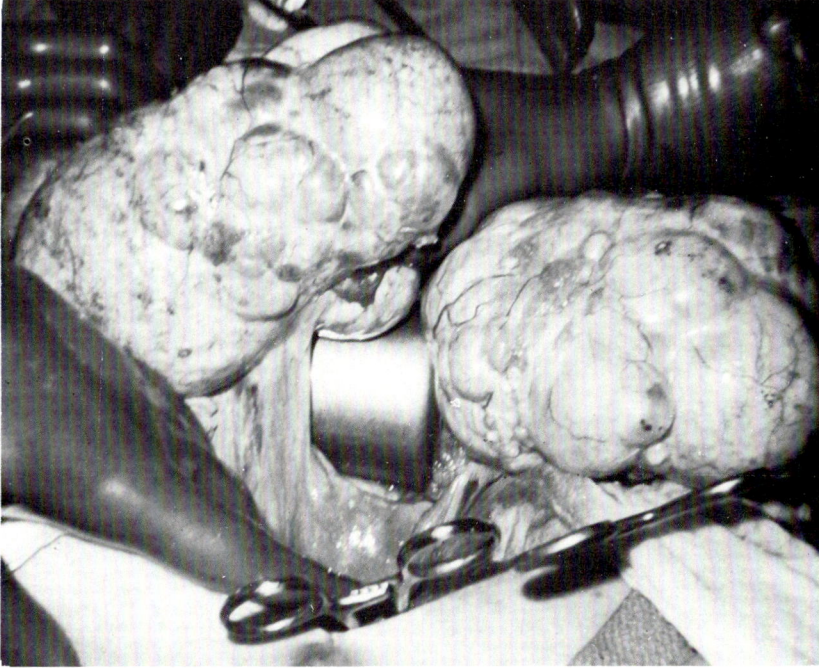

Fig. 5-15 Bilateral serous cystadenocarcinomas before removal at laparotomy. The posterior surface of the uterus is visible between the bladder blade and the clamp. Ascites and peritoneal seeding were absent. The irregular bossellations reflect the multilocular, partially solid structure and suggest that the neoplasms are malignant.

TABLE 5-9   RELATIVE
FREQUENCY OF PRIMARY
CARCINOMAS ACCORDING
TO EPITHELIAL CELL TYPE

Cell Type	Per Cent
Serous	50
Mucinous	15
Endometrioid	15
Mesonephroid	5
Undifferentiated	15

early spread throughout the peritoneal cavity. Approximately 60% of the neoplasms are incompletely resectable at the time of diagnosis. In general the prognosis is poor with an overall 5 year survival rate of about 25%.

Mucinous Carcinoma

Mucinous carcinoma comprises only 15% of ovarian epithelial malignancies. In contrast to serous carcinoma, it is more likely to be well-differentiated and confined to one ovary at the time of diagnosis (Table 5-10). Surface involvement is uncommon (Fig. 5-16). Approximately half of the patients with mucinous carcinoma survive for 5 years.

Endometrioid Carcinoma

Endometrioid ovarian carcinoma was first described by Sampson in 1925, but only in the last decade has it become widely recognized as a distinct entity. It accounts for about 15% of all ovarian carcinomas. Histologically the pattern is indistinguishable from that of adenocarcinoma of endometrial origin, and squamous differentiation is common (Fig. 5-17). Concomitant adenocarcinoma of the endometrium is reported in 15-30% of the cases. Approximately 10% of endometrioid ovarian carcinomas are accompanied by ovarian endometriosis, but it is unusual for malignant transformation of the endometriosis to be demonstrable. In the majority of cases the synchronous ovarian and endometrial carcinomas are independent primary tumors. Only 4% of all ovarian cancers are associated with adenocarcinoma of the endometrium. To be identified as such, endometrioid carcinomas must be reasonably well-differentiated, and this factor, along with the relatively slow growth rate, accounts for an overall survival rate of 50%.

TABLE 5-10 INCIDENCE OF STAGE I
CARCINOMAS IN EACH OF THE
EPITHELIAL CELL TYPES

Cell Type	Stage I Carcinomas (%)
Serous	20
Mucinous	50
Endometrioid	48
Mesonephroid	56
Undifferentiated	25

From Aure et al (1971a).

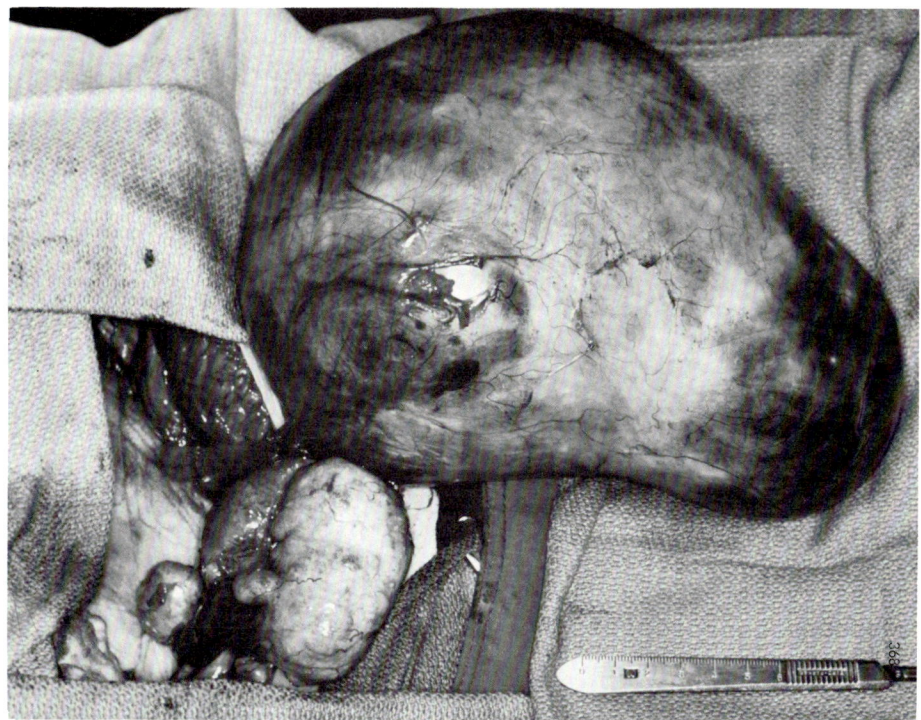

Fig. 5-16 Unilateral borderline mucinous carcinoma of the left ovary. Ascites without malignant cells was also present. The regular contour belies its multilocular composition.

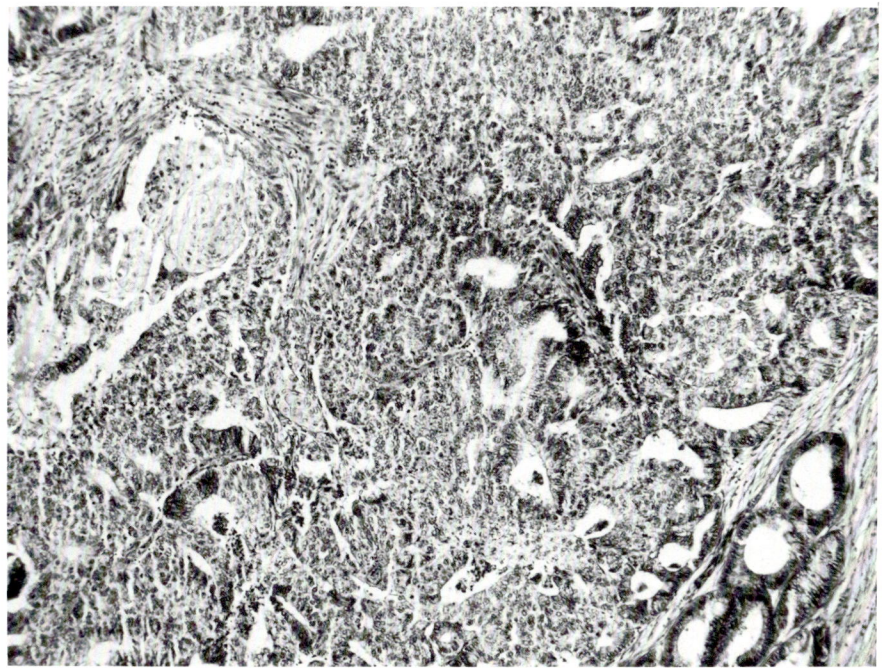

Fig. 5-17 Endometrioid ovarian carcinoma of the ovary. A focus of squamous metaplasia can be seen in the left upper quadrant of the photomicrograph. ×75.

Mesonephroid Carcinoma

Mesonephroid or clear cell carcinoma of the ovary (Fig. 5-18) accounts for 5% of all epithelial ovarian cancers. In more than 25% of cases pelvic endometriosis is observed, in contrast to an overall association with ovarian cancer of 8%. It is not uncommon to find areas of endometrioid pattern admixed with the mesonephroid carcinoma. Adenocarcinoma of the uterus is often associated with clear cell carcinoma of the ovary but does not seem to affect the prognosis adversely. The 5 year survival rate for all cases is approximately 50%.

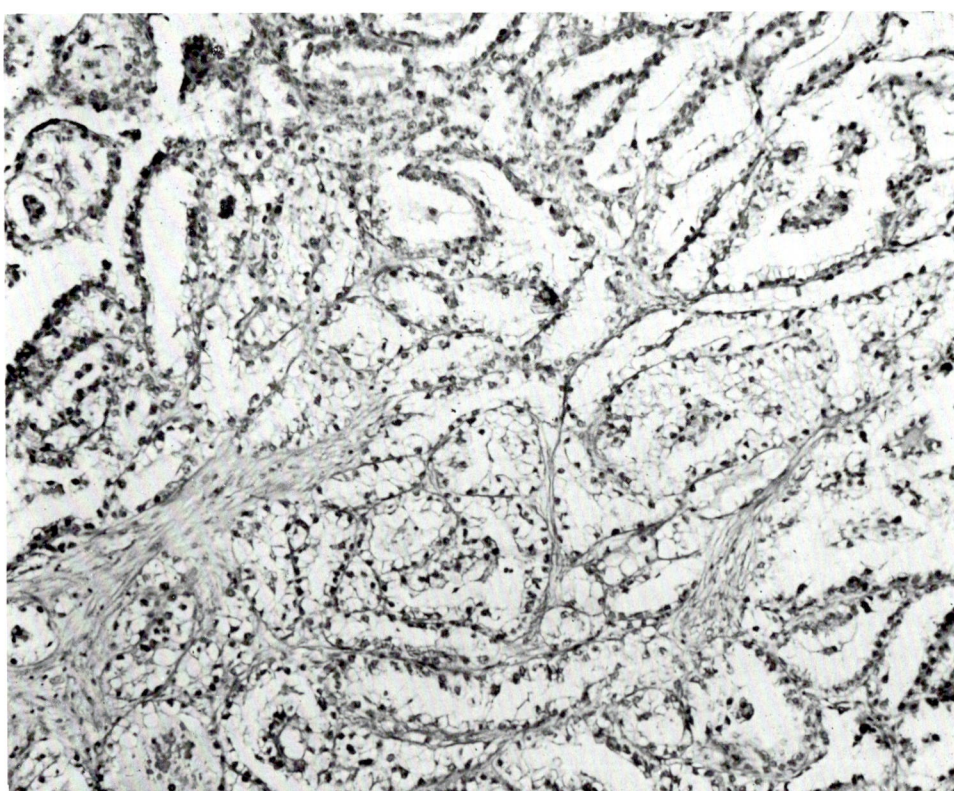

Fig. 5-18 Mesonephroid or clear cell carcinoma of the ovary. Characteristic microscopic features are the small cystic spaces lined by large cells with a clear cytoplasm. As the classification indicates, this neoplasm probably arises from the paramesonephric, celomic epithelium and not embryonic rests of mesonephric origin. ×80.

Carcinosarcoma and Mixed Mesodermal Tumors

Rarely ovarian tumors composed of carcinomatous and sarcomatous tissues occur. When the tumor contains sarcomatous elements such as rhabdomyosarcoma or chondrosarcoma representing tissues not normally present in the ovary (heterologous tissue), the designation mixed mesodermal tumor is appropriate. These are highly malignant neoplasms that occur predominantly in elderly women. There are usually pelvic and abdominal metastases at the time of diagnosis, and few patients survive more than 1 to 2 years.

Management of Malignant Epithelial Neoplasms

Factors in Management

Fundamental to the rational management of any malignant neoplasm is an understanding of its natural history. Ovarian carcinoma initially grows locally, invading the capsule and mesovarium. Adjacent organs are involved by contiguous growth and lymphatic spread. Once the malignancy has reached the external surface of the capsule, cells and tissue fragments are exfoliated into the peritoneal cavity, where they are free to circulate and implant. Local and regional lymphatic metastases may involve the uterus, fallopian tubes, and pelvic lymph nodes. Spread to the aortic nodes occurs via the lymphatic drainage of the ovarian vessels. The lymphatic route of metastases in ovarian carcinoma is less well appreciated than other pathways of spread, probably because it is relatively uncommon in the early stages of the disease and not readily detectable or greatly important in the advanced stages. In fatal cases lymphatic involvement is extensive according to the autopsy data of Bergman (1966) (Table 5-11). He found that nearly 80% of patients dying of ovarian carcinoma had metastases to the pelvic and aortic nodes and 50% had involvement of more distant nodal groups. Clinically, hematogenous dissemination is the least apparent mode of spread for ovarian carcinoma, and parenchymal liver and lung metastases are noted only infrequently. It is generally reported that ovarian carcinoma remains confined to the abdomen and pelvis, so that the majority of patients die from encasement of the abdominal viscera by tumor, which strangles the bowel and produces a state of inanition. According to Bergman's autopsy data, however, this concept of the pathophysiology of ovarian cancer is inaccurate, at least with regard to its terminal behavior. He found liver and lung metastases in one third of the cases and bone involvement in 14%.

The volume and the extent of the tumor at the time of diagnosis are the most important variables influencing prognosis in ovarian carcinoma. For purposes of comparing treatment results among different institutions, the extent of the disease is usually expressed in terms of stages. Although many staging systems have been devised, that adopted by FIGO in 1961 (Table 5-12) should be uniformly employed for reporting purposes. It should be emphasized that this is a surgical-pathologic staging and not a purely clinical staging system such as the ones used in cervical and vulvar carinoma. The basic divisions of this system are as follows: Stage I—the tumor is confined to the ovaries; Stage II—the tumor is confined to the pelvis; Stage III—the tumor is confined to the abdomen; and Stage IV—the tumor extends outside the abdominal cavity. In one of the largest and most detailed series of ovarian carcinoma reported, Aure et al (1971a) found

TABLE 5-11   LOCATION OF MESTATASES NOTED AT OPERATION AND AUTOPSY IN 86 CASES OF OVARIAN CARCINOMA

Location		Number of Cases	Per Cent
Peritoneum		75	87
Omentum		61	71
Opposite ovary		61	71
Uterus		16	19
Vagina		11	13
Lymph nodes			
Pelvic		69	80
Aortic		67	78
Mediastinal		43	50
Supraclavicular[a]	Left	23	50
	Right	21	46
Inguinal	Left	37	43
	Right	31	36
Axillary	Left	25	29
	Right	21	24
Pleura	Left	25	29
	Right	32	37
Lung		32	27
Liver		29	34
Bone		12	14
Spleen, kidney, adrenal, skin		5–7	6–8
Vulva, brain		1	1

[a]Examined in 46 cases only.

From Bergman (1966).

TABLE 5-12   FIGO STAGE-GROUPING FOR PRIMARY CARCINOMA OF THE OVARY (1974)

Stage I   Growth limited to the ovaries
  Stage Ia   Growth limited to *one* ovary; no ascites
          (i)   No tumor on the external surface; capsule intact
          (ii) Tumor present on the external surface or/and capsule ruptured
  Stage Ib   Growth limited to *both* ovaries; no ascites
          (i)   No tumor on the external surface; capsule intact
          (ii) Tumor present on the external surface or/and capsule(s) ruptured
  Stage Ic   Tumor either Stage Ia or Stage Ib, but with ascites* present or positive peritoneal washings
Stage II   Growth involving one or both ovaries with pelvic extension
  Stage IIa   Extension·and/or metastases to the uterus and/or tubes
  Stage ''', Extension to other pelvic tissues
  Stage IIc   Tumor either Stage IIa or Stage IIb, but with ascites* present or positive peritoneal washings
Stage III   Growth involving one or both ovaries with intraperitoneal metastases outside the pelvis and/or positive retroperitoneal nodes. Tumor limited to the true pelvis with histologically proven malignant extension to small bowel or omentum.
Stage IV   Growth involving one or both ovaries with distant metastases. If pleural effusion is present there must be positive cytology to allot a case to Stage IV.
          Parenchymal liver metastases equals Stage IV.
Special category. Unexplored cases which are thought to be ovarian carcinoma.

*Ascites is peritoneal effusion which in the opinion of the surgeon is pathological or/and clearly exceeds normal amounts.

TABLE 5-13
DISTRIBUTION OF 990
PATIENTS WITH
EPITHELIAL OVARIAN
CANCER BY STAGE

Stage	Per Cent	
I		43
Ia	29	
Ib	8	
Ic	6	
II		24
IIa	6	
IIb	18	
III		23
IV		10

From Aure et al (1971a).

that 43% of all cases were confined to the ovaries at the time of diagnosis (Table 5-13). If neoplasms of low potential malignancy are excluded, the proportion of Stage I cases drops to 37%. The 5 year survival gradient is apparent for the first three stages, but there was no real difference in survival rates between Stages III and IV. The prognosis for Stage Ia and Stage Ib subdivisions were significantly different, with survival rates of 70% and 45%, respectively. Survival for Stage Ic was essentially the same as for Stage Ib. Resectability had a measurable effect on survival in Stages II and III (Fig. 5-19), as did the volume of residual disease.

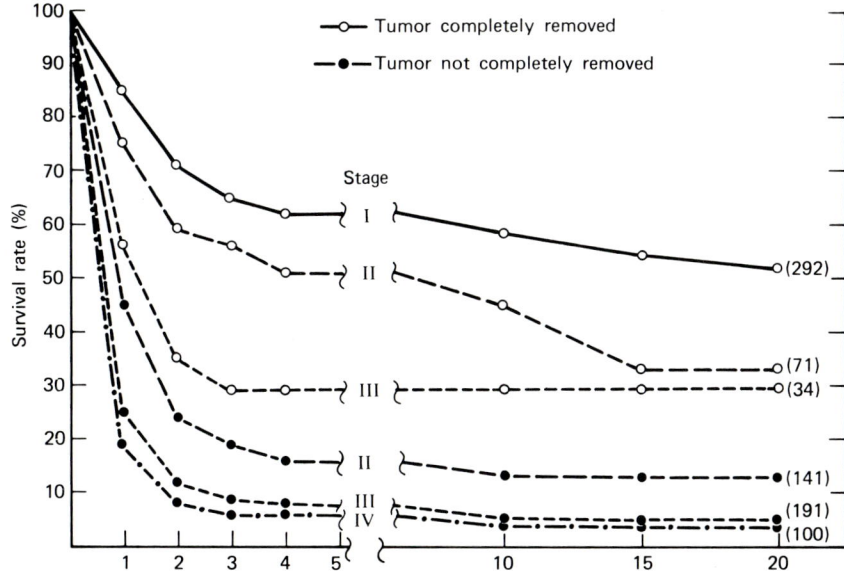

Fig. 5-19 Survival rate (life table technique) in ovarian carcinoma in relation to stage and operability (numbers of patients in parentheses). Stage III resectable carcinomas have a more favorable prognosis than Stage II incompletely resectable carcinomas. (Reprinted with permission from J.C. Aure, K. Hoeg, and P. Kolstad, Clinical and histologic studies of ovarian carcinoma: Long-term followup of 990 cases, *Obstet. Gynecol.* **37**:1, 1971.)

Accurate knowledge of the histologic type of ovarian malignancy is indispensable in assessing the prognosis and in planning treatment, but for epithelial tumors the degree of tissue differentiation and the stage are of greater prognostic importance than is the cell type. The biologic growth potential is far more limited for borderline tumors than for true carcinomas, and Grade 1 carcinomas are less aggressive than the more undifferentiated forms. The influence of grade on survival is more easily demonstrated for Stage I true carcinomas than for more advanced stages. Aure et al (1971a) reported a 95% five year survival rate for patients with Stage I borderline tumors, compared with 70% for those with true carcinomas. Munnell (1968) observed a 90% 5 year cure rate for Stage Ia borderline and Grade 1 lesions versus 50% for Grades 2 and 3 in the same stage.

Surgery

At the time of laparotomy a meticulous search must be made for evidence of extraovarian spread. This is crucial since the minimum scope of acceptable therapy must include all areas of known disease; there is no reasonable hope of cure if carcinoma resides outside the treatment field. Not only the location of the peritoneal metastases but also the size of the lesion should be noted. If there is no evidence of extension beyond the ovaries, washings are taken from the pelvis and abdomen for cytology and a piece of omentum is removed for pathologic examination. The retroperitoneal nodes should be palpated, and any suspicious lesion biopsied. The general plan of surgical therapy is to excise the uterus, tubes, and ovaries, as well as all readily resectable tumor. Removal of the uterus is an integral part of the treatment since it may be involved with tumor by direct extension, retrograde lymphatic flow, serosal implants, or transtubal spread. In addition, the endometrium may contain a separate primary cancer. The high incidence of bilateral ovarian involvement usually necessitates removal of both adnexae. Even when one ovary and tube appear normal, their preservation with few exceptions is unwarranted because of the incidence of occult tumor and the propensity for development of malignant disease in the retained ovary.

The principle of making a maximal surgical effort, espoused by Munnell (1968), to remove as much tumor as possible without risk of life-threatening complications appears to be valid. Numerous studies have indicated that the survival of patients is dependent to a greater degree on the amount of residual disease than on the initial stage. Fine judgment is necessary in determining how radical the surgery should be, but cases in which all visible disease can be removed, especially those without peritoneal implants, stand to gain the most by extended surgery. The therapeutic value of routine omentectomy in the management of epithelial ovarian carcinoma is debatable, but excision is clearly indicated when this organ is involved by tumor. If resection cannot be carried out because of advanced disease, an ovary should be biopsied or removed for histologic examination. In these cases it may be impossible to determine the origin of the intra-abdominal cancer.

Radiation Therapy

There is general agreement that epithelial carcinoma is responsive but not sensitive to ionizing radiations, although some clinical evidence indicates that mucinous tumors are resistent. The best techniques and the precise indications for radiation therapy remain controversial. Because of the propensity for ovarian cancer to disseminate intraperitoneally, the primary treatment field should encompass this entire anatomic region.

Unfortunately the kidneys and liver will not tolerate high doses of radiation, and treatment of the abdomen must be limited to marginally therapeutic doses. Furthermore, simultaneous treatment of a volume of tissue as large as the pelvis and abdomen is poorly tolerated, so that the rate at which the therapy proceeds must be reduced. To overcome the problems of the large treatment field, the abdomen and pelvis may be irradiated through separate ports or segmentally via the moving strip technique. The latter permits a more favorable time-dose relationship (Delclos and Fletcher, 1969). However, even when split fields are utilized, the liver and kidneys must be shielded. The literature most strongly supports a role for radiation therapy in the management of patients whose disease is limited to the pelvis. The collected series of Griffiths et al (1972) revealed a 5 year survival rate for Stage II cases of 19% for surgery alone, compared to 42% for surgery with postoperative irradiation.

Intraperitoneal radioactive colloidal gold (^{198}Au) has been widely used as a surgical adjunct in the management of resectable ovarian carcinoma since it was introduced by Muller in 1950. It is capable of delivering a higher dose of radiation to the peritoneal surfaces than can be achieved with external beam therapy. However, the superficial character of its radiations restricts its usefulness to cases with microscopic residual disease. A major disadvantage is the difficulty in obtaining a uniform distribution of the colloid within the peritoneal cavity. Nevertheless, the method is attractive because of its simplicity and its potential "treatment field." In a retrospective analysis, Aure et al (1971b) reported their experience with adjunctive radiation therapy in Stage I true ovarian carcinomas. They found that 89% of 51 patients treated with intraperitoneal colloidal gold and whole pelvis irradiation survived for 5 years, compared to 57% of 153 patients receiving whole pelvis irradiation alone. However, Decker et al (1973) were unable to demonstrate any advantage in using radioactive gold except in the case of intraperitoneal rupture of a malignant ovarian cyst. Recently, radioactive colloidal chromic phosphate (^{32}P) has been recommended (Hester and White, 1969) for intraperitoneal therapy. Since this isotope is a pure beta particle emitter, it poses less radiation hazard than radioactive gold, which has 10% gamma radiations. Although the therapeutic value of intraperitoneal radioactive isotopes remains open to question, the weight of evidence in the literature favors their beneficial effects.

Chemotherapy

Because ovarian carcinoma grows rapidly and disseminates early, the majority of cases are unresectable at the time of diagnosis. With the very limited success of radiation therapy, there has been an obvious need for a systemic approach to treatment. Ovarian carcinoma has proved to be one of the most drug responsive solid tumors, and cytotoxic agents have achieved an indispensable role in its management. The nitrogen mustard group of alkylating agents has demonstrated the greatest activity against the epithelial carcinomas, with melphalan, chlorambucil, cyclophosphamide, and thiotepa all effecting a 50% objective response rate according to several large series (Table 5-14). The average duration of response varies from 12 to 18 months in the different series, with the less differentiated tumors having more temporary responses. The antimetabolites methotrexate and 5-fluorouracil are active against ovarian carcinoma but apparently less so than the alkylating agents. Adriamycin, a new antineoplastic agent, has also demonstrated some activity in preliminary trials. Progestins have been recommended for the endometrioid and mesonephroid varieties of epithelial malignancies because of their

TABLE 5-14   REPORTED RESPONSE RATES OF PATIENTS WITH EPITHELIAL
OVARIAN CANCER (STAGES III AND IV) TREATED WITH CHEMOTHERAPY

Authors	Year	Drug	Schedule[a]	Number of Cases	(%) Response
Smith and Rutledge	1970	Melphalan	0.2 mg/kg/d X 5 q 4 wek PO or 1 mg/kg IV once q 3 wk	494	47
Masterson and Nelson	1965	Chlorambucil	0.2 mg /kg day PO	280	50
Wallach et al	1970	Thiotepa	10 mg/day IV X 15, then weekly	144	64
Beck and Boyes	1968	Cyclophosphamide	50-150 mg/d PO or 200 mg IV/d X 10	126	49

[a] PO = oral and IV = intravenous route of administration.

histologic similarity to the progestin-sensitive endometrial neoplasms, but their efficacy remains to be proved. Nevertheless, there are reports of these and other ovarian carcinomas responding to progestin therapy.

The therapeutic benefits of chemotherapy in advanced ovarian carcinoma are largely palliative, but survival time may also be extended. Masterson (1967) reported a double-blind study of 75 patients with advanced ovarian cancer in which the placebo group survived on the average 9.3 months verses 33.5 months for the chlorambucil group. Smith et al (1972) observed that 42% of 233 patients with Stage III and Stage IV ovarian carcinoma responding to melphalan survived for 2 years and 16% were alive at 5 years, compared to 10% and 0%, respectively, for 208 nonresponders with a similar stage-grouping.

Reported trials of combination chemotherapy in the management of ovarian cancer are sparse, and the results are inconclusive. Greenspan (1968) observed a 65% objective response rate among 86 ovarian carcinoma patients treated with methotrexate and thiotepa, but Wallach et al (1970) obtained an essentially identical response rate with thiotepa alone. In a randomized study comparing single agent to combination drug therapy, Smith et al (1972) found the response rate with actinomycin-D, 5-fluorouracil, and cyclophosphamide (Act Fu Cy) to be similar to that with melphalan alone. Because the toxicity of the combination regimen was significantly greater, the authors recommended the use of single agent therapy. The success of combination drug therapy in other tumors, however, and the solid theoretic basis for its superiority over single agent therapy assure that efforts will be continued to find more effective combinations.

The substantial recurrence rate of resectable ovarian carcinoma even with postoperative radiotherapy has logically led to the use of adjuvant drug therapy in early ovarian cancer. Patients with apparently resectable disease who have microscopic residual cancer should be more curable if adjuvant chemotherapy is begun soon after surgery than when the disease becomes clinically apparent. Many treatment centers are investigating the use of cytotoxic drugs in early ovarian carcinoma, but the results of these investigations have not been reported.

Combined Chemotherapy and Radiation Therapy

The responsiveness of ovarian epithelial carcinoma to radiation and drug therapy has led to efforts at combining these two treatments sequentially and concurrently. Griffiths et al (1972) in a retrospective analysis of nonrandomized Stage II and Stage III patients found that the radiation plus alkylating agent group had a significantly better survival time than the radiation-only group. They recommended administering the drug after the radiation is completed, however, because bone marrow depression required interruption of drug therapy when the two were administered concurrently. At the M. D. Anderson Hospital, one fourth of the patients who received melphalan drug therapy for 1 year and were then irradiated for residual disease were unable to complete their course of radiation therapy because of persistent bone marrow depression. Furthermore, there did not seem to be any improved survival in the irradiated group as compared to patients treated with melphalan alone (Smith et al, 1972). Decker et al (1967a), reporting from the Mayo Clinic, observed a better survival slope for patients with advanced ovarian cancer receiving cyclophosphamide and radiation therpay than for those treated with radiation alone. The drug was given during the course of radiation and on a maintenance basis afterwards. The authors noted, however, that the combination therapy was very strenuous for the patients. A point to be considered in the planning of sequential chemotherapy and radiation therapy is the ischemic effect of radiation induced vasculitis, which theoretically could prevent therapeutic levels of drug from reaching the tumor. Beck and Boyes (1968) noted a poorer response to cyclophosphamide in ovarian cancer recurrent after irradiation than in fresh cases.

Postoperative Treatment

Nearly every postoperative patient with ovarian carcinoma will require adjunctive irradiation or chemotherapy. If the malignancy is diagnosed after a unilateral salpingo-oophorectomy, removal of the residual ovary is generally advisable because it may contain microscopic disease or produce an independent primary tumor at a later time. Completion of the surgical therapy may be accomplished before or after the adjuvant chemotherapy or irradiation, but it should not delay the institution of adjuvant therapy. The primary determinants of additional postoperative treatment are the volume and the location of residual disease. The effectiveness of irradiation is inherently dependent on adequate oxygenation of tumor cells, regardless of the natural radiosensitivity of the tumor tissue. Since the pool of hypoxic cells increases as the mass size increases, the response to irradiation diminishes. Crowding and hypoxia undoubtedly become significant in relation to clinically feasible doses of irradiation when tumor nodules achieve a size of 1-2 cm. It is unreasonable to expect the limited dose of radiations that can be administered to the abdomen to eradicate disease of macroscopic dimensions. Although the pelvis can be treated with a higher dose of radiation than the abdomen, there are practical limitations to the size of tumor mass that can be managed radiotherapeutically. There is little value in subjecting a patient with tumor masses several centimeters in diameter to a prolonged course of pelvic irradiation.

Among the epithelial ovarian malignancies, the cell type will not usually influence the treatment plan since all have similar spread patterns and sensitivities to drugs and radiations. End results will be primarily a function of grade and stage, provided that the treatment is equivalent. Whatever therapeutic combination is selected, it should encompass the entire peritoneal cavity. The management of all but the best risk group (i.e., borderline tumors and Stage Ia, Grade 1, true carcinomas), should be aggressive since the prognosis is generally poor. The optimal time for initiating adjuvant therapy is the immediate postoperative period, and avoiding delay is critical when dealing with a rapidly growing malignancy.

The patient with Stage I ovarian carcinoma can be managed with postoperative intraperitoneal isotope therapy or systemic chemotherapy with an alkylating agent for 12-18 months. External beam abdominal and pelvic irradiation provides a better depth dose than isotope therapy, but it is more time consuming and not as well tolerated. There is no evidence that it is superior to intraperitoneal isotope therapy in the management of Stage I disease. For resectable Stage II and Stage III disease, as well as Stage I poorly differentiated tumors, a combination of radiation therapy followed by chemotherapy offers the maximum effort that can be directed against this group of poor prognosis malignancies.

When there is small residual disease confined to the pelvis, whole pelvis irradiation combined with external beam abdominal irradiation or intraperitoneal nuclide administration is indicated. After completion of the radiation therapy, long-term chemotherapy should be instituted. The management of the patient with large residual disease in the pelvis or with a macroscopic disease outside the pelvis (this will include nearly half the cases of ovarian carcinoma) should be initiated with chemotherapy. Drug therapy is continued as long as there is evidence of a beneficial effect. If no response is obtained after an adequate trial, or if an initial response is followed by disease progression, the therapy must be changed. Under these circumstances the feasibility of surgical excision and also radiation therapy should be reassessed. Occasionally the shrinkage of a tumor mass due to drug therapy will make an inoperable mass resectable or reduce its size sufficiently so that a good effect from irradiation can be anticipated. In general, however, changing to a different drug regimen is the only reasonable therapeutic alternative when the drug in use fails.

"Second-Look" Laparotomy

A small fraction of the patients treated with cytotoxic agents for advanced ovarian carcinoma will have a sustained response with all clinical evidence of disease having disappeared. Indefinite administration of alkylating agents is not always possible because of bone marrow toxicity. Even when the drug is well tolerated, continuing the therapy is undesirable if it is unnecessary. At the M. D. Anderson Hospital, 103 patients were subjected to a laparotomy after receiving melphalan for 1 year (Smith et al, 1972). Only patients having a complete or significant partial response were operated. Of the 103 cases, 23 were found to be free of disease and received no further therapy. The 2 and 5 year survival rates for this group of patients were 96% and 72%, respectively. The patients who may have benefited most from the "second-look" operation were those who had resectable residual disease that often was cliniically occult. The role of laparotomy before discontinuing chemotherapy in the management of ovarian carcinoma remains to be defined. Certainly patients with Stage I, well-differentiated carcinoma and borderline lesions should be excluded since their recurrence rate is low and the time of recurrence late.

Reproductive Conservation

The occurrence of ovarian cancer in a young woman threatens not only her life but also her reproductive faculties. When the tumor is a high grade malignancy or has achieved an advanced stage, the danger to life is so great that restricting therapy to unilateral salpingo-oophorectomy in order to preserve the childbearing potential is not a reasonable alternative. However, the risk-to-benefit ratio of conservative surgery is usually considered acceptable when the tumor is a low grade malignancy and is confined to one ovary. Among the epithelial cancers, borderline and Grade 1 lesions of all cell types are suitable for conservative surgical management provided that certain other requirements are met (Table 5-15). It is not known whether under these circumstances surgery alone is as effective as surgery plus adjuvant radiation therapy or chemotherapy, but a 5 year survival rate for Stage Ia borderline lesions of 95% and for Stage I, Grade 1, true carcinomas of 90% can be anticipated. Thus, although the degree of risk to the patient incurred by preserving the opposite ovary and withholding adjuvant radiotherapy or chemotherapy is unknown, it is judged to be small. There is an approximately 5% incidence of occult disease in the preserved ovary, but wedge biopsy at the time of initial surgery should reduce the magnitude of this threat. The probability of developing a malignancy in the preserved ovary at some later date is judged to be somewhat less than 5%. This contingency can be managed by removing the preserved ovary after the patient has completed her family.

The greatest danger of conservative therapy is the possibility that the disease has already produced microscopic metastases to the peritoneal surfaces. A detailed search for evidence of extraovarian spread at the time of surgery is important in every case of ovarian cancer, but when conservative surgical therapy is being considered it is absolutely imperative. Peritoneal washings and an omental biopsy will also help to reduce the possibility of selecting conservative therapy in the presence of extraovarian disease. If any of these investigations yields evidence that the cancer is not confined to one ovary, conservative management is no longer indicated. If there has been preoperative or intraoperative rupture of a malignant cyst, if surface excrescences are present, or if the malignancy is adherent to adjacent structures, conservative surgery does not seem to be justified even though all other criteria are satisfied. The prognosis under these conditions has already been compromised (Webb et al, 1973). Ascites associated with a malignant ovarian tumor always interdicts conservative therapy. Periodic cul-de-sac cytology may prove to be useful in the follow-up of patients managed conservatively. The safety of adjuvant chemotherapy, which presumably could eradicate occult residual disease while preserving fertility, has not been determined.

TABLE 5-15 REQUIREMENTS
FOR CONSERVATIVE
MANAGEMENT OF PATIENTS
WITH OVARIAN CANCER

1. Stage Ia carcinoma (no ascites)
2. Favorable histologic type
   a. Borderline or well-differentiated epithelial ovarian carcinoma
   b. Pure dysgerminoma; granulosa tumor; arrhenoblastoma
3. Young woman of low parity
4. Cancer encapsulated and unruptured
5. No surface excrescences or adhesions
6. No invasion of capsule, or mesovarium
7. Negative peritoneal washings
8. Negative ovarian wedge biopsy and omental biopsy
9. Close follow-up possible

Serous Effusions

Clinically apparent ascites is associated with ovarian carcinoma in about one third of cases and constitutes one of the most common side problems in the management of this disease. The more voluminous effusions are often obvious, but a large ovarian cyst, distended loops of bowel, and simple obesity can mimic the clinical picture of ascites. Ascites itself may be a manifestation of disease other than intra-abdominal malignancy, including cirrhosis of the liver, pancreatitis, tuberculous peritonitis, and Meigs's syndrome. When the cause of abdominal distension is unclear, radiographic and ultrasound studies may be helpful. The patient who presents with ascites should not be routinely subjected to abdominal paracentesis or cul-de-sac needle aspiration. If the patient has a large malignant cyst rather than ascites, rupture and seeding of the peritoneal cavity may occur. In addition, malignant cells may seed the paracentesis tract. The value of paracentesis in the presence of a pelvic or abdominal tumor is limited. Cytologic examination of the fluid may be negative in the presence of malignancy, but even a positive finding seldom provides a clue to the origin of the tumor. Withdrawal of the abdominal fluid should be carried out to relieve respiratory embarrassment or pain, and improved gastrointestinal function and relief of nausea, vomiting, and constipation may occur after paracentesis. The concept of removing ascites preoperatively to avert the complications of sudden decompression of the abdomen at surgery is fallacious and may even be harmful if the fluid reforms rapidly. There is no better way to do the initial paracentesis in a patient with ovarian cancer than at laparotomy. If the individual proves to have a large malignant cyst rather than ascites, it can be removed intact.

It has been a longstanding practice to instill an antineoplastic agent into the peritoneal cavity at the time of laparotomy if unresectable cancer is found. This is not, however, the optimal means of administering drugs to control ascites or treat cancer. These agents can be given more effectively and in a more controlled manner postoperatively. Other chemicals, such as atabrine and nitrogen mustard, produce an adhesive serositis that may partly obliterate the peritoneal cavity, making further surgical intervention difficult if not impossible. The reaccumulation of ascites after surgery is invariably associated with unresectable carcinoma, and in the great majority of these cases systemic chemotherapy will be the indicated treatment. Control of ascites is one of the most sensitive indicators of tumor response and can be expected in approximately 60% of cases. Chemotherapy can be initiated intraoperatively or at any time during the postoperative period if rapid ascites formation is a problem. Such an excessive production of intraperitoneal fluid may result in fluid and electrolyte imbalance with hypovolemia, oliguria, and protein depletion. However, in the majority of cases in which ascites cannot be adequately controlled by systemic chemotherapy, the rate of reaccumulation is sufficiently slow that the patients can be kept comfortable by periodic paracentesis. External irradiation is not recommended in the management of ascites, but intraperitoneal radioactive chromium phosphate or gold is frequently effective. Either can be used in concert with chemotherapy since these isotopes produce no bone marrow toxicity. Pleural effusions are especially suitable for this mode of therapy. A pleural effusion may represent the spread of ovarian cancer to the lung and pleural surfaces or simply a movement of ascitic fluid through the diaphragmatic lymphatics into the pleural cavity. Patients with symptomatic pleural effusions need immediate thoracentesis to relieve respiratory embarrassment and prevent life threatening cardiopulmonary complications. Recurrence on drug therapy is an indication for intrapleural radioactive gold or phosphorus.

5-4   NEOPLASMS DERIVED FROM GERM CELLS

Germ cell tumors constitute 15-20% of all primary ovarian neoplasms and are second only to epithelial tumors in frequency of occurrence. No other group of neoplasms encompasses such a wide range of biologic, pathologic, and clinical diversity. Their occurrence predominately in young women is another feature that serves to intensify the interest in this group of ovarian neoplasms. In order of decreasing frequency the ovarian germ cell tumors are subgrouped into teratoma, dysgerminoma, embryonal carcinoma, and choriocarcinoma. Mixtures of these types are not uncommon. Gonadoblastoma is included among the germ cell tumors because of its close structural relationship and its propensity to give rise to germ cell tumors.

Teratomas

Teratomas are presumably of germ cell derivation and are composed usually of elements from all three germ layers: ectoderm, mesoderm, and endoderm. Teratomas of the ovary are consistently chromatin positive, whereas testicular teratomas are chromatin negative, positive, or mixed. Teratomas are cystic or solid, and they are composed of immature (embryonal) or mature (adult) tissues. The malignant potential of these neoplasms is related to the presence of immature or partially differentiated tissues rather than to their morphologic cystic or solid composition.

Mature, "Solid" Teratoma

This rare variety of teratoma is composed entirely of mature or adult tissues. It is essential that adequate histologic study of the tumor be carried out to assure that no immature (embryonal or partially differentiated) tissues, including other germ cell elements such as embryonal carcinoma and choriocarcinoma, are present before rendering this diagnosis. Such a tumor composed entirely of adult tissues is benign.

Dermoid Cyst

The dermoid cyst or benign cystic teratoma is one of the most common ovarian neoplasms; it accounts for over 95% of all ovarian teratomas. It is composed entirely of mature (adult) tissues, usually representing all three germ layers. The typical dermoid cyst contains a prominent, unilocular cavity lined by skin and filled with hair and a sebaceous, oily liquid (Fig. 5-9). Teeth, occasionally embedded in a rudimentary jawbone, are present in nearly 50% of dermoid cysts. Rarely parts of extremities such as fingers and caricatures of fetuses called homunculi ("little men") are formed.

About 25% of benign cystic teratomas are discovered in postmenopausal women, and half occur between the ages of 30 and 50. It is the most common ovarian neoplasm of childhood. In one study 15% of married, postmenopausal women with the diagnosis of dermoid cysts were nulliparous. The cyst wall typically has one or more nodular thickenings known as dermoid processes or Rokitansky's protuberances. It is within this area that the greatest variety of tissue types is found.

The majority of dermoid cysts are asymptomatic, being discovered on routine pelvic examination, at the time of surgery for other diseases, or on x-ray films. Torsion and rupture are more frequent during pregnancy, the latter being almost exclusively associated with pregnancy. Rarely dermoids become infected. Rupture into a hollow viscus has been reported. Several instances of autoimmune hemolytic anemia associated with benign cystic teratoma are recorded in the literature. Clinically and hematologically this syndrome is indistinguishable from other causes of autoimmune hemolytic anemia, but it does not respond to steroids or splenectomy. The anemia is apparently cured by removal of the tumor.

Benign cystic teratomas frequently contain thyroid tissue on microscopic examination (Fig. 5-20), but occasionally the thyroid tissue predominates and these lesions are then referred to as struma ovarii. The thyroid tissue in ovarian struma is capable of functioning and concentrating radioactive iodine. A number of these patients have shown clinical and biochemical evidence of hyperthyroidism, but some also have had a coexistent cervical goiter. The degree of thyrotoxicosis correlates roughly with the amount of functioning thyroid tissue in the ovary.

Malignancies Arising in Dermoid Cysts

Secondary malignant change may develop in any of the mature tissues occurring in

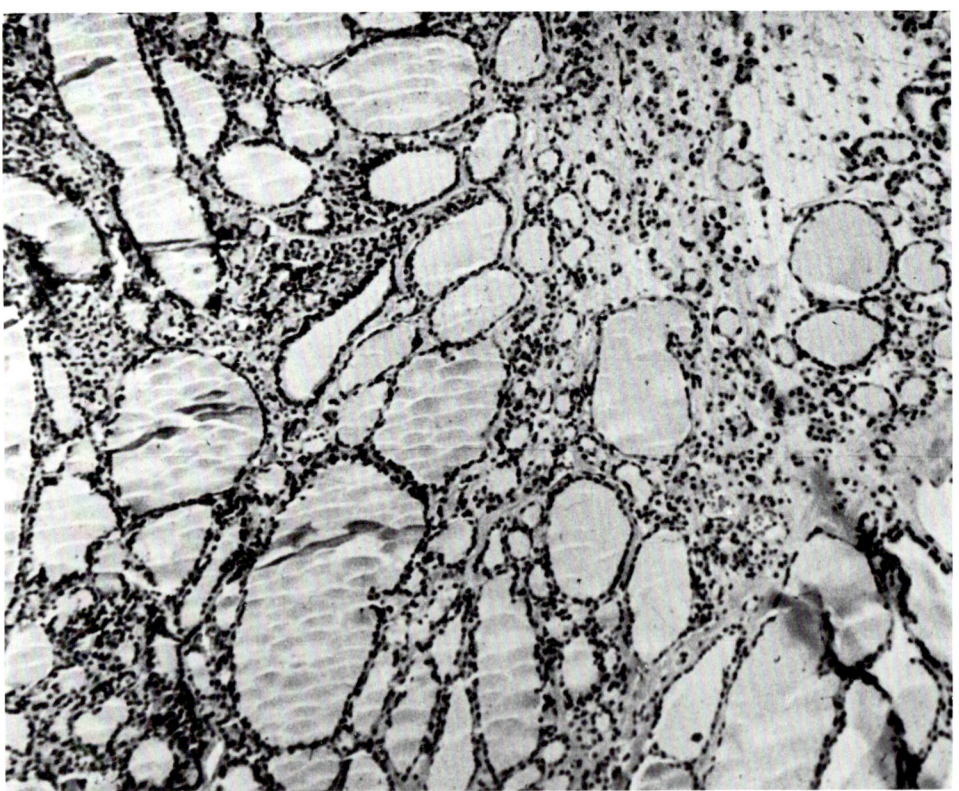

Fig. 5-20 Thyroid tissue from a benign cystic teratoma (dermoid cyst). When thyroid is the predominant tissue, the dermoid is properly called a struma ovarii. ×80.

dermoid cysts. The incidence of malignant change is reported in large series to be approximately 1%, and, as might be expected from the preponderance of skin in dermoids, the great majority of these malignancies are squamous carcinomas. Both *in situ* and invasive forms have been observed. Malignancy may develop in association with struma ovarii, and a high percentage of these patients demonstrate pleural effusion and ascites. Although the thyroid carcinomas are generally of low grade malignancy, hematogenous spread to lungs, bone, and liver, as well as peritoneal seeding, does occur. A variety of other cancers have been reported in dermoids, including adenocarcinoma, sarcoma, and melanoma.

The risk of malignancy occurring in a dermoid cyst increases with age, and most cases are found in postmenopausal women. It is important that every dermoid be thoroughly examined histologically, especially in the region of Rokitansky's knuckle, to detect any area of malignant change. Malignancy may be suspected at surgery if adhesions, thickened areas or solid nodules in the cyst wall, necrosis, or rupture is found.

Carcinoid Tumors

Over 30 cases of primary carcinoid tumor of the ovary have been recorded in the literature. Secondary lesions from gastrointestinal carcinoids are less frequently encountered. Ovarian carcinoids probably arise from argentiffin cells associated with gastrointestinal or bronchial mucosa occurring in teratomas. Approximately one third to one half of primary ovarian carcinoids are associated with the carcinoid syndrome. In contrast to intestinal carcinoids, metastases are not required for the occurrence of this syndrome with an ovarian primary. The syndrome results from the secretion of serotonin (5-hydroxytryptamine), bradykinin, and possibly other hormones, which produce cutaneous flushing, diarrhea, facial cyanosis, evidence of rightsided heart failure, and bronchospasm, either in combination or alone. Apparently the syndrome is not found in nonmetastatic intestinal carcinoids because the hormones are inactivated in the liver before entering the systemic circulation. The great majority of ovarian carcinoids reported were confined to one ovary at the time of diagnosis. The prognosis is excellent in these cases.

Immature Teratomas

About 1% of teratomas are composed entirely of partially or incompletely differentiated tissues resembling embryonic rather than adult structures. Commonly these are neuroectodermal derivatives. These tumors are usually solid (Fig. 5-21) with cystic areas, but the diagnosis of malignancy is essentially dependent on the histologic identification of immature tissue. The malignant potential and consequently the prognosis appear to correlate with the amount and degree of tissue immaturity (Fig. 5-22). Although numerous long-term survivals of individuals with immature or partially differentiated teratomas have been documented, at least one third of all cases reported in the literature have died of tumor. Mature glial implants seem to augur a good outcome (Robboy and Scully, 1970), but this finding does not guarantee a benign course (Albites, 1974). Serum gonadotropin and alpha-fetoprotein titers complement the histologic search for choriocarcinoma and embryonal carcinoma. The presence of these tissues worsens the prognosis.

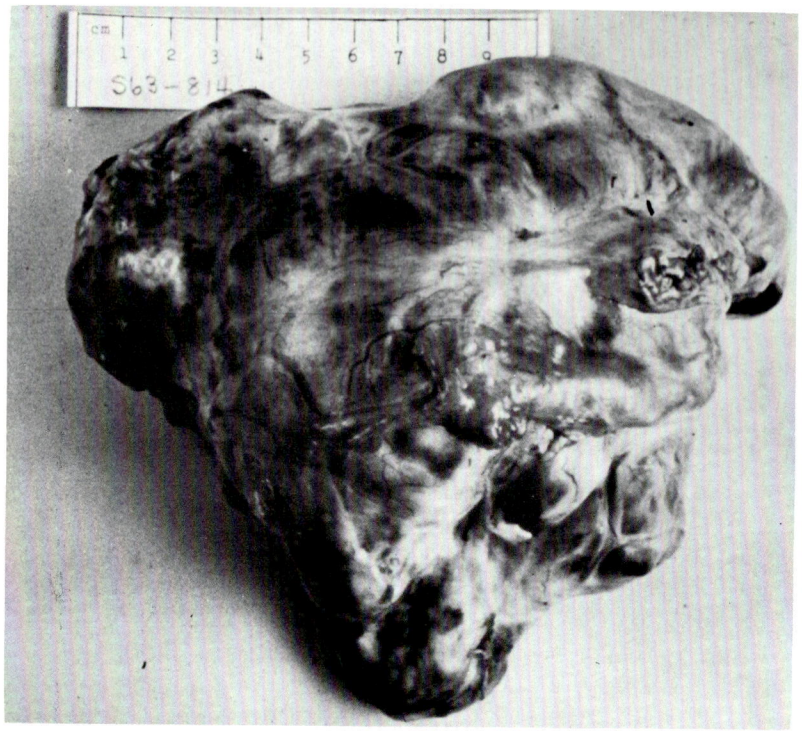

Fig. 5-21 Immature (malignant) teratoma of the ovary. Although a "solid" tumor, multiple cystic spaces which account in part for its irregular configuration are common.

Dysgerminoma

Dysgerminoma is a malignant germ cell tumor accounting for 1—2% of all ovarian neoplasms. It occurs predominately in children and young women with 80% found in females between the ages of 10 and 30 years. It rarely occurs after the menopause. Dysgerminoma is the most frequently occurring malignant neoplasm associated with intersex states and often develops in a gonadoblastoma. In the majority of cases the tumor is grossly confined to one ovary at the time of diagnosis. About 10% will involve both ovaries, and evidence of extraovarian extension will be present in one fourth of the cases at initial laparotomy. Approximately 15% of dysgerminomas are mixed (Figs. 5-23a and 5-23b) with other more malignant germ cell elements: endodermal sinus tumor, choriocarcinoma, or immature teratoma. The presence of these elements is suggested on gross examination of the tumor by areas of hemorrhage, cystic spaces, necrosis, and other regions with a consistency different from that of the main body of the tumor. Dysgerminoma has a strong proclivity for lymphatic spread but is also capable of intraperitoneal dissemination in the manner of other ovarian cancers. The pelvic and aortic nodes seem to be the most frequent targets for metastasis. Prognosis in cases of pure dysgerminoma confined to one ovary at the time of diagnosis is excellent, with 5 year survival rates in the range of 90—95%.

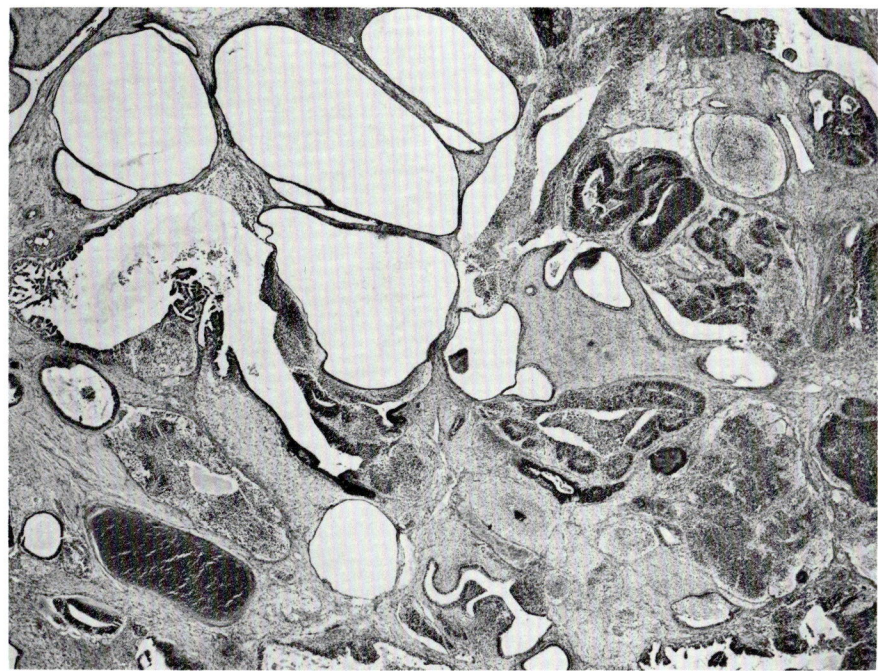

Fig. 5-22 Immature (malignant) teratoma. The immature or partially differentiated character of the abundant neural tissue (right half of photomicrograph) identifies the malignant potential of this tumor. Choroid plexus and cartilage can also be seen. This tumor recurred in the abdomen with essentially the same histologic pattern. No embryonal carcinoma or choriocarcinoma was present. ×20.

Embryonal Carcinoma

Embryonal carcinoma is one of the most malignant neoplasms arising in the ovary. It was originally described by Schiller, who mistakenly combined it with clear cell (mesonephroid) carcinoma and designated the two as "mesonephroma ovarii." We are indebted to Telium for recognizing embryonal carcinoma as a distinct entity. He noted the histologic similarity of this tumor and the endodermal sinus of Duval in the rodent placenta. For this reason he preferred the term *endodermal sinus tumor*, and this designation, as well as the name *yoke sac tumor*, is becoming increasingly more popular in the literature. Like other germ cell tumors, embryonal carcinoma occurs almost exclusively in children and young women with an average age of approximately 20 years. Most cases are confined to one ovary at the time of diagnosis. Often embryonal carcinoma is a portion of a mixed germ cell tumor containing dysgerminoma and/or choriocarcinoma. Frequently hemorrhagic ascitic fluid is present at the time of surgery, reflecting the friable nature of the tumor and its tendency toward necrosis. Alpha-fetoprotein is detectable in the serum in some patients with embryonal carcinoma. Elevated levels of chorionic gonadotropin occur if areas of trophoblastic differentiation are present in the tumor.

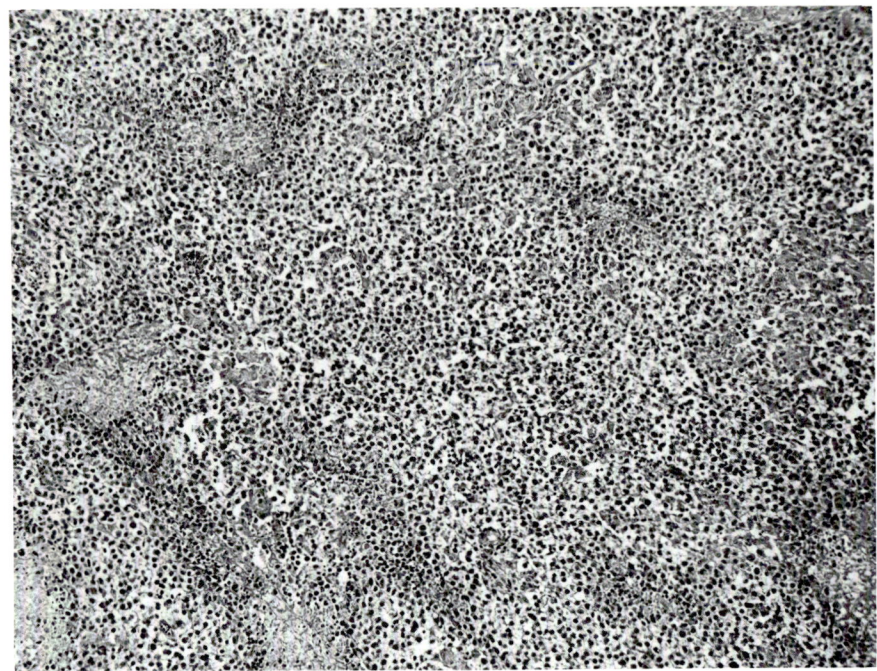

Fig. 5-23*a*   The dysgerminoma microscopically is composed of large, polygonal germ cells. The fibrous trabeculae are not prominent in this section but are marked by the characteristic infiltration with lymphocytes. ×75.

Choriocarcinoma

Teratomatous choriocarcinoma arising in the ovary is extremely rare and usually occurs as part of a mixed germ cell tumor. Gestational choriocarcinoma seldom involves the ovary, so that this is usually not a problem in the differential diagnosis. Like the gestational variety, teratomatous choriocarcinoma produces measurable levels of chorionic gonadotropin, which may serve as an aid to diagnosis, treatment, and follow-up. The excellent therapeutic achievements with antineoplastic drugs in gestational choriocarcinoma have not been realized in choriocarcinoma of germ cell origin. It is postulated that gestational choriocarcinoma, which develops from fetal tissue, is more curable because it incites a more intense immunologic host response than nongestational choriocarcinoma. Nevertheless, several cases of prolonged remission induced with chemotherapeutic agents have been reported for the teratomatous variety.

Gonadoblastoma

The gonadoblastoma is an unusual tumor of the ovary, described first by Scully in 1953. It is characterized by germ cells intimately mixed with indifferent sex cord elements resembling immature granulosa and Sertoli cells. In about two thirds of the cases, Leydig-like cells are present in the stroma. Gonadoblastomas are usually small tumors,

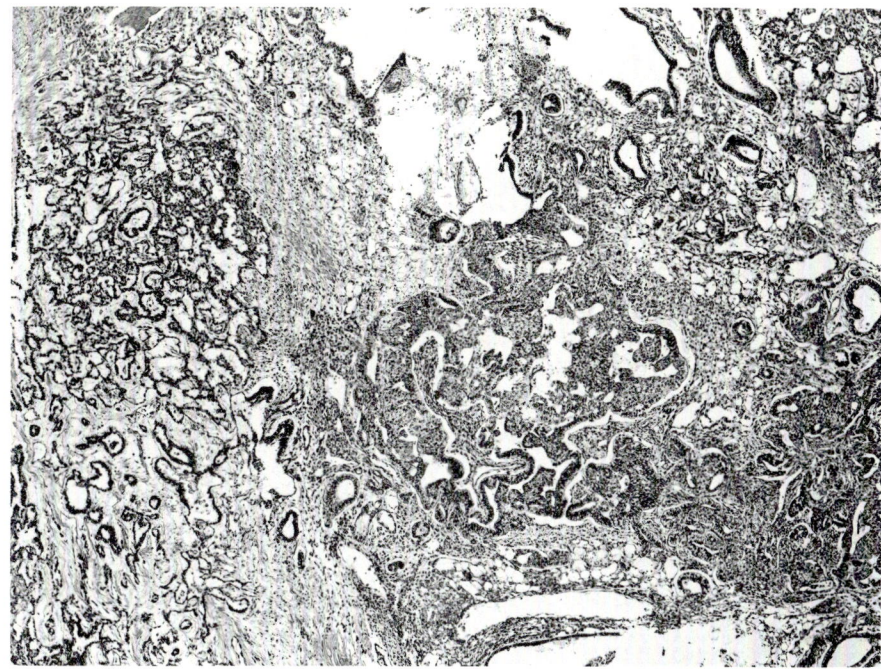

Fig. 5-23*b* Embryonal carcinoma. Section from a different area of the same tumor as in Fig. 5-23*a*. Typical microcystic pattern appears at the left of the photomicrograph. This finding drastically alters the generally good prognosis of pure dysgerminoma. X 35.

with the largest reported achieving a diameter of only 8 cm. Bilateral involvement occurs in about one third of the cases. Gonadoblastoma occurs almost exclusively in genetically abnormal individuals, who can usually be classified as examples of pure gonadal dysgenesis, mixed gonadal dysgenesis, or male pseudohermaphroditism. Nearly 90% of the cases are sex chromatin negative. The most common karyotypes are 46XY and 45X/46XY. About one fourth of the cases are phenotypic males. Ambiguous genitalia are common, and patients that are phenotypic females frequently show some evidence of masculinization. Calcifications often develop in gonadoblastomas and may be demonstrable on pelvic radiographs.

The importance of gonadoblastoma, in addition to its almost universal association with intersexual states, lies in its propensity for producing malignant germ cell tumors. Approximately half of the gonadoblastomas reported in the literature were associated with dysgerminoma. Occasional cases of choriocarcinoma, embryonal carcinoma, and mixed germ cell tumors have also been reported. Although a gonadoblastoma itself is benign, the frequency with which malignant germ cell neoplasms arise from this tumor justifies its being considered as a premalignant lesion. Germ cell tumors have arisen from gonadoblastoma as early as the first decade of life. This strong tendency to produce malignant tumors is sufficient reason for removal of gonadoblastomas as soon as they are discovered. Bilateral excision of the gonads should be done except in the rare patient who has a normal ovary on the contralateral side. Any patient with a diagnosis of a germ cell tumor should be scrutinized for evidence of gonadal dysgenesis because of the common association of these two conditions. Where doubt exists, a buccal smear or karyotype should be obtained.

Management of Germ Cell Tumors

The great majority of germ cell tumors are benign cystic teratomas. As with other cystic ovarian tumors, it is desirable to remove dermoids intact since benignity is established only by adequate microscopic examination. In addition, the sebaceous contents of dermoid cysts are irritating to the peritoneum and are capable of producing a chronic granulomatous inflammatory response. Whether cystectomy or salpingo-oophorectomy is performed will depend on the condition of the opposite adnexa and the surgeon's judgment regarding the salvageability of the involved ovary. Shelling out a dermoid does not always result in complete removal, and recurrences in the preserved ovary have been reported. Synchronous overt bilaterality occurs in 10% of the cases. In this circumstance bilateral cystectomy is indicated when preservation of ovarian function is an important consideration. Bivalving the apparently normal contralateral ovary in search of an occult dermoid frequently has been recommended, but neither the discovery rate of covert bilaterality nor the risk to the incised ovary has been assessed. Certainly, if the ovary is enlarged or nodular to palpation, it needs to be opened. Small cysts can be aspirated to identify the sebaceous contents of a dermoid as an alternative to bivalving the ovary. Randall (1962) found that 6% of patients undergoing a unilateral salpingo-oophorectomy for benign cystic teratomas required surgery for subsequent benign neoplasms, most of which were dermoids, in the preserved ovary.

Squamous carcinoma is the most common secondary malignancy encountered in dermoids, and the prognosis is largely contingent on the extent of disease at the time of diagnosis. If the cyst wall is intact and free of adhesions, and if there is no evidence of extraovarian spread, surgical excision of the involved adnexa seems to be adequate therapy. In the presence of rupture, ascites, or other evidence of spread, however, pelvic and abdominal irradiation should be administered postoperatively. The prognosis in such cases is poor.

Primary ovarian carcinoid has been reported to metastasize rarely. If a detailed search for evidence of extraovarian metastasis is negative, surgical excision is sufficient treatment for this malignancy. Periodic determinations of urinary 5-hydroxyindole acetic acid (5-HIAA), a metabolite of serotonin, are of limited value in the posttreatment surveillance program but may detect clinically occult disease. If the carcinoid is unresectable or recurrent, chemotherapy is indicated. Both 5-fluorouracil and actinomycin D have demonstrated activity against this malignancy.

Immature or partially differentiated teratomas are indications for adjunctive postoperative therapy unless only a microscopic focus of immature tissue is present. These tumors are generally regarded as radiation resistant, and the preferred mode of adjuvant treatment is with oncolytic drugs. Chemotherapy should be initiated in the postoperative period as soon as the patient has recovered from surgery. As a rule these malignancies grow rapidly, and unnecessary delay merely permits expansion of the residual tumor volume. Although three different drug regimens have been reported to be effective in the management of immature teratomas (Table 5-16), these tumors are so rare that response rates and cure rates have not been determined. Drug therapy is continued for 1–2 years. Consideration should be given to a second-look operation before discontinuing chemotherapy, particularly if there was disease spread at the time of diagnosis. The residual ovary should be excised.

Dysgerminoma can frequently be managed conservatively when it is confined to one ovary at the time of diagnosis. This is true despite the fact that 20% of the cases so

TABLE 5-16   COMBINATION CHEMOTHERAPY IN OVARIAN CANCER

Drug	Dosage	Schedule
Act Fu Cy		
Actinomycin D	0.01 mg/kg, not to exceed 0.5 mg/day	IV daily × 5 days and repeated every 4 weeks
5-Fluorouracil	5 mg/kg	IV daily × 5 days and repeated every 4 weeks
Cyclophosphamide	5 mg/kg	IV daily × 5 days and repeated every 4 weeks
VAC		
Vincristine	1.5 mg/M² body surface area, not to exceed 2 mg/week	IV weekly × 4-6 weeks; then every other week
Actinomycin D	0.01 mg/kg/day × 5	IV every 4-6 weeks
Cyclophosphamide	8 mg/kg/d × 5	IV every 4-6 weeks
MAC		
Methotrexate	0.3 mg/kg IV or IM, not to exceed 15 mg/day	Daily × 5 days every 2-3 weeks
Actinomycin D	0.01 mg/kg IV, not to exceed 0.5 mg/day	Daily × 5 days every 2-3 weeks
Chlorambucil [a]	0.2 mg/kg PO, not to exceed 12 mg/day	Daily × 5 days every 2-3 weeks

[a]Cyclophosphamide, 3-5 mg/kg IV (maximum 250 mg), may be given daily instead of chlorambucil.

Modified from Smith et al (1973) and Woodruff et al (1968).

managed will experience recurrence within 1—3 years, because the extraordinary radiosensitivity of this tumor permits therapeutic control of most recurrences. The requirements for conservative therapy (i.e., unilateral salpingo-oophorectomy), are listed in Table 5-15. Examination and selected sampling of the ipsilateral pelvic and aortic nodes will provide additional assurance that the disease is confined to the ovary. The tumor must be examined scrupulously by the pathologist for the presence of embryonal carcinoma or choriocarcinoma. The presence of these elements precludes therapeutic conservatism. Gonadotropin titers may be helpful in detecting occult malignant trophoblastic tissue. If the dysgerminoma is not confined to one ovary, the treatment of choice is bilateral salpingo-oophorectomy, excision of the uterus, and postoperative external irradiation to the pelvis and abdomen. If there is evidence of aortic nodal metastasis, the radiation field should be extended to include the mediastinal and supraclavicular nodes. As mentioned above, dysgerminoma, like testicular seminoma, is very radiosensitive, and the abdomen is able to tolerate doses in the therapeutic range. Recurrence after conservative surgery is also managed with radiation therapy, but first reexploration should be done to define the extent of disease, excise bulky tumor masses, and obtain adequate tissue for histologic examination. Apparently pure dysgerminoma may recur as the highly malignant embryonal carcinoma or choriocarcinoma, which is properly treated with chemotherapy, not radiation. The role of chemotherapy in the management of dysgerminoma has usually been limited to irradiation failures. However, Hittle believes that radiation therapy is so poorly tolerated in children that adjunctive therapy with drugs is preferable. He recommends a drug regimen of vincristine, actinomycin D, and cyclophosphomide (VAC).

Embryonal carcinoma of the ovary is an extremely malignant tumor with only occasional cures resulting from surgery alone or surgery with adjunctive irradiation. The reports of Neubecker and Breen (1962a), Santesson and Marrubini (1957), Woodruff et al (1968), and Abell et al (1965) deal with a total of 87 pure or mixed embryonal carcinomas. Only 6 of these patients survived for more than 2 years despite the fact that the tumor was often limited to one ovary at the time of diagnosis. Most patients were dead within 1 year of diagnosis. Adjunctive irradiation did not appear to alter the relentless progression of this malignancy. Of the 6 cases achieving a 2 year survival, 4 had only small foci of embryonal carcinoma occurring in dysgerminoma, a combination that seems to ameliorate an otherwise dismal prognosis. Intensive combination drug therapy, however, promises to enhance significantly the survival time for this disease. Smith et al (1973) at the M.D. Anderson Hospital treated 6 cases of embryonal carcinoma with Act Fu Cy or VAC. One patient (Stage Ia) was well 4½ years after operation and 2 years of chemotherapy, and 3 patients (Stages II, III, and III) were living at 21 or 22 months, at which time they were still receiving chemotherapy. Forney et al (1974) at the University of Southern California treated 2 cases of embryonal carcinoma with Act Fu Cy for 1 year after surgery. The patients were free of disease 33 months (Stage IIb) and 24 months (Stage Ia) after surgery. Drug administration should begin during the postoperative period and be continued for 1–2 years. A second laparotomy performed before discontinuing drug therapy will provide maximum assurance that no residual viable disease is present. It is recommended that the contralateral ovary and uterus be removed at this time if they were not excised at the initial operation. Although bilaterality is exceptional in embryonal carcinoma, few young women with this disease have lived long enough to assess the malignant potential of the apparently normal ovary. The serum alphafeto-protein level may prove to be a sufficiently sensitive and reliable indicator of tumor volume to guide therapy and posttreatment surveillance, but at the present time its role has not been established.

Primary ovarian choriocarcinoma occurs predominately as one component of a mixed germ cell tumor. When it coexists with embryonal carcinoma, as is the usual case, the prognosis and treatment are determined by the more malignant element, that is, the embryonal carcinoma. Therapy is specifically directed at the choriocarcinoma when it occurs in pure form or mixed with less malignant germ cell elements such as dysgerminoma. Teratomatous choriocarcinoma is not radiocurable, but it does respond to combination drug therapy. Although the early experience with chemotherapy in ovarian choriocarcinoma indicated that it was not as susceptible to drug control as gestational choriocarcinoma, several cases with prolonged remission induced by the combination of methotrexate, actinomycin D, and chlorambucil (MAC) have been reported (Wider et al, 1969; Goldstein and Piro, 1972; Smith et al, 1973). Treatment response is monitored by serial determination of hCG titers. It has been conventional in the management of gestational choriocarcinoma to discontinue therapy one to three drug cycles after a normal hCG titer has been achieved and maintained. This has proved inadequate for ovarian choriocarcinoma, however, and drug administration should be continued for several months after the hCG titer has returned to normal. Because of the extreme sensitivity and reliability of the gonadotropin radioimmunoassay in detecting small amounts of functioning trophoblastic tissue, there does not seem to be any role for a second-look operation in the management of this disease.

5-5 NEOPLASMS DERIVED FROM SPECIALIZED GONADAL STROMA

Approximately 5% of all ovarian neoplasms are derived from the specialized gonadal stroma. These are commonly referred to as "functioning" tumors because of their ability to synthesize gonadal and adrenal steroid hormones, including estrogens, progesterone, testosterone and other androgenic compounds, and certain corticosteroids. However, hormone production is not a feature exclusive to gonadal stromal tumors. Any ovarian neoplasm, primary or metastatic, may stimulate the nonneoplastic ovarian stroma to synthesize and secrete steroid hormones.

The embryonic gonad is sexually bipotential, and the parenchyma of the ovary and the testicle are derived from the same primitive gonadal stroma. Teilum has pointed out that granulosa and Sertoli cells are homologous, as are theca and Leydig cells. It is not too surprising, then, that both ovarian and testicular tumors can reproduce the histologic and hormonal features of male and female gonadal stroma. The anlagen of the adrenal gland and gonad develop in adjacent areas of the embryo. Together they have been called the "steroid ridge." This proximate embryologic origin probably accounts for some ovarian stromal tumors resembling adrenal neoplasms, although origin from adrenal rests may also occur in some instances. Gonadal stromal tumors are classified according to their differentiation toward ovarian follicles, testicular tubules, Leydig cells, or adrenal cortical cells. The majority are tumors of "female-directed" cells and are classified as granulosa-theca tumors. A smaller percentage of gonadal stromal tumors belong in the Sertoli-Leydig category and are considered to be tumors of "male-directed" cells. The gynandroblastoma contains elements of both male- and female-directed cells. The lipid cell tumors encompass a group of neoplasms consisting primarily of Leydig (hilus)-like cells or adrenal cortical-like cells or both. Not infrequently gonadal stromal tumors are not sufficiently well-differentiated to allow exact classification. Hormone production by gonadal stromal tumors is not consistent and has not proved to be a reliable means of classifying this group of neoplasms. Occasionally a tumor composed of apparently female-directed cells is associated with evidence of androgenic hormone production and vice versa. In addition 15% of these tumors are apparently hormonally inert. Gonadal stromal tumors have also been variously classified as sex cord tumors and mesenchymomas.

Granulosa-Theca Tumors

Granulosa and theca tumors occur with approximately equal frequency. Not uncommonly there is an admixture of granulosa and thecal elements, but these cases should be classified as granulosa tumors, which are malignant, and the designation theca cell tumor or thecoma reserved for neoplasms consisting entirely of theca cells. Although both granulosa and theca tumors are frequently associated with estrogen production, the clinical effects depend to a certain degree on the patient's age. The most dramatic alterations occur in children, who develop pseudoprecocious puberty in response to the estrogen stimulation. During the reproductive years menorrhagia and irregular bleeding are the most common symptoms, although amenorrhea may be experienced by some patients. In the postmenopausal age group, resumption of vaginal bleeding, breast enlargement and tenderness, vaginal cornification, and other evidence of estrogen stimulation are sequelae of functioning granulosa and theca tumors. Rarely virilization may be seen with a cystic granulosa tumor occurring in a young woman. About 50% of the granulosa-theca tumors occur in postmenopausal individuals, while less than 5% develop in prepubertal females. The thecoma is especially likely to occur after the menopause and is rare in children. An unusual feature of granulosa tumors is their propensity to rupture and produce intraperitoneal bleeding, which can be of major proportions. Pregnancy and labor apparently predispose to rupture, and such an event may simulate abruptio placentae. Such a bleeding event in the nonpregnant individual may mimic a ruptured tubal pregnancy. Adenocarcinoma of the endometrium is associated with granulosa and theca cell tumors in 15% of the cases. A similar percentage have endometrial hyperplasia or polyps, but this association is twice as common in the postmenopausal age group. Because of this relationship, any postmenopausal woman with endometrial hyperplasia not receiving medicinal estrogen should be suspected of having a functioning ovarian tumor of the granulosa-theca type until proved otherwise. Not infrequently such tumors are too small to be readily palpated on pelvic examination.

Granulosa tumors are low grade malignancies, the great majority of which are confined to one ovary at the time of diagnosis. Only 5% are reported to be bilateral. Metastases occur in 5-10% of the Stage I cases, but they usually appear more than 5 years after treatment. It is not uncommon for recurrences to be detected 15—20 years after removal of the primary tumor. Hence long-term follow-up of patients with granulosa tumors is essential. Lymphatic and hemotogenous dissemination are uncommon, and distant metastases rare. The prognosis is excellent, with corrected survival rates as high as 97% at 5 years and 93% at 10 years (Norris and Taylor, 1968). Other studies, however, have recorded mortality rates of 25% after 10 years' follow-up.

On gross examination granulosa tumors are usually solid with areas of hemorrhage and cystic degeneration. They may be entirely solid or consist wholly of a single or multiple thin walled cysts. Microscopically the hallmark of the granulosa tumor is the Call-Exner body (Fig. 5-24). A wide variety of cellular patterns is seen, but these bear no prognostic significance provided that the diagnosis of granulosa tumor can be made with certainty. Undifferentiated ovarian carcinoma and metastatic breast cancer may be misdiagnosed as granulosa cell tumors.

Thecomas are invariably unilateral and benign. They may be associated with ascites, producing Meigs's syndrome. Association with uterine fibroids, chronic cystic mastitis, and breast cancer also has been reported. Cortical stromal hyperplasia is commonly found in both ovaries, and some authorities believe there is an etiologic relationship with these hyperplastic areas.

Sertoli-Leydig Cell Tumors

Sertoli-Leydig tumors are characterized by differentiation toward testicular structures. These neoplasms are uncommon and constitute less than 1% of all ovarian tumors. The most frequently encountered type is best known by its trivial name, arrhenoblastoma (from Greek *arrhenos* = male), and contains mixtures of Sertoli and Leydig cells and

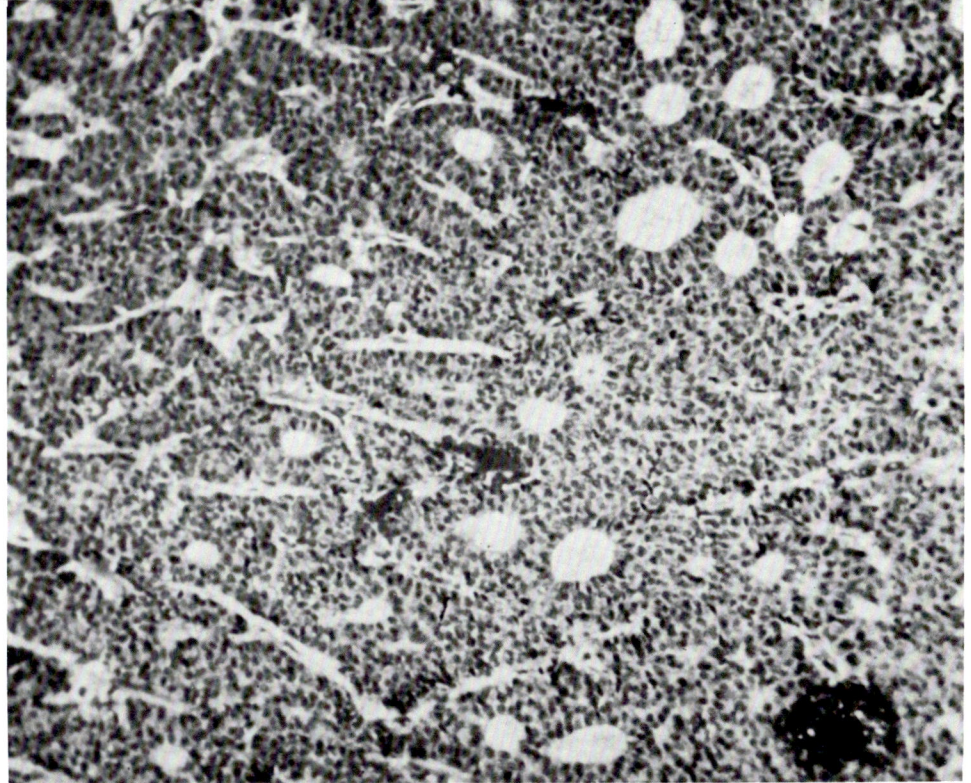

Fig. 5-24 Granulosa cell tumor. Numerous Call-Exner bodies, the hallmark of this neoplasm, are scattered throughout. ×140.

tissues similar to those of the fetal testis. The arrhenoblastoma, or Sertoli-Leydig cell tumor, is the prototype of the primary virilizing ovarian neoplasm. However, it is occasionally associated with estrogenic manifestations, and approximately 15% demonstrate no evidence of hormonal activity clinically.

The average age at diagnosis is 32 years, with half of the tumors occurring in women less than 25 years old. Clinical hormonal effects are less age dependent in masculinizing tumors than in estrogenic tumors, although the changes are less obtrusive in the postmenopausal woman. During the reproductive years defeminization usually precedes virilization, although these two features may occur in a disorderly fashion. The former process includes oligo-amenorrhea and atrophy of the breast tissue and genital organs. More reliable indicators of excess androgen production are the signs of virilization: clitoromegaly, hirsutism, acne, and hoarseness. Less often the body muscle mass increases and temporal balding occurs. These changes frequently occur over a period of several years before diagnosis. Although a rapid onset of virilization is considered characteristic of a neoplastic etiology, even in young women the symptoms and signs of an androgenic tumor may be insidious. Frequently an arrhenoblastoma is not palpable on clinical examination even though there is overt evidence of endocrine activity.

The diagnosis of a virilizing ovarian tumor is not difficult when the clinical evidence of excess androgen production is unequivocal and an adenexal mass is discovered on pelvic examination (Fig. 5-25). In the absence of a palpable ovarian mass, the major problem is

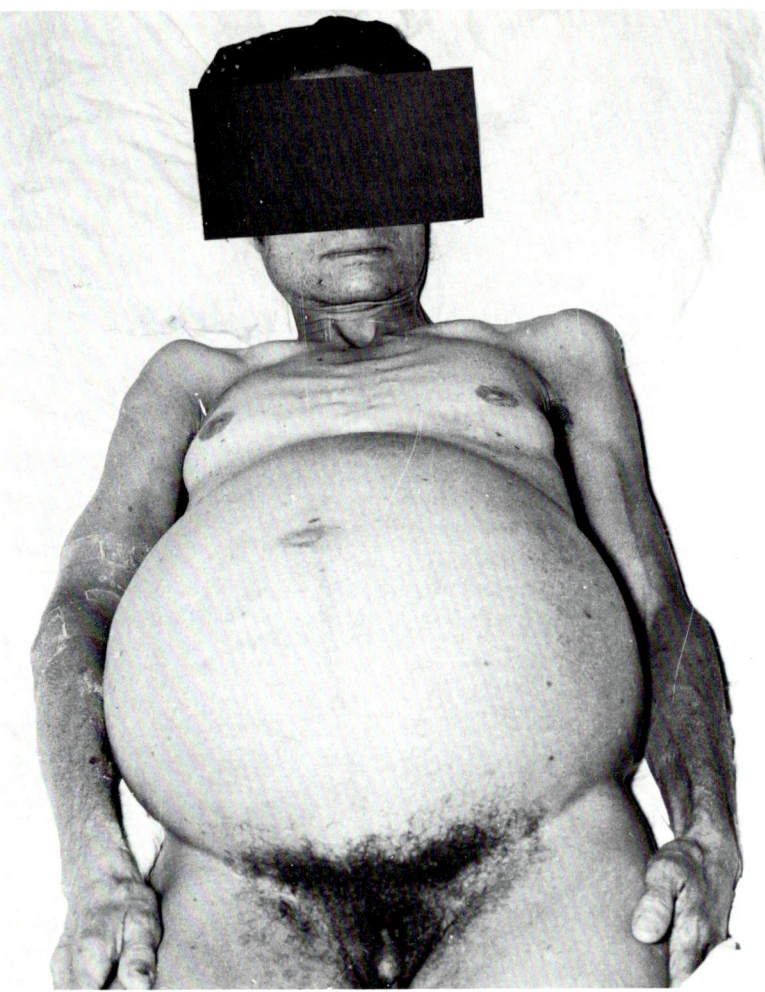

Fig. 5-25 Arrhenoblastoma. This 45 year old woman is obviously masculinized. In addition to clitoromegaly and facial hirsutism, she had developed hoarseness. The male body habitus is partially obscured by the abdominal distention due to ascites. Arrhenoblastoma usually occurs in younger women and seldom manifests overt malignant behavior.

to identify whether the androgen source is ovarian or adrenal. Certain investigative studies will usually locate the cryptic neoplasm. An occult ovarian tumor can be delineated by culdoscopy, laparoscopy, or pelvic pneumography, while an adrenal mass may be disclosed by intravenous pyelography or retroperitoneal air insufflation. Hormone assays may aid in the differential diagnosis of androgenic tumors since the steroidal biosynthetic pathways of the ovary and adrenal gland are different. The ovarian pathway favors the production of testosterone, an extremely potent androgen that contributes little to urinary levels of 17-ketosteroids. In contrast the adrenal pathway produces androstenedione, a relatively weak androgen, and a 17-ketosteroid. Consequently in the virilized patient high levels of urinary 17-ketosteroids point to an adrenal source of androgen. However, certain ovarian tumors may also produce high levels of 17-ketosteroids. Unfortunately stimulation-suppression tests are generally not of sufficient reliability to be decisive. The best diagnostic results are obtained by correlating the clinical data with relevant laboratory and x-ray studies.

Arrhenoblastomas are too rare to permit accurate predictions about their behavior. Prognosis cannot be reliably predicated on the histologic patterns, and classifications such as Meyer's are of little clinical value. Two large series of these tumors have been reported since 1960. In a group of 29 patients reported from the Armed Forces Institute of Pathology (O'Hern and Neubecker, 1962), only 1 developed metastasis. However, in a series reported from the Ovarian Tumor Registry (Novak and Long, 1965), 34% of 90 patients followed for at least 5 years died, presumably as a result of recurrent tumor. Unlike the situation with granulosa tumors, most deaths from arrhenoblastoma occur within 3 years of diagnosis.

The rare Sertoli tumor is generally associated with estrogen production. This neoplasm is composed entirely or predominantly of structures resembling fetal seminiferous tubules. Sertoli tumors have been discovered in young girls with pseudoprecocious puberty. The "sex cord tumors with annular tubules" described by Scully (1970c) and frequently associated with Peutz-Jeghers syndrome resemble Sertoli tumors, although others have interpreted them as granulosa tumors. Sertoli tumors are almost invariably benign.

Gynandroblastoma

Rarely a gonadal stromal tumor contains unequivocal granulosa cell elements combined with tubules and Leydig cells characteristic of the arrhenoblastoma. These tumors are designated as gynandroblastomas and may be associated with either androgen or estrogen production. They can be expected to behave as low grade malignancies similar to the individual components.

Lipid Cell Tumors

This is a heterogeneous group of tumors that have in common a parenchyma composed of polygonal cells containing lipid. Included are neoplasms that have been variously designated as hilus cell tumors, Leydig tumors, adrenal rest tumors, stromal luteomas, and masculinovoblastomas. Such appellations have been given to the various tumors in this group because of their anatomic position within the ovary, a microscopic likeness to the Leydig and adrenal cortical cells, or their endocrine effects. Lipid cell tumors are among the rarest functioning ovarian tumors and are usually virilizing. However, approximately 25% are associated with evidence of estrogenic activity. A Cushingoid syndrome, including obesity, impaired glucose tolerance, and hypertension, is found in about 10% of patients and can easily be mistaken for evidence of an adrenal disorder. The level of urinary 17-ketosteroids is usually elevated and often exceeds 30 mg/24 hours, a value more commonly associated with adrenal lesions than with ovarian neoplasms.

Reinke crystals, which normally occur in mature Leydig cells of the testis and in hilus cells of the ovary, are sometimes evident in ovarian lipid cell tumors. These tumors can be designated as hilus or Leydig cell tumors. Lipid cell tumors with Reinke crystals tend to occur in older women and to be smaller than their crystal-negative relatives. Their average size is about 3 cm, and frequently they are not palpable clinically, remaining undetected until the involved ovary is sectioned. Testosterone may be produced in sufficient quantities to cause virilization without elevating the level of urinary 17-ketosteroids.

Lipid cell tumors are unilateral and are commonly found in the medulla or hilar region of the ovary. On cut section they are often a bright yellow-orange because of the high lipid and lipochrome pigment content. The majority of lipid cell tumors are histologically and clinically benign. Tumors that have spread to contiguous organs or have microscopic cellular pleomorphism with a high mitotic activity should be considered malignant. However, a few large but histologically benign tumors have behaved in a malignant fashion. All ovarian lipid cell tumors with Reinke crystals are benign. Regardless of the presence or absence of Reinke crystals, neoplasms less than 8 cm in diameter can be expected to behave in a benign fashion.

Management of Gonadal Stromal Tumors

Ovarian neoplasms derived from the specialized gonadal stroma present few treatment problems provided that the diagnosis is accurate. Thecomas are benign and unilateral in nearly all cases, as are most lipid cell and Sertoli tumors. These lesions are adequately managed during the reproductive years by removing the involved ovary and ipsilateral tube. The uterus and the uninvolved adnexae should be excised in the peri- and postmenopausal age groups, as is the practice with other benign tumors. Granulosa cell tumors and arrhenoblastomas are low grade malignancies usually confined to one ovary at the time of diagnosis. If the peritoneal washings, omental biopsy, and wedge resection of the opposite ovary are normal, conservative surgery is sufficient therapy in the young woman provided that the tumor is intact (see Table 5-15). After removal of an arrhenoblastoma, menses usually resume within 1 or 2 months and the breasts rapidly return to normal. The acne is reversible, but the hirsutism, clitoromegaly, and hoarseness may be permanent or resolve only slowly. Fertility seems to be unimpaired. Patients whose disease is more advanced than Stage Ia should have both adnexae and the uterus removed along with all resectable tumor. Postoperatively adjunctive external pelvic and abdominal irradiation is indicated. Of course, when a granulosa tumor is complicated by adenocarcinoma of the endometrium, conservation of the uterus and uninvolved adnexa is no longer a consideration. Occasionally a lipid cell tumor will show histologic evidence of malignancy. In this case the uninvolved ovary cannot be preserved, and the surgical therapy should be followed by abdominal and pelvic irradiation. Many of the stromal tumors produce measurable levels of steroid hormones. Quantitative serial assays may prove useful in postoperative surveillance for recurrence. Determination of testosterone levels in serum or urine after therapy for arrhenoblastoma would seem to be the most promising. Estradiol and 17-ketosteroid values may reveal recurrent granulosa tumors and lipid cell tumors, respectively, before the disease is apparent clinically. The practical value of these studies has not been demonstrated, however.

5-6 NEOPLASMS DERIVED FROM NONSPECIFIC MESENCHYME

Benign and malignant tumors may arise in the ovary from the nonspecific supporting tissues that are common to most bodily organs. Such tumors include fibromas, hemangiomas, leiomyomas, soft tissue sarcomas, lymphomas, and other rare neoplasms. The fibroma and the lymphoma are the most common and most important in this category.

Fibroma

The fibroma is a benign connective tissue tumor composed of fibroblasts and collagen. It is one of the most common ovarian neoplasms and accounts for 20% of all solid ovarian tumors. It is not readily distinguished from the thecoma clinically or histologically, and some authorities prefer to categorize these lesions together. The average age of diagnosis is 48 years. The usual fibroma is 6 cm in diameter, 10% are bilateral, and areas of calcification are common.

The fibroma has been immortalized because of its role in Meigs's syndrome. In 1937 Meigs and Cass reported and emphasized the occasional coexistence of ovarian fibroma, ascites, and hydrothorax, at times complicated by cachexia. Since this clinical picture was considered diagnostic of advanced ovarian carcinoma, some women were permitted to die without therapeutic intervention. The ascites and hydrothorax are reversible after removal of the fibroma or other benign ovarian stromal neoplasm. Less than 5% of fibromas are associated with ascites and pleural effusion, which occur almost exclusively with tumors greater than 10 cm in diameter. The hydrothorax is usually on the right side and results from ascitic fluid traversing the diaphragm through congenital perforations or via lymphatics. The etiology of the ascites is unknown, but two theories have been proposed: (1) the tumor "irritates" the peritoneum, inducing it to produce the ascitic fluid; and (2) the tumor twists on its pedicle, obstructing the lymphatic outflow from the ovary. The resultant ovarian edema leads to fluid leaking from the tumor into the peritoneal cavity.

Lymphoma

Ovarian enlargement is rarely the initial clinical manifestation of lymphoma, and when the ovaries are involved there is usually disease in the regional lymph nodes or other organs. Burkitt's lymphoma, a form of stem cell lymphoma occurring primarily in children, has a predilection for involving the ovaries. Although this disease is found primarily in Africa, it occurs also in the United States. Among disseminated malignancies Burkitt's lymphoma is second only to gestational choriocarcinoma in its curability with chemotherapy. A 15% 5 year survival rate has been achieved using cyclophosphamide.

5-7 CARCINOMA METASTATIC TO THE OVARY

Virchow has been quoted as saying that the organs that most frequently produce malignant neoplasms are rarely the site of metastases. Certainly, the ovary is an exception to this dictum. Approximately 30% of women dying of cancer are found to have ovarian metastases at autopsy, and one fifth of those undergoing palliative oophorectomy for metastatic breast cancer have microscopic evidence of metastases to the ovaries. At least 5% of patients explored for ovarian cancer have a secondary rather than a primary lesion. The most common sources of metastases to the ovary are the gastrointestinal tract, breast, and pelvic organs; however, the last two sites seldom produce clinically significant ovarian metastases. In 75% of the cases of ovarian secondaries, both ovaries are grossly involved by metastases, and, with rare exception, when metastases are present in the ovary there is metastatic disease in other parts of the body also.

Kruckenberg Tumor

In 1896 Kruckenberg described an ovarian neoplasm that he designated as "fibrosarcoma ovarii mucocellulare (carcinomatodes)." He considered this to be a primary ovarian sarcoma. In 1902, Schlaggenhoffer established the metastatic nature of this tumor. Although the appellation *Kruckenberg tumor* has been used often to describe any secondary ovarian cancer, its application should be restricted to ovarian tumors that fit Kruckenberg's original description. Grossly these tumors are solid, kidney shaped, and usually bilateral. There is a tendency to retain the contour of the normal ovary. Adhesions and other intra-abdominal disease are usually absent. The average size is 10—15 cm, and on cut section hemorrhage and necrosis may be present. The cut surface often displays a gelatinous consistency. Microscopically there is a florid hyperplasia of the ovarian stroma, which tends to obscure the mucus-secreting, signet ring cells.

Nearly all tumors of the ovary fitting this description are metastases from a primary cancer in the stomach, although other primary sites such as the gallbladder, breast, and colon have been reported. Rarely, no primary site can be identified, and apparent cures have been produced after excision of the ovarian tumor. The route of spread from stomach to ovary is probably retrograde dissemination via the aortic lymphatics. Other proposed, but less likely, routes include the hematogenous and the transperitoneal. The occurrence of metastases to the ovary seems to be disproportionately common in premenopausal women, presumably because of the vascularity of the functioning ovary. However, the average age of women with Kruckenberg tumors is 45—50 years.

Carcinoma of the colon metastatic to the ovary may simulate primary mucinous cystadenocarcinoma of the ovary, and a thorough investigation of the colon must be made in all cases of mucinous ovarian cancer. Large areas of hemorrhage and necrosis are characteristic, and spontaneous rupture with intraperitoneal hemorrhage may occur. Because of the frequency with which carcinomas of the colon metastasize to the ovary, some authors recommend prophylactic bilateral ovariectomy as part of the surgical therapy for carcinoma of the colon in older women.

5-8 OVARIAN TUMORS IN PREGNANCY

Approximately once in every 1,000 consecutive pregnancies an ovarian tumor is diagnosed. This apparently coincidental occurrence poses a threat to both mother and fetus because of the necessity of therapeutic intervention or because of complications resulting from the tumor itself. There is an increased probability of an ovarian tumor twisting or rupturing during pregnancy. Furthermore, an ovarian tumor may cause obstruction of labor and necessitate cesarean section. According to some series reported in the literature, 1 of every 10 ovarian masses diagnosed during pregnancy is a large, cystic corpus luteum. These are invariably discovered and removed during the first half of pregnancy, when the normal corpus luteum may achieve a size of 8—10 cm. The majority of ovarian neoplasms complicating pregnancy are dermoid cysts and benign cystadenomas. Malignant tumors comprise only 3—6% of the neoplastic lesions of the ovary observed during pregnancy. From the small number of cases available for analysis, the incidence, stage, and histogenetic type of lesion do not seem to be different from what would be expected in a nonpregnant population of the same age group. The great majority of ovarian cancers discovered during pregnancy are Stage Ia, despite the fact that during the second and third trimesters the pregnant uterus may obscure the presence of an ovarian mass. The risk to the fetus from ovarian cancer is primarily that resulting from treatment, since metastasis to the placenta is rare and spread to the fetus has not been documented.

Management of an ovarian mass will depend to a certain degree on the stage of gestation. During the first trimester it is important to confirm the presence of an intrauterine pregnancy to avoid unnecessary delay in investigating the mass. Some circumspection is required, however, since a positive pregnancy test may be the result of gonadotropin produced by an ovarian germ cell tumor containing choriocarcinoma, rather than a pregnancy coexistent with an adnexal mass. If the mass is unilateral, mobile and cystic operation should be delayed until the pregnancy enters the second trimester, when surgery may be less likely to result in abortion. A corpus luteum may regress during the interval of observation. When an adnexal mass is discovered during the third trimester of pregnancy, surgery should be delayed until the stage of fetal viability or term, depending on the age of gestation. Operation in the postpartum period may be more advantageous to the patient and the fetus than cesarean section with removal of the tumor unless the tumor obstructs the birth canal.

Ovarian cancer diagnosed during pregnancy is treated as in the nonpregnant patient.

5-9 OVARIAN TUMORS IN CHILDREN

Ovarian neoplasms in children are quite unusual, although they account for two thirds of genital tract cancers in this age group. They are of special importance, however, since the malignancy rate is 50%. In the newborn period nearly all ovarian enlargements are functional or nonneoplastic cysts. Ovarian neoplasms of any type are decidedly rare before puberty (Table 5-17). The relative frequency of ovarian neoplasms during childhood and adolescence is the reverse of that in adults. Abell et al (1965) found that 90% of 35 ovarian neoplasms diagnosed before menarche were of germ cell origin and half of these were malignant. The remaining benign germ cell tumors were mature cystic teratomas. By comparison, only 15—20% of ovarian neoplasms in adults have a germ cell origin, and over 95% of these are benign. Neoplasms of epithelial origin are exceedingly rare before puberty, and nearly all of them are benign. When the series of Norris and Jensen (1972) is combined with that of Abell and Holtz (1965), the 120 epithelial ovarian tumors reported accounted for only 22% of the neoplasms in females less than 20 years of age. Only 10% of these were malignant, including borderline lesions.

Stromal tumors comprise about 15% of ovarian neoplasms reported in childhood and adolescence. However, they may be reported more frequently than other neoplasms because their hormonal effects make them especially interesting. It is estimated that only 2% of all cases of pseudoprecocious puberty are due to ovarian tumors. A few well documented examples of pseudoprecocious puberty occurring secondary to follicular cysts have been reported in the literature, but precocious puberty of ovarian origin is more commonly associated with a true neoplasm: granulosa tumor, Sertoli tumor or chorio-carcinoma. The granulosa tumors, like other non-germ cell tumors, are less inclined to manifest malignant behavior in this age group, than in older individuals. Thecomas and arrhenoblastomas are extremely rare before puberty.

Management of gynecologoic tumors in the pediatric age group poses some special problems. The incomplete physical and psychological development of children makes

TABLE 5-17   DISTRIBUTION OF 353 CASES OF OVARIAN TUMORS OF CHILDHOOD
BY AGE OF PATIENT

Type of Tumor	Age of Patient (years)			Total Number of Cases
	0—9	10-14	15-19	
Germ cell				
Benign cystic teratoma	5	14	52	71
Solid teratoma, immature	3	11	8	22
Solid teratoma, mature	2	2	2	6
Mixed teratoma, dysgerminoma, embryonal carcinoma, or choriocarcinoma	10	5	11	26
Dysgerminoma (pure)	7	17	24	48
Embryonal carcinoma (predominating)	5	16	11	32
Subtotal	32	65	108	205
Epithelial				
Cystadenoma and adenofibroma	1	4	54	59
Borderline tumors	0	0	5	5
Cystadenocarcinoma	0	1	2	3
Subtotal	1	5	61	67
Stromal				
Fibrothecoma	4	1	18	23
Arrhenoblastoma	1	1	12	14
Granulosa	5	2	5	12
Nonspecific	7	2	4	13
Subtotal	17	6	39	62
Miscellaneous				
Malignant, unclassified	4	2	8	14
Germinoma arising in gonadoblastoma	0	1	1	2
Lymphoma	0	2	0	2
Lymphangioma	0	1	0	1
Subtotal	4	6	9	19
Total, all cases	54	82	217	353

Modified from Norris and Jensen (1972).

them more vulnerable to permanent, crippling injuries from all modalities of cancer therapy. The immature tissues of the child are especially susceptible to radiation injury, and damage to bone growth centers can result in significant deformities in long-term survivors. The liver, kidney, and small bowel are less tolerant of radiation therapy in children than in the adult, necessitating lower doses or a reduced dose rate when treating the abdomen or pelvis. Radiation enterocolitis is particularly troublesome in infants and children because of the ease with which they develop fluid and electrolyte imbalance. With regard to chemotherapy, children tolerate a number of drugs better than adults, but the synergistic effect of drugs used with irradiation, especially actinomycin D, may be seriously exaggerated. The immediate and long-term effects of pelvic surgery are more predictable than those of radiotherapy and chemotherapy.

Frequently sterilization is an unavoidable sequel to pelvic cancer therapy. Although the importance of reproductive integrity in the development of the young woman's self-image must not be lightly regarded, conservatism is often not the best course. No individual has more to lose by inadequate treatment than a child, at least in terms of longevity and fulfillment. Any disease that threatens both the life of a child and her sexual-reproductive faculties invariably produces an intensely emotional atmosphere. Under these circumstances assessment of the risks and benefits becomes more difficult, but there should be no hesitation to remove or irradiate the reproductive organs in the course of cancer therapy if there is a reasonable expectation that doing so will contribute to a cure. In the face of disease that can be palliated only, the deleterious effects on the reproductive tract cannot be considered a major impediment to therapy.

5-10 OVARIAN CANCER—EPIDEMIOLOGY AND ETIOLOGY

Epidemiology

From the viewpoints of morbidity and mortality ovarian malignancies are the most important group of neoplasms in the field of gynecologic oncology. In the United States only 25% of all women diagnosed as having ovarian cancer survive for 5 years. The mortality rate from this malignancy has increased 250% since 1930, elevating it to the fourth leading cause of death among cancers in women; only cancers of the breast, colon, and lung account for more fatalities. In New York State the risk of death from ovarian cancer has apparently surpassed the combined risks from cervical cancer and corpus cancer (Randall, 1970). According to the statistics of the American Cancer Society, approxiamtely 14,000 new cases of ovarian cancer are diagnosed in the United States each year, and 10,500 deaths due to this malignancy occur during the same interval.

Ovarian cancer is predominantly a disease of peri- and postmenopausal women with an average age at diagnosis of 52 years. Both the histologic type of neoplasm and the overall frequency of occurrence vary significantly with age. In children and women less than 20 years old nearly 60% of ovarian neoplasms are of germ cell origin, whereas over 80% of tumors occurring in postmenopausal women are derived from the surface epithelium of the ovary. Before age 20 less than 1 case of ovarian cancer is diagnosed per 100,000 females per year. The occurrence rate increases to 27 at age 55 and continues to rise thereafter, achieving a level of approximately 75 cases per 100,000 females per year at age 75 (Table 5-18). The age adjusted annual death rates vary widely on an international basis, ranging from a low of 2 per 100,000 population in Japan and Chile to 13 in the Scandinavian countries. In the United States the annual death rate from ovarian cancer among Caucasian women is 7 per 100,000, compared to 6 for non-Caucasians.

TABLE 5-18   INCIDENCE RATES OF
OVARIAN CANCER PER 100,000 WOMEN

Age (years)	Oakland Kaiser Hospital (1958-63)	New York State (1960)
0-19	0	0.1
20-44	7.2	5.9
45-54	27.6	26.3
55-65	28.1	38.1
65-74	72.6	73.5
75+	158	131

From Bennington et al (1968).

Some epidemiologic studies have demonstrated that the incidence of ovarian cancer increases with a rise in social class. Age adjusted death rates of ovarian cancer are higher for single than married women, and the percentage of single women in many reported series of ovarian cancer appears to be disproportionately high. Wynder et al (1969) noted a significantly heavier menstrual flow during the later years of reproductive life and a greater occurrence of dysmenorrhea in 150 patients with ovarian cancer than in a matched control group. Other studies have shown a positive correlation of ovarian cancer and a history of endometrial cancer. A familial occurrence has been reported for dysgerminoma, arrhenoblastoma, mature cystic teratoma, and ovarian carcinoma. However, a genetic prediposition to the development of ovarian cancer could not be confirmed by a study of identical twins (Harvald and Hauge, 1963). Ovarian tumors are common in women with certain genetic diseases. For example, in Peutz-Jegher syndrome approximately 5% of the cases develop a gonadal stromal tumor. Individuals with XY gonadal dysgenesis have a predilection for developing gonadoblastoma, which often gives rise to a malignant germ cell tumor.

Etiology

There is no known cause of any of the numerous ovarian cancers, but several observations suggest that hormones may be involved in the genesis of certain tumors. Granulosa cell tumors can be induced experimentally in rodents by irradiating the ovaries and also by transplanting ovarian tissue into the spleen of an ovariectomized rat. Both of these manipulations result in increased levels of pituitary gonadotropins. In women the postmenopausal state is associated with elevated pituitary gonadotropins; however, granulosa tumors comprise a very small portion of ovarian cancers occurring in that age group. Furthermore, granulosa tumors occur with about the same frequency before and after the menopause. Nevertheless, the infrequency of ovarian cancer before puberty and the relatively high rate of occurrence after the menopause support some relationship of tumorogenesis to hormonal influences. The known association of mesotheliomas and asbestosis has suggested a possible etiology for epithelial tumors of the ovary, which are derived from a modified mesothelium. Graham and Graham (1967) found birefringent crystalline particles in 6 of 12 human ovarian lesions which they interpreted as borderline or microinvasive adenocarcinoma. The nature of the crystals was not identified. Using electron microscopy, Henderson (1971) was unable to find asbestos in any of 13 ovarian malignancies, but he identified talc in 10 of the specimens. The significance of these findings has not been elucidated.

5-11 OVARIAN CANCER - DETECTION AND PREVENTION

Detection

The natural history of ovarian cancer mitigates against dramatic improvements in therapy. The cryptic early development, rapid growth, and propensity for intraperitoneal spread frequently result in massive and unresectable disease at the time of diagnosis. It is unlikely that therapeutic advances will provide a means of eradicating any cancer in such an advanced state of development. A more reasonable prospect for improving the prognosis of ovarian cancer is earlier diagnosis. Routine pelvic examinations are ill suited to mass screening for ovarian carcinoma, but when pelvic examination is performed, its value can be enhanced by a more critical assessment of the findings. Barber and Graber (1971) have pointed out that a palpable ovary in any woman more than 3 years postmenopausal undoubtedly harbors an ovarian neoplasm. There is no role for "watchful expectency" or delay under any other disguise in this age group. Immediate investigation of an adnexal mass in a postmenopausal woman and also in prepubertal girls is mandatory. During the reproductive years delay is warranted only when the mass fulfills the criteria of a functional ovarian cyst.

The greatest hope for early diagnosis of ovarian cancer lies in the development of a sufficiently sensitive and reliable laboratory test that is suited to repetitive screening of the vast population at risk. Search for such a diagnostic test has resulted in a number of encouraging possibilities. The success of mass cytologic screening for cervical carcinoma and related premalignant lesions logically led to attempts at detection of ovarian cancer by cytologic means. It is clear that well established ovarian cancer sheds cells which are detectable in ascitic fluid as well as cervical-vaginal smears. However, it is rare that an ovarian neoplasm is initially detected by a cervical-vaginal smear obtained during a routine pelvic examination. Culdocentesis, which provides convenient access to the peritoneal cavity, has been utilized to obtain fluid for cytology in the hope of detecting early, asymptomatic ovarian cancer. Although early reports of this technique were encouraging, the overall results have been disappointing, in terms of both the frequency of unsatisfactory specimens and the yield of asymptomatic, early ovarian carcinomas.

The best prospect for developing a diagnostic screening test for ovarian cancer seems to lie in the field of tumor immunology. Tumor specific and tumor associated antigens have been identified for many human cancers, including serous carcinoma of the ovary (Levi et al 1968). Serum radioimmunoassay of these antigens could prove to be sufficiently sensitive and specific to detect preclinical ovarian cancer. The prototype of such measurable tumor markers is the polypeptide hormone human chorionic gonadotropin (hCG), produced by trophoblastic tumors of gestational and teratomatous origin. Recently a tumor associated antigen, alpha-fetoprotein (AFP), has been identified in the serum of women with embryonal carcinoma and other malignant germ cell tumors (Masopust et al, 1968); AFP determination could prove suitable as a diagnostic test and therapeutic monitor for embryonal carcinoma. Other serum factors, including lactic dehydrogenase, haptoglobin, and fucose frequently have abnormal values in patients with ovarian cancer. The titer of these substances roughly reflects the size of the viable tumor cell population. Whether such measurements will be of practical use has yet to be demonstrated.

Prevention

Prevention is another approach to reducing the morbidity and mortality resulting from ovarian cancer. However, the only known method of prevention is surgical castration. Since the risk of any woman developing ovarian cancer during her lifetime is only 1%, the probability of prophylactic ovariectomy benefiting the individual is small. Operating solely for the purpose of cancer prophylaxis cannot be seriously considered, but routine ovariectomy at the time of pelvic surgery could reduce the occurrence of ovarian cancer.

According to published series of ovarian cancer, 5-10% of cases occur in women who have previously undergone hysterectomy for benign disease (deNeef and Hollenbeck, 1966). There seems to be no valid objection to preventive ovariectomy in postmenopausal women since the ovaries have neither a reproductive nor an indispensable endocrine function at this time of life. Because the ovary is essential to conception, prophylactic ovariectomy during the reproductive years is reserved for patients undergoing hysterectomy for benign gynecologic disease. However, it is generally agreed that the relatively small risk of developing ovarian cancer does not justify sacrificing the endocrine function of the ovaries without respect to the patient's age. Most commonly the minimum age recommended for routine ovariectomy falls within the fifth decade of life, although some recommendations (Gibbs, 1971) extend down to age 35. The availability of medicinal estrogens has engendered the belief that the ovaries can be removed with impunity even in young women; but this is to a great extent speculative, and only long-term follow-up of large numbers of patients will decide the issue.

Paloucek (1970) investigated the risk of developing ovarian cancer after hysterectomy for benign disease. He reported a 25-40 year follow-up of 7299 women who had one or both ovaries preserved and found no evidence that hysterectomy or the indication for hysterectomy either increased or decreased the risk of developing an ovarian malignancy, nor did there seem to be any difference if one ovary or both ovaries were preserved. The ovaries apparently function normally after hysterectomy in the great majority of instances.

REFERENCES

Abell, M. R.: The nature and classification of ovarian neoplasms. *Can. Med. Assoc. J.* **94**:1102, 1966.

Abell, M. R., and Holtz, F.: Ovarian neoplasms in childhood and adolescence. II. Tumors of non-germ cell origin. *Am. J. Obstet. Gynecol.* **93**:850, 1965.

Abell, M. R., Johnson, V. J., and Holtz, F.: Ovarian neoplasms in childhood and adolescence. I. Tumors of germ cell origin. *Am. J. Obstet. Gynecol.* **92**:1059, 1965.

Acosta, A., Kaplan, A. L., and Kaufman, R. H.: Gynecologic cancer in children. *Am. J. Obstet. Gynecol.* **112**:944, 1972.

Albites, V.: Solid teratoma of the ovary with malignant gliomatosis peritonei. *Int. J. Gynaec. Obstet.* **12**:59, 1974.

Allan, M. S., and Hertig, A. T.: Carcinoma of the ovary. *Am. J. Obstet. Gynecol.* **58**:640, 1949.

American Cancer Society: *Cancer Facts and Figures*, 1973.

Anderson, W. R., Levine, A. J., and MacMillan, D.: Granulosa-theca cell tumors: Clinical and pathologic study. *Am. J. Obstet. Gynecol.* **110**:32, 1971.

Arey, L. B.: Origin and form of Brenner tumor. *Am. J. Obstet. Synecol.* **81**:743, 1961.

Arias-Bernal, L., and Jones, H. W.: Chromosomes of a malignant ovarian teratoma. *Am. J. Obstet. Gynecol.* **100**:785, 1968.

Asadourian, L. A., and Taylor, H. B.: Dysgerminoma: An analysis of 105 cases. *Obstet. Gynecol.* **33**:370, 1969.

Aure, J. C., Hoeg, K., and Kolstad, P.: Radioactive colloidal gold in the treatment of ovarian carcinoma. *Acta Radiol.* **10**:399, 1971b.

Aure, J. C., Hoeg, K., and Kolstad, P: Radioactive colloidal gold in the treatment of ovarian carcinoma. *Acta Radiol.* **10**:399, 1971b.

Aure, J. C., Hoeg, K., and Kolstad, P.: Psammoma bodies in serous carcinoma of the ovary: A prognostic study. *Am. J. Obstet. Gynecol.* **109**:113, 1971c.

Aure, J. C., Hoeg, K., and Kolstad, P.: Carcinoma of the ovary and endometriosis. *Acta Obstet. Gynecol.* **50**:63, 1971d.

Azoury, R. S., and Woodruff, J. D.: Primary ovarian sarcomas: Report of 43 cases from the Emil Novak Ovarian Tumor Registry. *Obstet. Gynecol.* **37**:920, 1971.

Bagley, C. M., Jr., Young, R. C., Canellos, G. P., and DeVita, V. T.: Treatment of ovarian carcinoma: Possibilities for progress. *N. Engl. J. Med.* **287**:856, 1972.

Barber, H. R. K., and Graber, E. A.: The PMPO syndrome (postmenopausal palpable ovary syndrome). *Obstet. Gynecol.* **38**:921, 1971.

Barber, H. R. K., and Graber, E. A.: Gynecological tumors in childhood and adolescence. *Obstet. Gynecol. Surv.* **28**:357, 1973.

Barlow, J. J., Piver, M. S., Chuang, J. T., Cortes, E. T., Ohnuma, T., and Holland, J. F.: Adriamycin and bleomycin, alone and in combination, in gynecologic cancers. *Cancer* **32**:735, 1973.

Barnes, P. H.: Oophorectomy in primary carcinoma confined to one ovary. *Can. Med. Assoc. J.* **79**:416, 1958.

Beck, R. E., and Boyes, D. A.: Treatment of 126 cases of advanced ovarian carcinoma with cycophoshamide. *Can. Med. Assoc. J.* **98**:539, 1968.

Bennington, J. L., Ferguson, B. R., and Haber, S. L.: Incidence and relative frequency of benign and malignant ovarian neoplasms. *Obstet. Gynecol.* **32**:627, 1968.

Bergman, F.: Carcinoma of the ovary: A clinicopathological study of 86 autopsied cases with special reference to mode of spread. *Acta Obstet. Gynecol. Scand.* **45**:211, 1966.

Blackwell, W. J., Dockerty, M. B., Masson, J. C., and Mussey, R. D.: Dermoid cysts of the ovary: Their clinical and pathologic significance. *Am. J. Obstet. Gynecol.* **51**:151, 1946.

Boivin, Y., and Richart, R. M.: Hilus cell tumors of the ovary: A review with a report of 3 new cases. *Cancer* **18**:231, 1965.

Braun, P. A., and Richart, R. M.: Functioning ovarian carcinoid tumors. *Obstet. Gynecol.* **34**:390, 1969.

Breen, J. L., and Neubecker, R. D.: Ovarian malignancy in children with special reference to the germ cell tumors. *Ann. N. Y. Acad. Sci.* **142**:208, 1962.

Breen, J. L., and Neubecker, R. D.: Malignant teratoma of the ovary: An analysis of 17 cases. *Obstet. Gynecol.* **21**:669, 1963.

Brody, S.: Clinical aspects of dysgerminoma of the ovary. *Acta Radiol.* **56**:209, 1961.

Burns, B. C., Jr., Rutledge, F. N., Smith, J. P., and Delclos, L.: Management of ovarian carcinoma: Surgery, irradiation and chemotherapy. *Am. J. Obstet. Gynecol.* **98**:374, 1967.

Carlson, D. H., and Griscom, N. T.: Ovarian cysts in the newborn. *Am. J. Roentgenol. Radium Ther. Nucl. Med.* **116**:664, 1972.

Chalvardjian, A., and Scully, R. E.: Sclerosing stromal tumors of the ovary. *Cancer* **31**:664, 1973.

Christian, C. D.: Ovarian tumors: An extension of the Peutz—Jeghers syndrome. *Am. J. Obstet. Gynecol.* **111**:529, 1971.

Chung, A., and Birnbaum, S. J.: Ovarian cancer associated with pregnancy. *Obstet. Gynecol.* **41**:211, 1973.

Classification and staging of malignant tumours in the female pelvis. *Acta Obstet. Gynecol. Scand.* **50**:1, 1971.

Climie, A. R. W., and Heath, L. P.: Malignant degeneration of benign cystic teratomas of the ovary: Review of the literature and report of a chondrosarcoma and carcinoid tumor. *Cancer* **22**:824, 1968.

Counseller, V. S., Hunt, W., and Haigler, F. H.: Carcinoma of the ovary following hysterectomy. *Am. J. Obstet. Gynecol.* **69**:538, 1955.

Creasman, W. T., and Rutledge, F. N.: The prognostic value of peritoneal cytology in gynecologic malignant disease. *Am. J. Obstet. Gynecol.* **110**:773, 1971.

Creasman, W. T., Rutledge, F. N.: and Smith, J. P.: Carcinoma of the ovary associated with pregnancy. *Obstet. Gynecol.* **38**:111, 1971.

Cruikshank, D. P., and Buchsbaum, H. J.: Effects of rapid paracentesis: Cardiovascular dynamics and body fluid composition. *J. Am. Med. Assoc.* 225:1361, 1973.

Czernobilsky, B., and LaBarre, G.C.: Carcinosarcoma and mixed mesodermal tumor of the ovary: A clinicopathologic analysis of 9 cases. *Obstet. Gynecol.* 31:21, 1968.

Czernobilsky, B., Silverman, B. B., and Enterline, H.T.: Clear-cell carcinoma of the ovary: A clinicopathologic analysis of pure and mixed forms and comparison with endometrioid carcinoma. *Cancer* 25:762, 1970.

Czernobilsky, B., Silverman, B. B., and Mikuta, J. J.: Endometrioid carcinoma of the ovary: A clinicopathologic study of 75 cases. *Cancer* 26:1141, 1970.

De Alvarez, R. R., Mendelson, E. G., Castellanos, H., and Lundy, L. E.: Virilizing lipoid tumors of the ovary. *Obstet. Gynecol.* 35:956, 1970.

Decker, D. G., Malkasian, G. D., Jr., Mussey, E., and Johnson, C. E.: Cyclophosphamide: Evaluation in recurrent and progressive ovarian cancer. *Am. J. Obstet. Gynecol.* 97:656, 1967a.

Decker, D. G., Mussey, E., Malkasian, G. D., and Johnson, C. E.: Adjuvant therapy for advanced ovarian malignancy. *Am. J. Obstet. Gynecol.* 97:171, 1967b.

Decker, D. G., Webb, M. J., and Holbrook, M. A.: Radiogold treatment of epithelial cancer of ovary: Late results. *Am. J. Obstet. Gynecol.* 115:751, 1973.

Dehner, L. P., Norris, H. J., and Taylor, H. B.: Carcinosarcomas and mixed mesodermal tumors of the ovary. *Cancer* 27:207, 1971.

Delclos, L., and Fletcher, G. H.: Postoperative irradiation for ovarian carcinoma with the cobalt-60 moving strip technique. *Clin. Obstet. Gynecol.* 12:993, 1969.

Delclos, L., and Quinlan, E. J.: Malignant tumors of the ovary managed with postoperative megavoltage irradiation. *Radiology* 93:659, 1969.

DeNeef, J. C., and Hollenbeck, Z. J. R.: The fate of ovaries preserved at the time of hysterectomy. *Am. J. Obstet. Gynecol.* 96:1088, 1966.

Dinnerstein, A. J., and O'Leary, J. A.: Granulosa-theca cell tumors: A clinical review of 102 patients. *Obstet. Gynecol.* 31:654, 1968.

Dockerty, M. B.: Primary and secondary ovarian adenoacanthoma. *Surg. Gynecol. Obstet.* 99:392, 1954.

Dockerty, M. B., and Masson, J. C.: Ovarian fibromas: A clinical and pathological study of 283 cases. *Am. J. Obstet. Gynecol.* 47:741, 1944.

Dunnihoo, D. R., Grieme, D. L., and Woolf, R. B.: Hilar-cell tumors of the ovary: Report of two new cases and review of the world literature. *Obstet. Gynecol.* 27:703, 1966.

Emig, O. R., Hertig, A. T., and Rowe, F. J.: Gynandroblastoma of the ovary: Review and report of a case. *Obstet. Gynecol.* 13:135, 1959.

Fathalla, M. F.: Factors in the causation and incidence of ovarian cancer. *Obstet. Gynecol. Surv.* 27:751, 1972.

Felmus, L. B., and Pedowitz, P.: Clinical malignancy of endocrine tumors of the ovary and dysgerminoma. *Obstet. Gynecol.* 29:344, 1967.

Fenn, M. E., and Abell, M. R.: Carcinosarcoma of the ovary. *Am. J. Obstet Gynecol.* 110:1066, 1971.

Ferenczy, A., Okagaki, T., and Richart, R. M.: Para-endocrine hypercalcemia in ovarian neoplasms: Report of mesonephroma with hypercalcemia and review of literature. *Cancer* 27:427, 1971.

Forney, J. P., DiSaia, P. J., and Morrow, C. P.: Endodermal sinus tumor. *Obstet. Gynecol.*, in Press, 1974.

Gentil, F., and Junqueira, A. C., Eds.: Ovarian Cancer, UICC Monograph Series, Vol. 2. Springer-Verlag, New York, 1968.

Gibbs, E. K.: Suggested prophylaxis for ovarian cancer. *Am. J. Obstet. Gynecol.* 111:756, 1971.

Gillibrand, P. N.: Granulosa-theca cell tumors of the ovary associated with pregnancy: Case report and review of the literature. *Am. J. Obstet. Gynecol.* 94:1108, 1966.

Goldstein, D. P., and Piro, A. J.: Combination chemotherapy in the treatment of germ cell tumors containing choriocarcinoma in males and females. *Surg. Gynecol. Obstet.* 134:61, 1972.

Goldston, W. R., Johnston, W. W., Fetter, B. F., Parker, R. T., and Wilbanks, G. D.: Clinicopathologic studies in feminizing tumors of the ovary. *Am. J. Obstet. Gynecol.* 112:422, 1972.

Graham, J., Burstein, P., and Graham, R.: Prognostic significance of pleural effusion in ovarian cancer. *Am. J. Obstet. Gynecol.* 106:312, 1970.

Graham, J. B., and Graham, R. M.: Ovarian cancer and asbestosis. *Environ. Res.* 1:115, 1967.

Graham, J. B., Graham, R. M., and Schueller, E. F.: Preclinical detection of ovarian cancer. *Cancer* 17:1414, 1964.

Gray, L. A., and Barnes, M. L.: Endometrioid carcinoma of the ovary. *Obstet. Gynecol.* 29:694, 1967.

Greene, R. R.: Feminizing tumors of the ovary and carcinoma of the endometrium. *Obstet. Gynecol. Ann.* 1973, p. 393.

Greenspan, E. M.: Thio-tepa and methotrexate chemotherapy of advanced ovarian carcinoma. *J. Mt. Sinai Hosp.* 32:52, 1968.

Griffiths, C. T., Grogan, R. H., and Hall, T. C.: Advanced ovarian cancer: Primary treatment with surgery, radiotherapy, and chemotherapy. *Cancer* 29:1, 1972.

Groeber, W. R.: Ovarian tumors during infancy and childhood. *Am. J. Obstet. Gynecol.* 86:1027, 1963.

Grogan, R. H.: Accidental rupture of malignant ovarian cysts during surgical removal. *Obstet, Gynecol.* 30:716, 1967.

Gusberg, S. B., and Kardon, P.: Proliferative endometrial response to theca-granulosa cell tumors. *Am. J. Obstet. Gynecol.* 111:633, 1971.

Hale, R. W.: Krukenberg tumor of the ovaries: A review of 81 records. *Obstet. Gynecol.* 22:221, 1968.

Halpin, R. F., and McCann, T. O.: Dynamics of body fluids following the rapid removal of large volumes of ascites. *Am. J. Obstet. Gynecol.* 110:103, 1971.

Hart, W. R., and Norris, H. J.: Borderline and malignant mucinous tumors of the ovary: Histologic criteria and clinical behavior. *Cancer* 31:1031, 1973.

Harvald, B., and Hauge, M.: Heredity of cancer elucidated by a study of unselected twins. *J. Am. Med. Assoc.* 186:749, 1963.

Henderson, W. J., Joslin, C. A. F., Turnbull, A. C., and Griffiths, K.: Talc and carcinoma of the ovary and cervix. *J. Obstet. Gynaecol. Brit. Commonw.* 78:266, 1971.

Hertig, A. T., and Gore, H.: *Tumors of the Female Sex Organs.* Part 3: Tumors of the Ovary and Fallopian Tube. In *Atlas of Tumor Pathology*, Sect. 9, Fasc. 33. Armed Forces Institute of Pathology, Washington D.C.; 1961.

Hester, L. L., and White, L.: Radioactive colloidal chromic phosphate in the treatment of ovarian malignancies. *Am. J. Obstet. Gynecol.* 103:911, 1969.

Hirabayashi, K., and Graham, J.: Genesis of ascites in ovarian cancer. *Am. J. Obstet. Gynecol.* 106:492, 1970.

Hittle, R. E., Associate Radiologist, Head of Radiotherapy, Children's Hospital of Los Angeles: Personal communication.

Hughesdon, P. E.: Thecal and allied reactions in epithelial ovarian tumors. *J. Obstet. Gynaec. Brit. Emp.* 65:702, 1958.

Huntington, R. W., and Bullock, W. K.: Yolk sac tumors of the ovary. *Cancer* 25:1357, 1970.

Javert, C. T., and Finn, W. F.: Arrhenoblastoma: The incidence of malignancy and the relationship to pregnancy, to sterility, and to treatment. *Cancer* 4:60, 1951.

Jensen, R. D., and Norris, H.J.: Epithelial tumors of the ovary. *Arch. Pathol.* 94:29, 1972.

Johansson, H.: Clinical aspects of metastatic ovarian cancer of extragenital origin. *Acta Obstet. Gynecol. Scand.* 39:681, 1960.

Joshi, V. V.: Primary Krukenberg tumor of ovary: Review of literature and case report. *Cancer* 22:1199, 1968.

Julian, C. G., and Woodruff, J. D.: The role of chemotherapy in the treatment of primary ovarian malignancy. *Obstet. Gynecol. Surv.* 24:1307, 1969.

Julian, C. G., and Woodruff, J. D.: The biologic behavior of low-grade papillary serous carcinoma of the ovary. *Obstet. Gynecol.* **40**:860, 1973.

Kase, N.: Steroid synthesis in abnormal ovaries. II. Granulosa cell tumor. *Am. J. Obstet. Gynecol.* **90**:1262, 1964.

Kase, N., and Conrad, S.: Steroid synthesis in abnormal ovaries. I. Arrhenoblastoma. *Am. J. Obstet. Gynecol.* **90**:1251, 1964.

Keettel, W. C., Fox, M.R., Longnecker, D. S. and Latourette, H. B.: Prophylactic use of radioactive gold in the treatment of primary ovarian cancer. *Am. J. Obstet. Gynecol.* **94**:766, 1966.

Kelley, R. R., and Scully, R. E.: Cancer developing in dermoid cysts of the ovary. *Cancer* **14**:989, 1961.

Kempers, R. D., Dockerty, M. D., Hoffman, D. L., and Bartholoman, L. G.: Struma ovarii—ascitic, hyperthyroid, and asymptomatic syndromes. *Ann. Intern. Med.* **72**:883, 1970.

Kistner, R. W.: Intraperitoneal rupture of benign cystic teratomas: Review of the literature with a report of two cases. *Obstet. Gynecol. Surv.* **7**:603, 1952.

Koller, O., and Gjonnaess, H.: Dysgerminoma of the ovary: A clinical report of 20 cases. *Acta Obstet. Gynecol. Scand.* **43**:268, 1964.

Koss, L. G., Rothschild, E. O., Fleisher, M., and Francis, J. E.: Masculinizing tumor of the ovary apparently with adrenocortical activity. *Cancer*, **23**:1345, 1969.

Kottmeier, H. L.: The classification and treatment of ovarian tumors. *Acta Obstet. Gynecol. Scand.* **31**:313, 1952.

Kottmeier, H. L.: Problems relating to classification and stage-grouping of malignant tumors in the female pelvis. In *Cancer of the Uterus and Ovary*, a collection of papers presented at the Eleventh Annual Clinical Conference on Cancer, The University of Texas, M.D. Anderson Hospital and Tumor Institute. Year Book Medical Publishers, Chicago, 1966, p. 17.

Kottmeier, H. L.: Clinical staging in ovarian carcinoma. In *Ovarian Cancer*, F. Gentil and A. C. Junqueira, Eds. UICC Monograph Series, Vol. 2. Springer-Verlag, New York, 1968a, p. 146.

Kottmeier, H. L.: Surgical management-conservative surgery. In *Ovarian Cancer*, F. Gentil and A. C. Junqueira, Eds., UICC Monograph Series, Vol. 2. Springer-Verlag, New York, 1968b, p. 157.

Kottmeier, H. L.: Treatment of ovarian cancer with thiotepa. *Clin. Obstet. Gynecol.* **11**:428, 1968c.

Koven, B. J., Dollinger, M. R., and Nadel., M. S.: Response to actinomycin D of malignant carcinoid arising in an ovarian teratoma. *Am. J. Obstet. Gynecol.* **101**:267, 1968.

Kurman, R. J., and Craig, J. M.: Endometrioid and clear cell carcinoma of the ovary. *Cancer* **29**:1653, 1972.

Levi, M. M.: Antigenicity of ovarian and cervical malignancies with a view toward possible immunodiagnosis. *Am. J. Obstet. Gynecol.* **109**:689, 1971.

Levi, M. M., Parshley, M. S., and Mandl, I.: Antigenicity of papillary serous cystadenocarcinoma tissue culture cells. *Am. J. Obstet. Gynecol.* **102**:433, 1968.

Li, F. P., Rapoport, A. H., Fraumeni, J. F., and Jensen, R. D.: Familial ovarian carcinoma. *J. Am. Med. Assoc.* **214**:1559, 1970.

Long, M. E., and Taylor, H. C., Jr.: Endometrioid carcinoma of the ovary. *Am. J. Obstet. Gynecol.* **90**:936, 1964.

Lyon, F. A., Sinykin, M. B., and McKelvey, J. L.: Granulosa-cell tumors of the ovary: Review of 23 cases. *Obstet. Gynecol.* **21**:67, 1963.

Malkasian, G. D., Jr., Decker, D. G., Mussey, E., and Johnson, C. E.: Observations on gynecologic malignancy treated with 5-fluorouracil. *Am. J. Obstet. Gynecol.* **100**:1012, 1968.

Malkasian, G. D., Jr., Dockerty, M. B., and Symmonds, R. E.: Benign cystic teratomas. *Obstet. Gynecol.* **29**:719, 1967.

Malkasian, G. D., Jr., and Symmonds, R. E.: Treatment of the unilateral encapsulated ovarian dysgerminoma. *Am. J. Obstet. Gynecol.* **90**:379, 1964.

Malloy, J. J., Dockerty, M. B., Welch, J. S., and Hunt, A. B.: Papillary ovarian tumors. I. Benign tumors and serous and mucinous cystadenocarcinomas. *Am. J. Obstet. Gynecol.* **93**:867, 1965a.

Malloy, J. J., Dockerty, M. B., Welch, J. S., and Hunt, A. B.: Papillary ovarian tumors. II. Endometrioid cancers and mesonephroma ovarii. *Am. J. Obstet. Gynecol.* **93**:880, 1965b.

Marshall, J. R.: Ovarian enlargements in the first year of life: Review of 45 cases. *Ann. Surg.* **161**:372, 1965.

Masopust, J., Kithier, K., Radl, J., Kouteck, Y. G., and Kotal, L.: Occurrence of fetoprotein in patients with neoplasms and nonneoplastic diseases. *Int. J. Cancer* **3**:364, 1968.

Masterson, J. G.: Discussion of paper by Burns, B. C., Rutledge, F. N., et al: Management of ovarian carcinoma. *Am. J. Obstet. Gynecol.* **98**:374, 1967.

Masterson, J. G., and Nelson, J. H., Jr.: The role of chemotherapy in the treatment of gynecologic malignancy. *Am. J. Obstet. Gynecol.* **93**:1102, 1965.

McGowan, L., Stein, D. B., and Miller, W.: Cul-de-sac aspiration for diagnostic cytologic study. *Am. J. Obstet. Gynecol.* **96**:413, 1966.

Meigs, J. V., and Cass, J. W.: Fibroma of the ovary with ascites and hydrothorax with a report of 7 cases. *Am. J. Obstet. Gynecol.* **33**:249, 1937.

Moore, J. G., Schifrin, B. S., and Erez, S.: Ovarian tumors in infancy, childhood, and adolescence. *Am. J. Obstet. Gynecol.* **99**:913, 1967.

Morrow, C. P., and Hart, W. R.: The ovaries. In *Gynecology and Obstetrics: The Health Care of Women*, Seymour Romney et al., Eds. McGraw-Hill, New York, In press.

Munnell, E. W.: The changing prognosis and treatment in cancer of the ovary: A report of 235 patients with primary ovarian carcinoma, 1952-1961. *Am. J. Obstet. Gynecol.* **100**:790, 1968.

Munnell, E. W.: Is conservative therapy ever justified in stage I (Ia) cancer of the ovary? *Am. J. Obstet. Gynecol.* **103**:641, 1969.

Neubecker, R. D., and Breen, J. L.: Embryonal carcinoma of the ovary. *Cancer* **15**:546, 1962a.

Neubecker, R. D., and Breen, J. L.: Gynandroblastoma: A report of five cases, with a discussion of the histogenesis and classification of ovarian tumors. *Am. J. Clin. Pathol.* **38**:60, 1962b.

Nieminen, V., and Purola, E.: Stage and prognosis of ovarian cystadenocarcinomas. *Acta Obstet. Gynecol. Scand.* **49**:49, 1970.

Norris, H. J., and Jensen, R. D.: Relative frequency of ovarian neoplasms in children and adolescents. *Cancer* **30**:713, 1972.

Norris, H. J., and Robinowitz, M.: Ovarian adenocarcinoma of mesonephric type. *Cancer* **28**:1074, 1971.

Norris, H. J., and Taylor, H. B.: Nodular theca-lutein hyperplasia of pregnancy (so-called "pregnancy luteoma"): A clinical and pathological study of 15 cases. *Am. J. Clin. Pathol.* **47**:557, 1967.

Norris, H. J., and Taylor, H. B.: Prognosis of granulosa-theca tumors of the ovary. *Cancer* **21**:255, 1968.

Norris, H. J., and Taylor, H. B.: Virilization associated with cystic granulosa tumors. *Obstet. Gynecol.* **34**:629, 1969.

Novak, E. R., Kutchmeshgi, J., Mupas, R. S., and Woodruff, J. D.: Feminizing gonadal stromal tumors: Analysis of the granulosa-theca cell tumors of the Ovarian Tumor Registry. *Obstet. Gynecol.* **38**:701, 1971.

Novak, E. R., and Long, J. H.: Arrhenoblastoma of the ovary: A review of the Ovarian Tumor Registry. *Am. J. Obstet. Gynecol.* **92**:1082, 1965.

Novak, E. R., and Mattingly, R. F.: Hilus cell tumor of the ovary. *Obstet. Gynecol.* **15**:425, 1960.

O'Hern, T. M., and Neubecker, R. D.: Arrhenoblastoma. *Obstet. Gynecol.* **19**:758, 1962.

O'Neill, R. T., and Mikuta, J. J.: Hypoglycemia associated with serous cystadenocarcinoma of the ovary. *Obstet. Gynecol.* **35**:287, 1970.

Pàloucek, F. P.: Quoted by C. L. Randall. In Gynecologic Oncology, H. R. K. Barber and E. A. Graber, Eds. Williams and Wilkins, Baltimore, 1970, p. 211.

Parker, R. T., Parker, C. H., and Wilbanks, G. D.: Cancer of the ovary: Survival studies based upon operative therapy, chemotherapy, and radiotherapy. *Am. J. Obstet. Gynecol.* **108**:878, 1970.

Pedowitz, P., and O'Brien, F. B.: Arrhenoblastoma of the ovary: Review of the literature and report of 2 cases. *Obstet. Gynecol.* **16**:62, 1960.

Pedowitz, P., Felmus, L. B., and Mackles, A.: Precocious pseudo-puberty due to ovarian tumors. *Obstet. Gynecol. Surv.* **10**:633, 1955.

Perez, C. A. and Bradfield, J. S.: Radiation therapy in the treatment of carcinoma of the ovary. *Cancer* **29**:1027, 1972.

Peterson, W. F., Prevost, E. C., Edmunds, F. T., Hundley, M. Jr., and Morris, F. K.: Benign cystic teratomas of the ovary: A clinicostatistical study of 1,007 cases with a review of the literature. *Am. J. Obstet. Gynecol.* **70**:568, 1955.

Peterson, W. F.: Solid histologically benign teratomas of the ovary. *Am. J. Obstet. Gynecol.* **72**:1094, 1956.

Peterson, W. F.: Malignant degeneration of benign cystic teratomas of the ovary. A collective review of the literature. *Obstet. Gynecol. Surv.* **12**:793, 1957.

Piver, M. S.: Radioactive colloids in the treatment of stage IA ovarian cancer. *Obstet. Gynecol.* **40**:42, 1972.

Purola, E., and Nieminen, U.: Does rupture of cystic carcinoma during operation influence the prognosis? *Ann. Chir. Gynaecol. Fenn.* **57**:615, 1968.

Purola, E.: Serous papillary ovarian tumors: A study of 233 cases with special reference to the histological type of tumor and its influence in prognosis. *Acta Obstet. Gynecol. Scand.* **42**:7, 1963.

Randall, C. L., Hall, D. W., and Armenia, C. S.: Pathology in the preserved ovary after unilateral oophorectomy. *Am. J. Obstet. Gynecol.* **84**:1233, 1962.

Robboy, S. J., and Scully, R E.: Ovarian teratoma with glial implants on the peritoneum: An analysis of 12 cases. *Hum. Pathol.* **1**:643, 1970.

Roth, L. M., and Sternberg, W. H.: Proliferating Brenner tumor. *Cancer* **27**:687, 1971.

Rothman, L. A., Cohen, C. S. and Astarloa, J.: Placental and fetal involvement by maternal malignancy: A report of rectal carcinoma and a review of the literature. *Am. J. Obstet. Gynecol.* **116**:1023, 1973.

Rubin, P.: A critical analysis of current therapy of carcinoma of the ovary: Introduction to symposium. *Am. J. Roentgenal., Radium Ther. Nucl. Med.* **88**:833, 1962.

Rubin, P., Grise, J. W., and Terry, R.: Has postoperative irradiation proved itself? *Am. J. Roentgenol., Radium Ther. Nucl. Med.* **88**:849, 1962.

Salerno, L. J.: Feminizing mesenchymomas of the ovary. *Am. J. Obstet. Gynecol.* **84**:731, 1962.

Samanth, K. K., and Black, W. C.: Benign ovarian stromal tumors associated with free peritoneal fluid. *Am. J. Obstet. Gynecol.* **107**:538, 1970.

Sampson, J. A.: Endometrial carcinoma of ovary arising in endometrial tissue in that organ. *Arch. Surg.* **10**:1, 1925.

Santesson, L., and Marrubini, G.: Clinical and pathological survey of ovarian embryonal carcinomas, including so-called "mesonephromas" (Schiller) or "mesoblastomas" (Teilum), treated at the Radiumhemmet. *Acta Obstet. Gynecol. Scand.* **36**:399, 1957.

Schellhas, H. F., Trujillo, J. M., Rutledge, F. N., and Cork, A.: Germ cell tumors associated with XY gonadal dysgenesis. *Am. J. Obstet. Gynecol.* **109**:1197, 1971.

Schiller, W.: Mesonephroma ovarii. *Am. J. Cancer* **35**:1, 1939.

Schueller, E. F., and Kirol, P. M.: Prognosis in endometrial carcinoma of the ovary. *Obstet. Gynecol.* **27**:850, 1966.

Scully, R. E.: Gonadoblastoma: A gonadal tumor related to the dysgerminoma (seminoma) and capable of sex hormone production. *Cancer* **6**:455, 1953.

Scully, R. E.: Ovarian tumors of germ cell origin. In *Progress in Gynecology*, Vol. 5, S. H. Sturgis and M. L., Taymor, Eds. Grune and Stratton, New York, 1970a.

Scully, R. E.: Recent progress in ovarian cancer. *Hum. Pathol.* **1**:73, 1970b.

Scully, R. E. Sex cord tumor with annular tubules: A distinctive ovarian tumor of the Peutz-Jeghers syndrome. *Cancer* **25**:1107, 1970c.

Scully, R. E.: Gonadoblastoma. *Cancer* **25**:1340, 1970d.

Scully, R. E., Richardson, G. S., and Barlow, J. F.: The development of malignancy in endometriosis. *Clin. Obstet. Gynecol.* **9**:384, 1966.

Shanks, H. G. I.: Pseudomyxoma peritonei. *J. Obstet. Gynaecol Brit. Commonw.* **68**:212, 1961.

Shuster, M., Mendoza-Divino, E., and Joselson, H.: Carcinoid tumor metastasizing to the ovaries. *Obstet. Gynecol.* **36**:515, 1970.

Simmons, R. L., and Sciarra, J. J.: Treatment of late recurrent granulosa cell tumors of the ovary. *Surg. Gynecol. Obstet.* **124**:65, 1967.

Sjostedt, D., and Wahlen, T.: Prognosis of granulosa cell tumours. *Acta Obstet. Gynecol. Scand.* (Suppl. 6) **40**:1, 1961.

Skipper, H. E., Schabel, F. M., and Wilcox, W. S.: On the criteria and kinetics associated with "curability" of experimental leukemia. *Cancer Chemother. Rep.* **35**:1, 1964.

Smith, J. P., and Rutledge, F. N.: Chemotherapy in the treatment of cancer of the ovary. *Am. J. Obstet. Gynecol.* **107**:691, 1970.

Smith, J. P., Rutledge, F. N.: and Sutow, W. W.: Malignant gynecologic tumors in children: Current approaches to treatment. *Am. J. Obstet. Gynecol.* **116**:261, 1973.

Smith, J. P., Rutledge, F. N.: and Wharton, J. T.: Chemotherapy of ovarian cancer: New approaches to treatment. *Cancer* **30**:1565, 1972.

Sobrinho, L. G., Levine, R. A., and DeConti, R. C.: Amenorrhea in patients with Hodgkin's disease treated with antineoplastic agents. *Am. J. Obstet. Gynecol.* **109**:135, 1971.

Spanos, W. J.: Preoperative hormonal therapy of cystic adnexal masses. *Am. J. Obstet. Gynecol.* **116**:551, 1973.

Sternberg, W. H., and Barclay, D. L.: Luteoma of pregnancy. *Am. J. Obstet. Gynecol.* **95**:165, 1966.

Sternberg, W. H., and Gaskill, C. J.: Theca-cell tumors: With a report of twelve new cases and observations on the possible etiologic role of ovarian stromal hyperplasia. *Am. J. Obstet. Gynecol.* **59**:575, 1950.

Symmonds, R. E., and Tauxe, W. N.: Gallium-67 scintigraphy of gynecologic tumors. *Am. J. Obstet. Gynecol.* **114**:356, 1972.

Talerman, A., Huyzinga, W.T., and Kuipers, T.: Dysgerminoma: Clinicopathologic study of 22 cases. *Obstet. Gynecol.* **42**:137, 1973.

Taylor, H. B., Barter, R. H., and Jacobson, C. B.: Neoplasms of dysgenetic gonads. *Am. J. Obstet. Gynecol.* **96**:816, 1966.

Taylor, H. B., and Norris, H. J.: Lipid cell tumors of the ovary: An analysis of 30 cases. *Cancer* **20**:1953, 1967.

Taylor, H. C., Jr., and Alsop, W. E.: Spontaneous regression of peritoneal implantations from ovarian papillary cystadenoma. *Am. J. Cancer* **16**:1305, 1932.

Taylor, H. C., Jr.: Malignant and semimalignant tumors of the ovary. *Surg. Gynecol. Obstet.* **48**:204, 1929.

Teilum, G.: Classification of testicular and ovarian androblastoma and Sertoli cell tumors. *Cancer* **11**:769, 1958.

Teilum, G.: Classification of endodermal sinus tumor (mesoblastoma vitellinum) and so-called "embryonal carcinoma" of the ovary. *Acta Pathol. Microbiol. Scand.* **64**:407, 1965.

Teilum, G.: Endomdermal sinus tumors of the ovary and testis: Comparative morphogenesis of the so-called mesonephroma ovarii (Schiller) and extra-embryonic (yolk sac allantoic) structures of the rat placenta. *Cancer* **12**:1029, 1959.

Teilum, G.: Histogenesis and classification of mesonephric tumors of female and male genital system and relationship to so-called benign adenomatoid tumours (mesotheliomas): Comparative histological study. *Acta Pathol. Microbiol. Scand.* **34**:431, 1954.

Terz, J. J., Barber, H. R. K., and Brunschwig, A.: Incidence of carcinoma in the retained ovary. *Am. J. Surg.* **113**:511, 1967.

Teter, J.: Prognosis, malignancy, and curabilty of the germ-cell tumor occurring in dysgenetic gonads. *Am. J. Obstet. Gynecol.* **108**:894, 1970.

Teter, J., and Boczkowski, K.: Occurrence of tumors in dysgenetic gonads. *Cancer* **20**:1301, 1967.

Thompson, J. P., Dockerty, M. B., Symmonds, R. E., and Hayles, A. B.: Ovarian and parovarian tumors in infants and children. *Am. J. Obstet. Gynecol.* **97**:1059, 1967.

Thurlbeck, W. M., and Scully, R. E: Solid teratoma of the ovary: A clinicopathological analysis of 9 cases. *Cancer* **13**:804, 1960.

Turner, H. B., Douglas, W. M., and Gladding, T. C.: Choriocarcinoma of the ovary. *Obstet. Gynecol.* **24**:918, 1964.

Villasanta, U., and Bloedorn, F. G.: Operation, external irradiation, radioactive isotopes and chemotherapy in treatment of metastatic ovarian malignancies. *Am. J. Obstet. Gynecol.* **102**:531, 1968.

Wallach, R. C., Kabakow, B., Blinick, G., and Antopol, W.: Thiotepa chemotherapy for ovarian carcinoma: Influence of remission and toxicity on survival. *Obstet. Gynecol.* **35**:278, 1970.

Walton, P. D., Jamieson, A. D. and Shingleton, H. M.: The expanding role of diagnostic ultrasound in obstetrics and gynecology. *Surg. Gynecol. Obstet.* **137**:753, 1973.

Webb, M. J., Decker, D. G., Mussey, E., and Williams, T. J.: Factors influencing survival in Stage I ovarian cancer. *Am. J. Obstet. Gynecol.* **116**:222, 1973.

White, K. C.: Ovarian tumors in pregnancy: A private hospital ten year survey. *Am. J. Obstet. Gynecol.* **116**:544, 1973.

Wider, J. A., Marshall, J. R., Bardin, C. W., Lipsett, M. B., and Ross, G. T.: Sustained remissions after chemotherapy for primary ovarian cancers containing choriocarcinoma. *N. Engl. J. Med.* **280**:1439, 1969.

Wider, J. A., and O'Leary, J. A.: Dysgerminoma: A clinical review. *Obstet. Gynecol.* **31**:560, 1968.

Wilkinson, E. J., Friedrich, E. G., and Hosty, T. A.: Alpha-fetoprotein and endodermal sinus tumor of the ovary. *Am. J. Obstet. Gynecol.* **116**:711, 1973.

Williams, T. J., Symmonds, R. E., and Litwak, O.: Management of unilateral and encapsulated ovarian cancer in young women. *Gynecol. Oncol.* **1**:143, 1973.

Wisniewski, M., and Deppisch, L. M.: Solid teratomas of ovary. *Cancer* **32**:440, 1973.

Woodruff, J. D., Bie, L. S., and Sherman, R. J.: Mucinous tumors of the ovary. *Obstet. Gynecol.* **16**:699, 1960.

Woodruff, J. D., and Julian, C. G.: Histologic grading and morphologic changes of significance in the treatment of semi-malignant and malignant ovarian tumors. *Proc. Nat. Cancer Conf.* **6**:346, 1970.

Woodruff, J. D., Murthy, Y. S., Bhaskar, T. N., Bordbar, F., and Tseng, S. S.: Metastatic ovarian tumors. *Am. J. Obstet. Gynecol.* **107**:202, 1970.

Woodruff, J. D., Noli Castillo, R. D., and Novak, E. R.: Lymphoma of the ovary: A study of 35 cases from the Ovarian Tumor Registry of the American Gynecological Society. *Am. J. Obstet. Gynecol.* **85**:912, 1963;

Woodruff, J. D., and Novak, E. R.: Papillary serous tumors of the ovary. *Am. J. Obstet. Gynecol.* **67**:1112, 1954.

Woodruff, J. D., and Novak, E. R.: The Krukenberg tumor: Study of 48 cases from the Ovarian Tumor Registry. *Obstet. Gynecol.* **15**:351, 1960.

Woodruff, J. D., Protos, P., and Peterson, W. F.: Ovarian teratomas: Relationship of histologic and ontogenic factors to prognosis. *Am. J. Obstet. Gynecol.* **102**:702, 1968.

Woodruff, J. D., Rauh, J. T., and Markley, R. L.: Ovarian struma. *Obstet. Gynecol.* **27**:194, 1966.

Wynder, E. L., Dodo, H., and Barber, H. R. K.: Epidemiology of cancer of the ovary. *Cancer* **23**:352, 1969.

CHAPTER SIX

Cancer
of the Vagina

Although cancer of the vagina has always been overshadowed in importance by the more frequently occurring malignant neoplasms of the cervix and vulva, it accounts for 1-4% of all gynecologic malignancies. These lesions may be more frequent than suspected, but because of the intermediate position of the vagina and the greater frequency of cancer in the cervix and the vulva, an advanced vaginal lesion would often be considered as an extension of cancer in one of these sites. Historically there is a prevailing feeling of hopelessness about this lesion. This has its origin in the writings of Taussig (1935), whose pessimism was stated as follows: "Primary cancer of the vagina is rare and most universally fatal." Recent reports on the outcome of this disease, however, have been less discouraging.

Nearly all primary vaginal tumors are squamous in type. Adenocarcinoma, sarcoma, and melanoma of the vagina have been reported, but collectively comprise less than 8% of all vaginal cancer.

6-1 LOCATION OF PRIMARY LESION

The vagina is a thin walled structure with a rich lymphatic drainage. This may account for early lymph mode metastasis and the poor survial rates recorded by early authors. When one considers the different pathways for lymphatic drainage from various areas of the vagina, the specific location of vaginal neoplasms may be quite important. The lymphatic efferents of the vault are similar to those of the cervix and lead to lateral and posterior pelvic nodes. The lymphatics from the central portion of the vagina form collecting trunks laterally. The lateral trunks from the anterior portion of the vagina terminate in nodes at the lateral pelvic wall or in the paravesicle nodes. The lateral trunks from the posterior wall of the vagina drain to the deep pelvic nodes and the area of the inferior gluteal artery. The lower portion of the vagina, especially around the vestibule, connects with a network of lymphatics that drains to the regional nodes in the femoral triangle (see Fig. 6-1).

A large majority of vaginal lesions are found on the posterior wall of the upper third of the vagina. The fact that slightly more than half of all primary vaginal cancers occur in this upper third of the vagina on the posterior wall has led to some speculation concerning the etiology of vaginal cancer, and many have suggested the probability that accumulation of irritating or macerating material in the posterior fornix may produce chronic irritation and thereby give rise to the malignant change. This hypothesis has of course, never been substantiated and is made doubtful by the fact that the second most common site for carcinoma of the vagina appears to be the anterior aspect of the lower third, where no such pooling of material can occur. Reports have been written concerning possible predisposing factors, such as pessary, prolapse, repeated pregnancies, irritating chemicals, syphilis, leukorrhea, and leukoplakia, but nothing definite has ever been uncovered. It is fairly well established that lesions of the lower third of the vagina are spread by way of the femoral nodes, as one would expect in view of the lymphatic drainage of this area. Positive inguinal nodes have also been documented in cases of

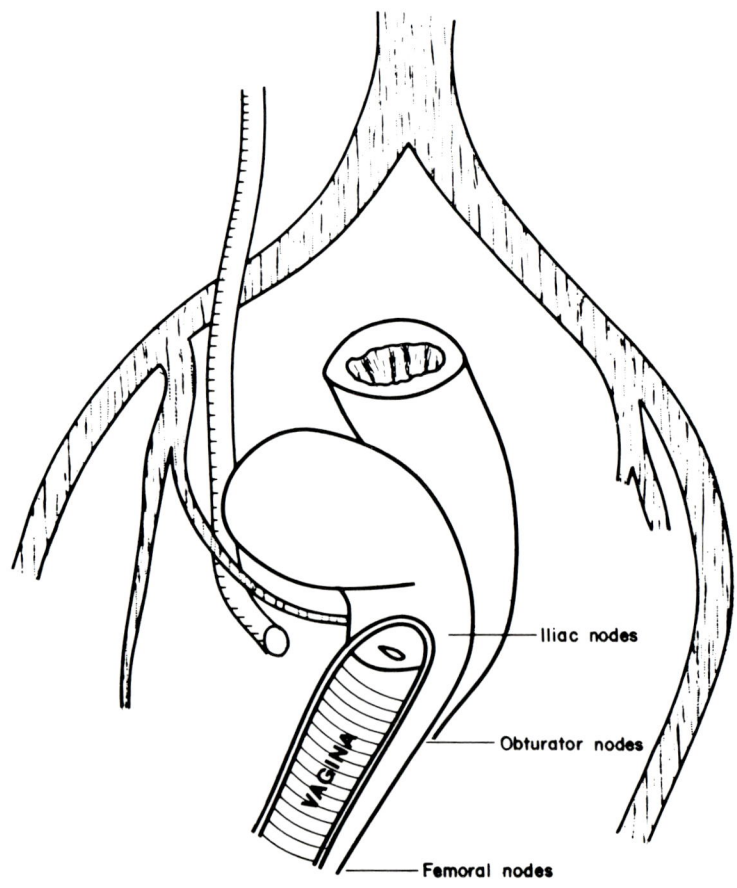

Fig. 6-1 Lymphatic drainage of the individual thirds of the vagina.

carcinoma of the vagina arising in the middle and upper thirds; these are problably explained by the very rich anastomoses between the lymphatics of this organ.

In general, it has been found that patients with lesions limited to the upper third of the posterior vagina have a much better prognosis than those with tumors located elsewhere. In a review of 104 patients, Smith (1955) found 6.8% survivors among 29 patients with cancer in the lower third of the vagina, 25.0% in 48 patients with middle third tumors, and 37.0% in 27 patients with upper third lesions. Merrill and Bender (1958) contrasted 28.6% cures in 14 upper third tumors with 11.1% in 9 tumors located in the distal third. It appears that cancers located on the posterior aspects of the upper third of the vagina do not metastasize as readily as those arising elsewhere. Moreover, they lend themselves more easily to currently available conventional forms of therapy applicable in like manner to the much more common cancer of the cervix.

6-2   STAGING CLASSIFICATION

Stage I   Carcinoma is limited to the vagina.
Stage II   Carcinoma has involved the subvaginal tissue but has not extended onto the pelvic wall.
Stage III   Carcinoma has extended onto the pelvic wall.
Stage IV   Carcinoma has extended beyond the true pelvis or has involved the bladder or the rectum. Bullous edema or tumor bulge into the bladder or rectum is not acceptable evidence of invasion of these organs.

As with other pelvic malignancies, staging is done in a manner that gives consideration both to the bulk of the primary lesion and to the involvement of neighboring structures.

The symptoms of cancer of the vagina are similar in some respects to those of cervical cancer. Vaginal bleeding and discharge are the most frequent symptoms in most series. Most patients with invasive lesions have had vaginal bleeding, and gross lesions are found on examination (Fig. 6-2). *In situ* lesions are usually found by the use of vaginal Papanicolaou smears. Bladder pain and frequent voiding are more common as early symptoms of vaginal cancer than of cervical cancer. This is not surprising since a lower growth in the vagina would be nearer the vesicle neck with resulting compression of the bladder at an earlier stage of the disease. Continuing to spread, such a cancer quite commonly involves the paracolpos, bladder, rectum, and vulva. Involvement of the cervix is more or less precluded because of the restriction imposed by the criteria for case selection, those involving the cervix ordinarily being deemed to have arisen in that organ.

Special charcteristics appear to apply with reference to spread to adjacent structures according to the location of the tumor in the vagina. Anterior vaginal tumors penetrate relatively early into the subjacent bladder wall, whereas posterior tumors merely displace and distend the more elastic vagina in that location. It appears that the posterior wall can be distended considerably by the rapidly growing tumor before deep layers are invaded. By contrast, the anterior wall tends to be fixed and the tumor penetrates earlier in its course to the mucosa of the bladder, creating early bladder symtomatology. The elasticity of the posterior vaginal wall favors local growth. It is noted that tumors of the upper posterior vagina grow to a rather large size, filling the upper vagina, without necessarily penetrating the muscularis or involving the lymphatics or areolar tissue in the rectovaginal septum. Decreased distensibility and elasticity of the anterior vaginal mucosa favors the

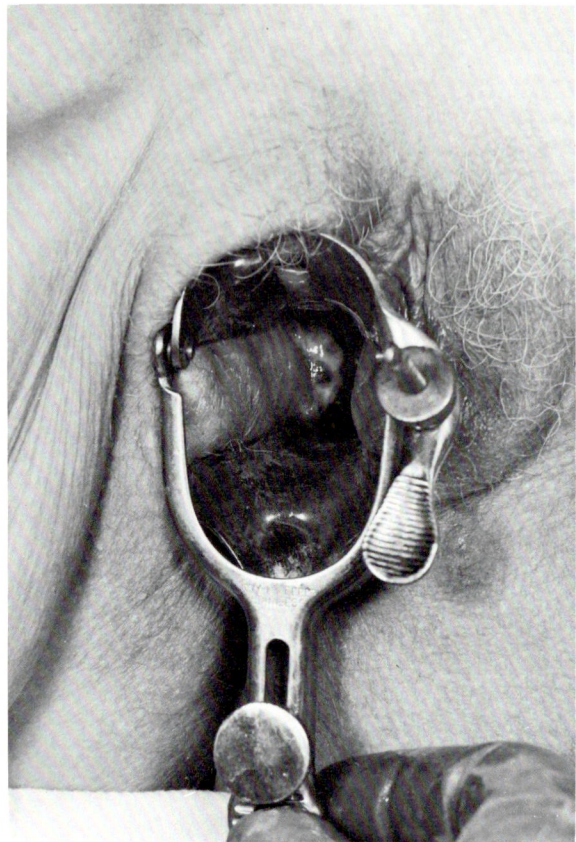

Fig. 6-2 Stage I squamous cell carcinoma of the middle third of the vagina, presented as postmenopausal bleeding.

spread of tumors located in the vicinity of the bladder neck and urethra relatively early in the course of their natural history and accounts for the poor prognosis.

6-3 THERAPY

Unfortunately these lesions are often well advanced before symptoms appear. Also physician error apprears not uncommon, lesions being either missed or misdiagnosed. Frick et al (1968) found that the diagnosis had been missed on first examination in 10 of the 52 patients he reviewed. Palmer and Biback (1954) reported doctor delay in diagnosis of 10 months on the average in 25 of their patients, with delays as long as 36 months in 3 of them. In 19, no pelvic examination was done at all in spite of the presenting complaint referrable to this area; in 6 others, local ineffectual treatment was given without first establishing the diagnosis. The special anatomy of the vagina favoring early spread, particularly its thin wall, loose areolar investiture, and rich lymphatic system, has been discussed above. Also, the rarity of vaginal cancer mitigates against this consideration as a likely diagnosis.

The technical difficulties of applying satisfactory radiation dosage to tumors of the vagina, especially those located in the lower aspects, are great. Therefore it is not uncommon to find irradiation dosage of inadequate amounts. Surgical approach to this area may have to be ultraradical and therefore not applicable to most patients because of advanced age. Almost half of the patients are 60 years of age or older, with a peak incidence of disease in the 50-70 year age group.

Because of the close proximity of the bladder and the rectum to the vagina, the treatment of invasive squamous cell carcinoma of the vagina with surgery usually involves radical procedures, including exenteration. Radiation therapy is therefore the treatment of choice with many individuals since it allows for both preservation of the vagina and markedly less risk to the patient's life. The only question that remains, of course, is whether irradiation therapy can provide comparable survivals. As one reviews the series of vaginal cancers, it is difficult to find any institution that has alternately treated its patients with either surgery or irradiation therapy. However, it would appear from analysis of several series that irradiation therapy results in survival rates that are comparable to those in the best of surgical series. A report by Rutledge (1967) listed 3 and 5 year survival rates of 42 and 44%, respectively, for patients treated primarily with radiotherapy. A recent report by Brown et al (1971) gives more details on survival with regard to stage (Table 6-1).

The treatment plan with regard to irradiation therapy must consider the depth of invasion of the lesion. Lesions with significant invasion of the paracolpos are treated with whole pelvis irradiation followed by interstitial implantation of the tumor bed. Many have preferred vaginal applicators to deliver the radium portion of the therapy. However, these applicators have their limitations in that the depth dose obtained is seldom effective for more than a half centimeter below the vaginal mucosa. Therefore, unless there are multifocal lesions, it seems more appropriate to utilize interstitial implantation of the tumor bed with radium needles (Fig. 6-3a). This type of treatment plan has resulted in excellent survivals in the series reviewed by Brown et al from M. D. Anderson Hospital. Vaginal applicators such as the Bloedorn applicator are, on the other hand, an excellent treatment device for carcinoma *in situ* of the vagina, where depth dose is not a consideration.

The limitations imposed by the radiotherapeutic index, referred to in Chapter 7 on vulvar cancer, is applicable here as well. Although we are not dealing with radioresistant neoplasms in a radiosensitive bed, real limitations exist nonetheless. The proximity of relatively radio-sensitive tissues, such as the bladder and rectum, provides a challenge especially in treating tumors located in the lower thirds of the vagina. Similar limitations

TABLE 6-1   5 YEAR SURVIVAL RATES
FOR PATIENTS WITH INVASIVE
SQUAMOUS CELL CARCINOMA OF VAGINA

Stage	Absolute	Corrected[a]
I	11/16 (69%)	11/13 (85%)
II	13/19 (68%)	13/17 (76%)
III	4/15 (27%)	4/10 (40%)
IV	0/11	0/9

[a]Corrections for intercurrent disease taken from Brown et al (1971).

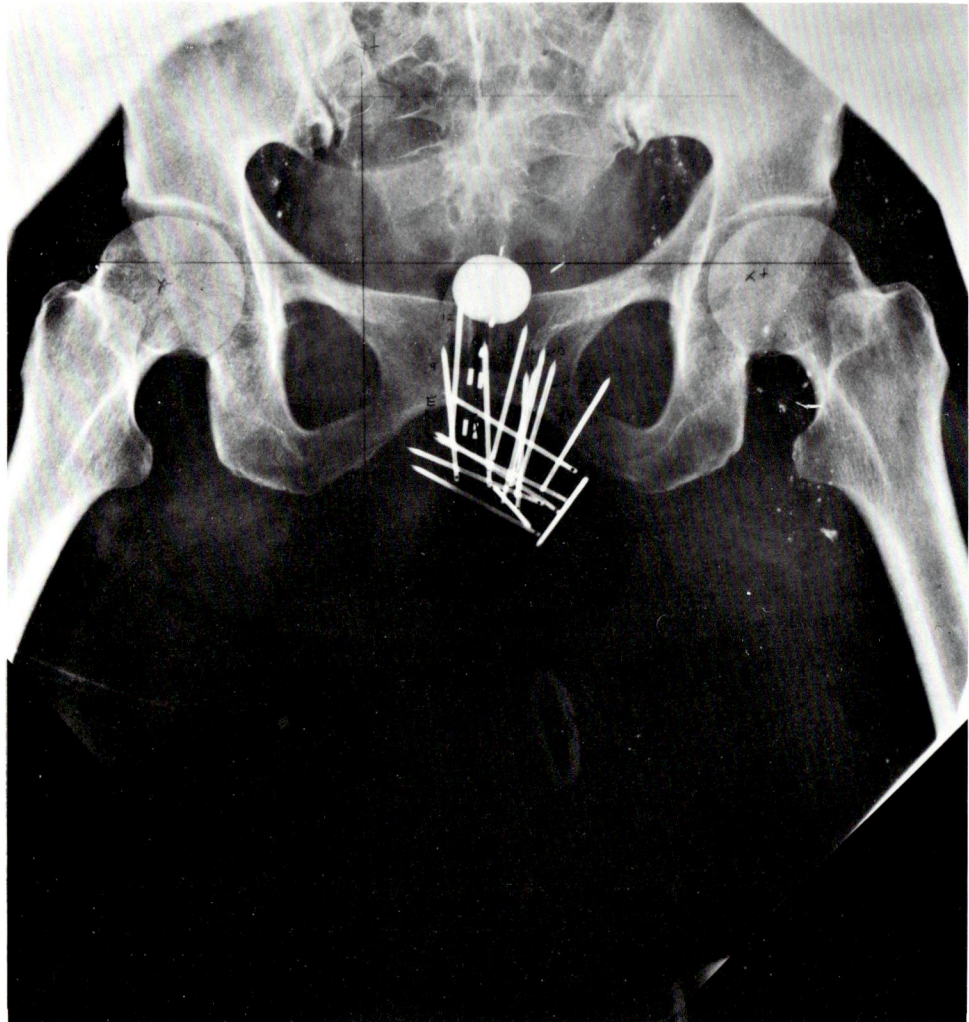

Fig.Fig. 6-3a Volume implant with radium needles in a patient with squamous cell carcinoma of the lower one third of the vagina.

apply, of course, to radiotherapy for carcinoma of the cervix but to a lesser degree. It is assumed that with judicious selection of radiation dosage (Table 6-2), placement of sources, filters, and so forth it should be possible to minimize the more serious complications of acute radiation reactions of these organs. Careful use of therapy is necessary in the treatment of vaginal carcinoma, especially when it involves the lower two thirds of the vagina (Fig. 6-3b).

The difficulty in applying radiation systems to vaginal lesions has led some to advocate a surgical approach. As early as 1905, Wertheim treated several patients with carcinoma of the vagina with radical hysterecomy and vaginectomy. He performed a radical hysterectomy, using the technique developed for cervical cancer together with complete isolation of the vaginal tube down to the introitis. He then completed the procedure with a perineal approach, making a circular incision at the introitis and removing the rest of the vagina from below. It is a tribute to his skill that two of the four patients he operated

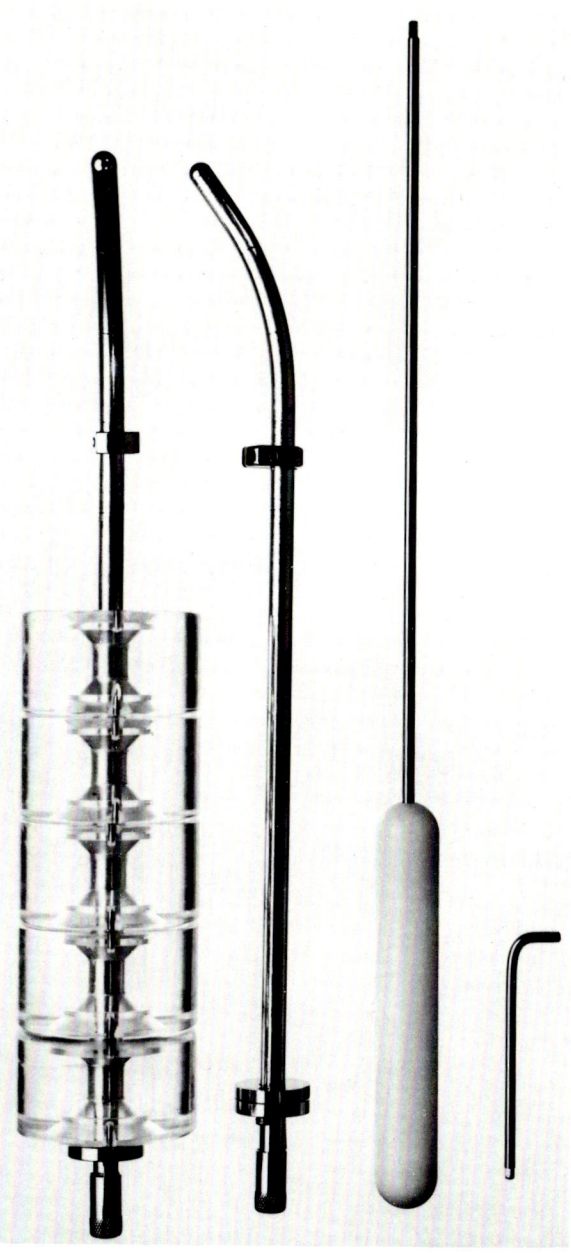

Fig. 6-3*b* Delclos uterine-vaginal afterload applicator. Centrally loaded Lucite cylinders range from 2.0 to 4.5 cm and will fit tandems with varying curves.

on were still alive and apparently free of disease 5 years after their operations. In 1948, Stanley Way attempted to approach this lesion by performing an anterior exenteration. His technique was adopted by Alexander Brunschwig, who utilized exenteration consistently for the treatment of carcinoma of the vagina. The complications associated with these procedures, especially in this older group of patients, constitute the limiting factor to the surgical approach.

TABLE 6-2   RADIATION THERAPY—SUGGESTED TREATMENT PLANS

Stage	External	Local
0	None	6000-9000 rads to mucosa
I (thick)	4000-5000 rads whole pelvis	Intersititial implant, 3000-4000 rads
(thin)	None	Interstitial implant, 6000-7000 rads
II	4000-5000 rads whole pelvis	Interstitial implant, 3000-4000 rads
III	5000 rads whole pelvis 2000 rads (10 X 10 cm. field)	None
IV	5000 rads whole pelvis and individualize	

Some have expressed doubts, questioning the value of ultraradical surgery for vaginal carcinoma specifically. Merrill and Bender (1958), for example, note that few authors have reported any success with the surgical management of vaginal carcinoma. Their experience is that the procedure is often incomplete. It can be said that the superiority of radical surgery to the radiation treatment of cancer of the vagina is yet to be demonstrated. However, it has been shown that radical operations can be curative, especially in selected cases. The difficulty is that the disease often involves the levator ani muscles, especially when the tumor is located in the middle or lower third of the vagina. This necessitates removal of most, if not all, of the levator ani sling, thus contributing considerably to the morbidity of these radical procedures. The most ardent supporters of radiation therapy, however, suggest that surgery may be useful in the treatment of radiation failures. Similarly, supporters of the surgical approach, such as Palumbo et al (1969), utilize radiation for recurrences after surgery.

6-4   THREE RARE VAGINAL CANCERS

Adenocarcinoma of the Vagina

Adenocarcinoma arising in the vagina is one of the rarest gynecologic malignancies. Origin from paramesonephric (müllerian) epithelium, mesonephric remnants (Gartner's duct), and endometriosis has been postulated. In 1971 Herbst et al reported several cases of clear cell adenocarcinoma of the vagina (Fig. 6-4). This dramatic clustering of cases prompted an epidemiologic study that demonstrated an association of this malignancy with maternal ingestion of diethylstilbestrol (DES), a nonsteroidal estrogenic substance that was commonly used in the management of threatened abortion, habitual abortion, diabetic pregnancies, and other high risk obstetrical problems. This association has been confirmed by the national registry established by these investigators. By the end of 1973, almost 200 cases of clear cell carcinoma of the vagina and cervix were registered. Nearly all of the females with DES associated vaginal and cervical adenocarcinomas have been

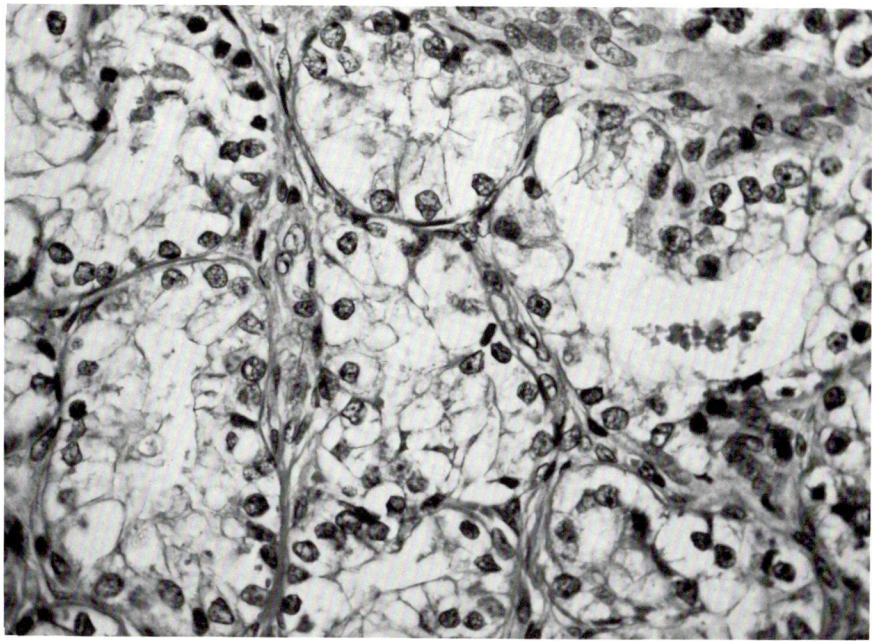

Fig. 6-4 Photomicrograph of a clear cell carcinoma of the vagina occurring in a 14 year old girl who was a stilbestrol exposed offspring.

postmenarchial and less than 30 years of age, with an average age of 17½. The primary symptoms are abnormal bleeding and vaginal discharge. Because of the threat posed by this malignancy, it is no longer acceptable to manage abnormal perimenarchial vaginal bleeding and vaginal discharge without a gynecologic examination. Pap smears alone are not reliable to exclude the presence of adenocarcinoma in these individuals.

The optimum therapy for clear cell carcinoma of the vagina and cervix has not been established. The incidence of lymph node metastasis is fairly high, approximately 18% in Stage I and 30% or more in Stage II. The neoplasm tends to remain superficial, suggesting the possibility that this disease can be treated locally, especially if the lesion is small. However, one instance of pelvic node metastasis has been reported in a patient with less than 3 mm of invasion. If the growth is confined to the cervix, radical hysterectomy and pelvic lymphadenectomy are the recommended therapy, with retention of the ovaries More extensive tumors and lesions involving the vagina are more suitable for irradiation, which should include the pelvic nodes and parametrial tissues. Survival is stage related, but 5 year follow-up data are not available at this time.

Systematic examinination of DES exposed offspring, whether symptomatic or not, has disclosed that at least 60% have vaginal adenosis, that is, endocervical-like epithelium in the vagina. A smaller portion of cases has minor anomalies of the cervix and vagina. The origin of clear cell adenocarcinoma from adenosis remains to be established. It is not known whether only offspring with adenosis are at risk for developing adenocarcinoma. Diethylstilbestrol exposed offspring also may have an increased risk of developing squamous neoplasia because of the large transformation zone (see Section 2-1 on preinvasive disease of the cervix and Chapter 3 on colposcopy). Although a few cases of dysplasia and carcinoma *in situ* associated with adenosis have been reported, the risk of developing squamous lesions remains speculative at the present time since no DES exposed offspring have entered the age group for which squamous cell carcinoma is most prevalent.

All DES exposed females should undergo a gynecologic examination on a semiannual basis begining at age 14 or at menarche, whichever occurs first. Examination should include a careful inspection of the cervix and vagina before and after Lugol's stain. Cytology is obtained by scraping the cervix and any suspicious area in the vagina. Palpation of the vagina, including the rectovagingal septum, should be performed. Colposcopic examination helps to identify areas for biopsy and is recommended as part of the routine evaluation. Regular examination hopefully will permit detection of adenocarcinoma and squamous neoplasia during their earliest stages of development. No active management is recommended for vaginal adenosis, which, like normal columnar epithelium on the ectocervix, will be physiologically transformed into squamous epithelium. To date, DES exposed male offspring have shown no adverse effects.

Stilbestrol and related compounds (hexestrol, dienestrol) are absolutely contraindicated in pregnancy. Whether steroidal estrogens administered exogenously are capable of inducing similar abnormalities is unknown.

Sarcoma of the Vagina

Spindle cell sarcomas of the vagina such as leiomyosarcoma and fibrosarcoma have been reported but are quite rare. These malignancies tend to behave in a manner similar to their corresponding cell types on the vulva in that well differentiated lesions have a good prognosis with clinical removal of the area and pleomorphic lesions have a poor prognosis regardless of therapy.

Like soft tissue sarcomas of the vulva and elsewhere in the genital tract, lymphatic system involvement is an integral aspect of the natural history of sarcomas of the vagina. This is probably due to the rich network of lymphatics surrounding the vagina. Hematogenous dissemination appears to occur relatively late in the course of this disease, so that the very grave prognosis for sarcomas encountered elsewhere and the hopelessness of local therapy are perhaps not entirely applicable here. There are several reports of patients with long-term survival after local excision of the lesion and local radiation therapy postoperatively. In some cases local growth is encountered with death from urinary complications before distant metastatic dissemination can occur. In 1967 Rutledge reported four patients, one of whom had leiomyosarcoma. Two were treated with only interstitial irradiation; one died after 1 year, and the other was living and well 4 years later. The patient with leiomyosarcoma was treated by external radiation only and survived for 1 year before she was lost to follow-up. The fourth was treated by a combination of external x-ray and actinomycin D therapy; she died in less than 1 year.

Another rare and tragic lesion predominately of childhood is sarcoma botryoides. Such lesions are usually multicentric and tend to arise on the anterior wall at the apex of the vagina. They are quite immature histologically and resemble embryonic mesenchymal tissue. Rhabdomyoblastic elements are not uncommon. In contrast to the histologic appearance of other mixed mesodermal lesions, cartilage and bone are generally not found. Delay in diagnosis is common; there have been several reports of delays of up to 4 years before instituting definitive therapy. Diagnosis of any vaginal polypoid lesion in a child and prompt investigation of genital bleeding are mandatory in order to avoid these costly delays. These lesions are deceptively superficial, arising as they do from epithelial tissues in several sites simultaneously to give the appearance of simple polyps. These patients present most frequently with vaginal bleeding or discharge. Although the upper anterior vaginal wall is the most common site, these tumors may arise from other locations. They grow very rapidly and fill the vagina, protruding through the introitis, where grapelike tumors become apparent externally. Generally, it has been accepted that these lesions do not metastasize as widely in children in the early stages; however, they have been reported in the femoral, parametrial, pelvic, and paraaortic lymph nodes, as well as the vulva, the lung, and extensively in the abdominal viscera. Huffman (1968) reviewed 150 cases and found 19 patients surviving for more than three years and twelve for more than five years. Six of them had been treated by exenteration, two by radical hystero-vaginectomy, 5 by lesser operative procedures, 4 by combined surgery and irradiation, one by x-ray alone, and three by unknown means. In 1967 Rutledge and Sullivan reported four survivors among five children with sarcoma botryoides treated by exenteration, although follow-up at the time of their report was not prolonged, extending for six months, two, four, and five years, respectively. Since the actual extent of the disease cannot be readily determined on a clinical basis, these extremes of radicality in the surgical approach appear justified, no matter how reluctant one might be to undertake such procedures with young patients.

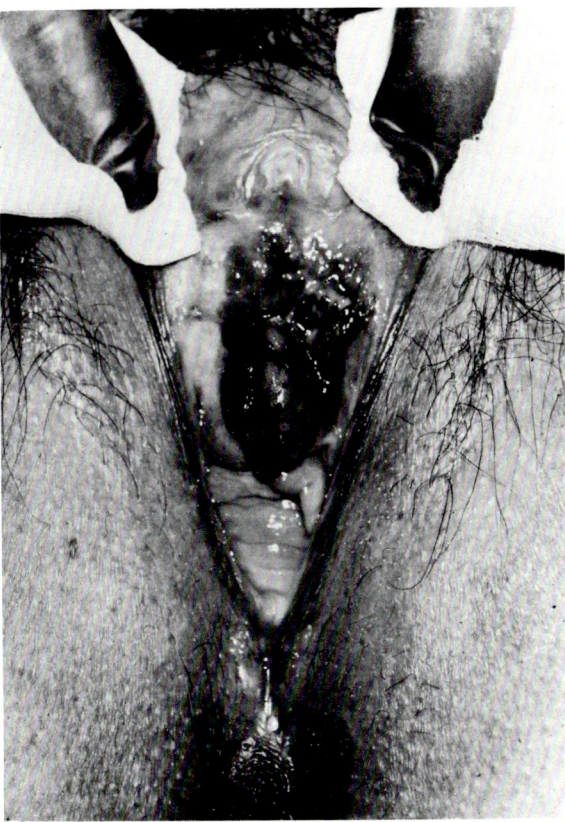

Fig. 6-5 Melanoma occurring on the lower one third of the vagina and involving the periurethral tissue.

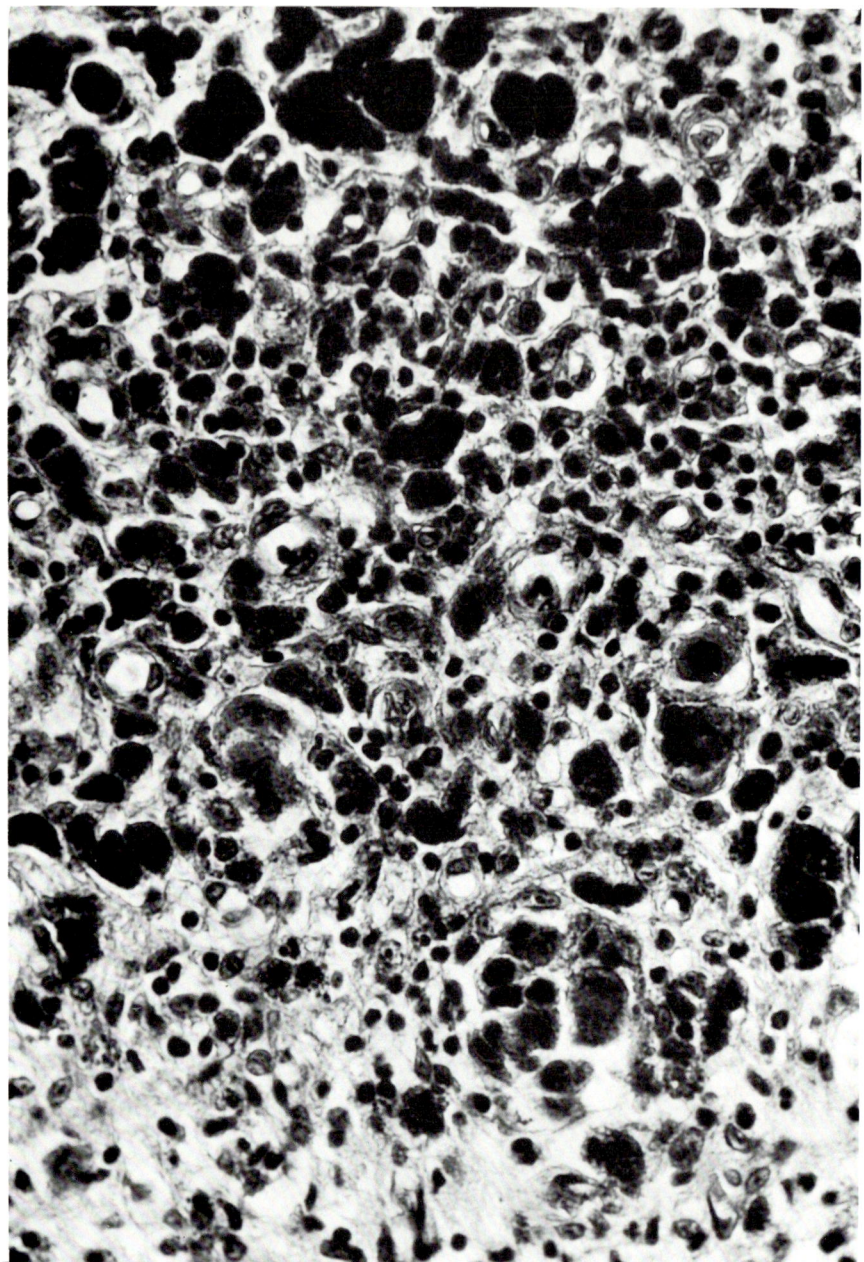

Fig. 6-6 Photomicrograph of lesion seen in Fig. 6-5. Note the heavy, dark staining pigment in many of the cells.

Malignant Melanoma

The extreme rarity of this lesion is indicated by the incidence of only 2 cases among over 116 patients with vaginal carcinoma collected from a cumulative study (Fricke et al,

1954). The developmental characteristics of this neoplasm appear to be the same in the vagina as in the vulva, and rapid progression with hematogenous dissemination is common, producing distant metastasis and death in most cases. The site of origin is usually difficult to determine since these lesions grow rapidly. They are recognized readily by their color (Fig. 6-5 and 6-6). By infiltrating the surface of the vagina they often cause ulceration of the vaginal membrane. They may extend exophytically into the vagina to produce a fungating lesion or may grow directly into the bladder or rectum and spread cephalically to invade the cervix, cardinal ligament, and peritoneum. In the vagina, unlike the vulva, hematogenous dissemination appears to be common.

Surgery appears to be the treatment of choice, and the extent of the surgery depends on the location of the lesion. Lesions involving the lower third of the vagina usually are treated with vulvectomy and groin and deep node dissection in addition to radical hysterectomy and vaginectomy. For lesions involving the upper two-thirds of the vagina, some form of exenteration with pelvic lymphadenectomy is the usual treatment. Experience with this disease is so scattered that survival rates are not available. The outlook for these patients is poor, however, since the lesion is often quite advanced at the time when therapy is begun.

REFERENCES

Brown, A. R., Fletcher, G. H., and Rutledge, F. N.: Irradiation of *"in situ"* and invasive squamous cell carconoma of the vagina. *Cancer* 28:1278, 1971.

Dunn, L. J., et al: Primary carcinoma of vagina. *Am. J. Obstet Gynecol.* 96:1112, 1966.

Frick, H. C. et al: Primary carcinoma of vagina. *Am. J. Obstet. Gynecol.* 101:695, 1968.

Fricke, R. E., VanHerik, M., and Soule, E. H.: Treatment of rare lesions on the uterus and vagina. Radiology 63:353, 1954.

Gray, L. et al: *In situ* and early invasive carcinoma of vagina. *Obstet. Gynecol.* 34:226, 1969.

Greenwald, P., et al: Vaginal cancer after maternal treatment with synthetic estrogens *N. Eng. J. Med.* 285:390, 1971.

Herbst, A. L.: Current data from the clear cell adenocarcinoma registry. Presented at the 5th Annual Meeting of the Society of Gynecolgic Oncologists, Key Biscayne, Fla. January 9, 1974.

Herbst, A. L., Green, T. H., and Ulfelder, H.: Primary carcinoma of vagina. *Am. J. Obstet. Gynecol.* 106:210, 1970.

Herbst, A. L., Ulfelder, H., and Poskanzer, E. C.: Adenocarcinoma of the vagina: Association of maternal stilbestrol therapy with tumor appearance in young women. *N. Engl. J. Med.* 284:878, 1971.

Herbst, A. L., et al: Clear cell adenocarcinoma of the genital tract in young females: Registry Report. *N. Engl. J. Med.* 287:1259, 1972.

Huffman, J. W.: *The Gynecology of Childhood and Adolescence*. W. B. Saunders, Philadelphia, 1968.

Latourette, H. B.: End results of treatment of cancer of vagina. *Ann. N. Y. Acad. Sci.* 114:1020, 1964.

Merrill, J. A., and Bender W. T.: Primary carcinoma of the vagina. *Obstet. Gynecol.* 11:3, 1958.

Nolan, J., and Weaver, P.: Unpublished data.

Palmer, J. P., and Biback S. M.: Primary cancer of the vagina. *Am. J. Obstet. Gynecol.* 67:377, 1954.

Palumbo, L., et al: Primary carcinoma of vagina. South. Med. J. 62:1048, 1969.

Rutledge, F. N. Cancer of vagina. *Am. J. Obstet. Gynecol.* 97:635, 1967.

Rutledge, F. N. and Sullivan, M.: Sarcoma botryoides. *Ann. N. Y. Sci.* 142:694, 1967.

Single, B. D.: Primary carcinoma of vagina. *Cancer*, September 1951, p. 1073.

Smith, F. R., Primary carcinoma of vagina. *Am. J. Obstet. Gynecol.* 69:525, 1955.

Taussig, F. J.: Primary cancer of the vulva, vagina and female urethra. *Surg. Gynecol. Obstet.* **60**:477, 1935.

Way, S.: Primary carcinoma of the vagina. *J. Obstet. Gynaecol. Brit. Emp.* **55**:739, 1948.

Wertheim, E.: Abdominal exstirpierte schiedenkarzinome. Zbl. gynäk **29**:1218, 1905.

Whitehouse, W. L.: Primary carcimona of vagina. *J. Obstet. Gynaecol. Brit. Commonw.* **69**:481, 1962.

CHAPTER SEVEN

Cancer of the Vulva

Vulvar carcinoma is the fourth most common of primary pelvic cancers, being exceeded in frequency by cervix, corpus, and ovarian cancer, and accounts for 3-4% of all primary malignancies of the genital canal. It is preeminently a disease of elderly women, the incidence being highest in the seventh decade.

In the past three decades, a number of reports have confirmed that radical vulvectomy and inguinal lymphadenectomy constitute the appropriate treatment for invasive carcinoma of the vulva. Pelvic lymphadenectomy has been utilized by some surgeons, but recently most gynecologic oncologists have selected the cases for inclusion of this procedure. Here, as with other gynecologic malignancies, individualization of treatment has resulted in the best overall results, considering both the intention of cure and the quality of life. Neoplasms occurring on the vulva differ quite distinctly from skin cancers arising elsewhere in the body in terms of their malignant potential. Treatment philosophy, therefore, must be more aggressive. Cancer of the vulva is recognized as a serious disease that requires radical weapons to effect cure. The treatment plan can bring success only if it is based on a logical approach, designed to result in eradication of the disease locally and in all sites of spread.

7-1 VULVAR INTRAEPITHELIAL CARCINOMA

A confusing issue is the classification and role of vulvar dystrophies in the etiology of vulvar cancer. Table 7-1 categorizes vulvar dystrophy into distinct groups that have varying premalignant potentials. Although vulvar cancer has been reported coexistently with each of these conditions, it is more commonly associated with dystrophies heralded by dysplasia and/or epithelial atypia.

A primary determining factor in management is the demonstration of invasion through the basement membrane into the connective tissue stroma.

TABLE 7-1   VULVAR DYSTROPHIES

1. Hyperplastic
   a. Benign epithelial hyperplasia
      (neurodermatitis or lichen simplex chronicus)
   b. Atypical epithelial hyperplasia (dysplasia)
2. Atrophic—lichen sclerosus et atrophicus (LSA)
3. Mixed—LSA with foci of epithelial hyperplasia
   a. Without atypia
   b. With atypia

At times the malignancy remains intraepithelial, spreading in the epidermis and persisting within its confines. Intraepithelial carcinoma is regarded as a preinvasive lesion and is often referred to as Bowen's disease or carcinoma *in situ* of the vulva (Fig. 7-1). Treatment of this disease is simply local removal. However, since the disease is often multifocal or diffuse (Fig. 7-2), local removal usually means removal of the entire vulvar skin. In young individuals this can be combined with placement of a skin graft over the surgical defect (Rutledge & Sinclair 1968). This is removed from the medial aspect of the thigh or buttock, and the result is cosmetically quite satisfactory. Others have treated this disease with either local excision of the lesion or with topical 5-fluorouracil (5-FU) ointment; the latter treatment is investigational, however, and requires extremely close observation of the patient. In general, the standard treatment at the present time for multifocal Bowen's disease of the vulva is a simple vulvectomy with or without the application of a skin graft.

Another form of intraepithelial neoplasia of the vulva is Paget's disease (Fig. 7-3). This relatively rare condition manifests itself as a red, moist, slightly elevated patch that remains unchanged for long periods and is of doubtful malignancy to the observer. The

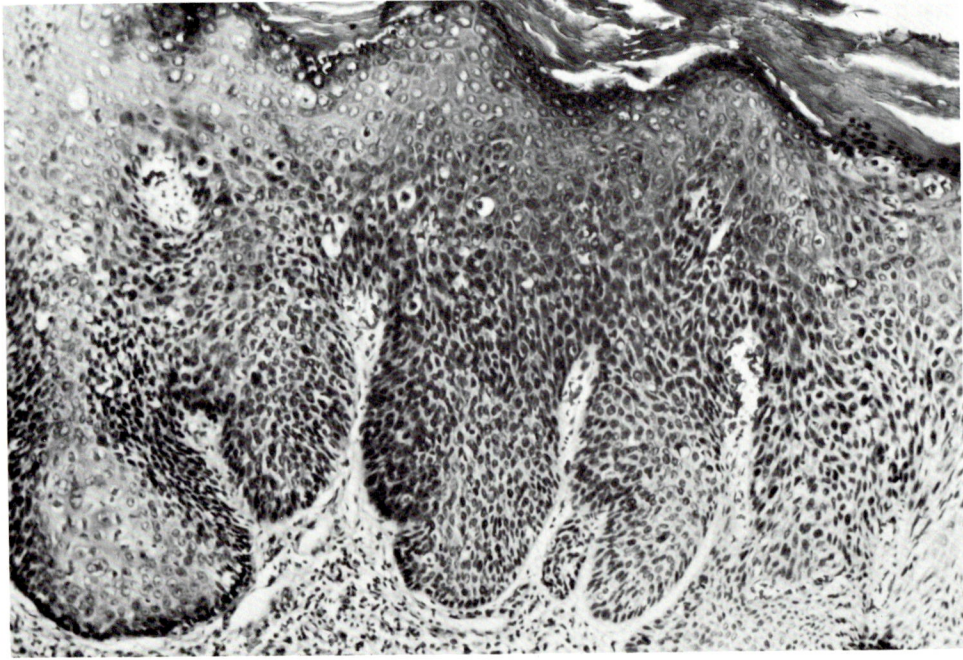

Fig. 7-1 Photomicrograph of carcinoma *in situ* (Bowen's disease) of the vulva.

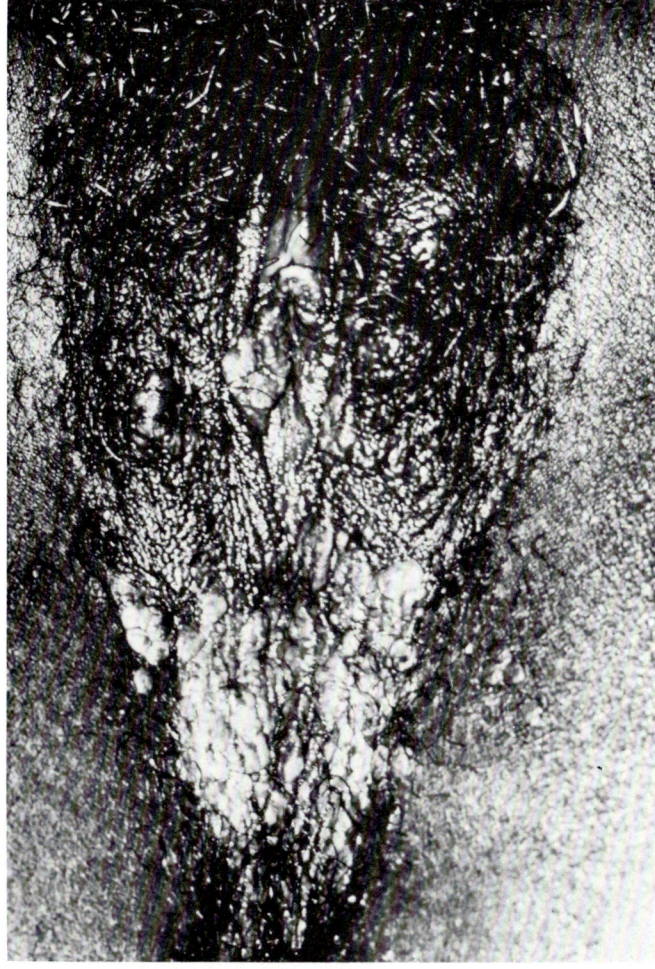

Fig. 7-2 Extensive carcinoma *in situ* of the vulva in a black patient with extension of the disease onto the labia majora and around the anus.

histologic picture is quite classic and is similar to that of Paget's disease of the mammary gland. Paget's disease of the vulva is associated with an underlying apocrine carcinoma in approximately 20-25% of the cases. Treatment is radical vulvectomy and then careful histologic study of the specimen. If an underlying apocrine gland carcinoma is uncovered, lymphadenectomy is warranted as a second stage procedure. It has been reported that patients with positive lymph nodes have a poor prognosis. The apocrine gland carcinoma associated with Paget's disease seems to metastasize in a manner similar to other vulvar cancers, and therefore lymphadenectomy appears logically indicated.

7-2 INVASIVE SQUAMOUS CELL CARCINOMA OF THE VULVA

Recognizing that malignant neoplasms of the vulva are not uniform histologically and that fine pathological distinctions are often difficult, we shall consider them in four categories:

1. Squamous cell carcinoma
2. Melanoma.
3. Sarcoma.
4. Adenocarcinoma.

With rare exceptions, most histologic variances behave about the same, so that treatment need not dwell exclusively on the matter of histologic consideration.

Location of the Primary Lesion

Although the primary lesion may appear anywhere on the vulva, certain sites are more commonly involved. Approximately 70% of the lesions occur on the labia, the labia majora being 3 times more frequently involved than the labia minora. Next in frequency is the clitoris, which is involved in roughly 13% of the cases. Either the urethra or the perineum can also be the site of a primary lesion. The lymphatics of the labia drain upward to the inquinal lymph nodes. Although the lymphatics of the perineum and posterior fourchette drain similarly to the vulva, the proximity to the anus allows for posterior drainage into the anal region and pelvic nodes. Obviously, the closer the lesion is to the anus the more likely the occurrence of this posterior drainage.

Sites and Manner of Spread (Fig. 7-4)

Cancer originating in the vulva generally spreads along the predictable pathways of the lymphatic system. Except possibly in association with melanoma, it is rare for such

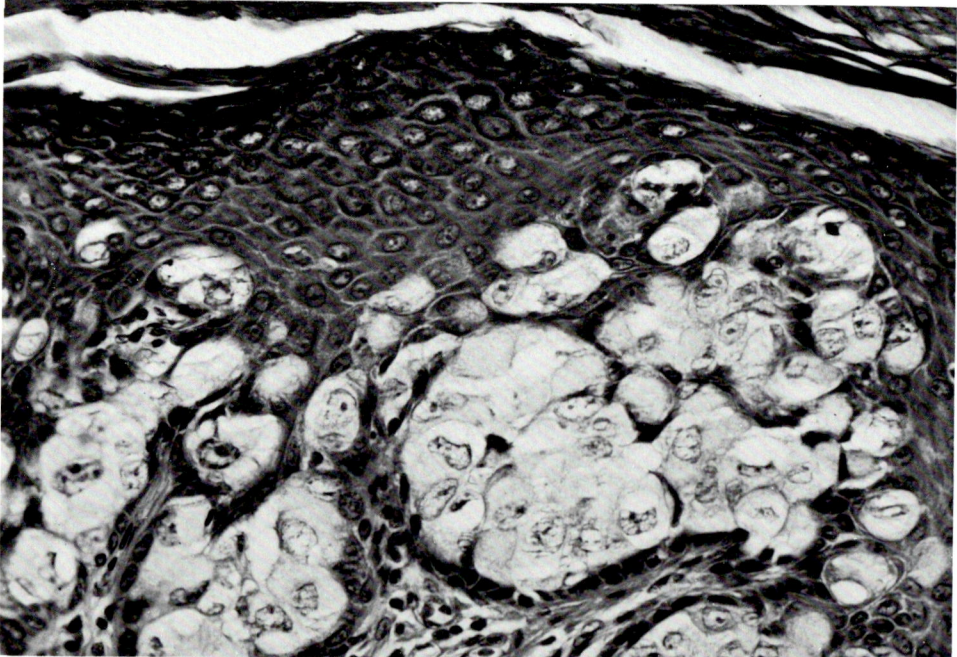

Fig. 7-3 Photomicrograph of Paget's disease of the vulva. Note the large, hyperchromatic cells surrounded by a clear zone of halo—these are known as Paget cells.

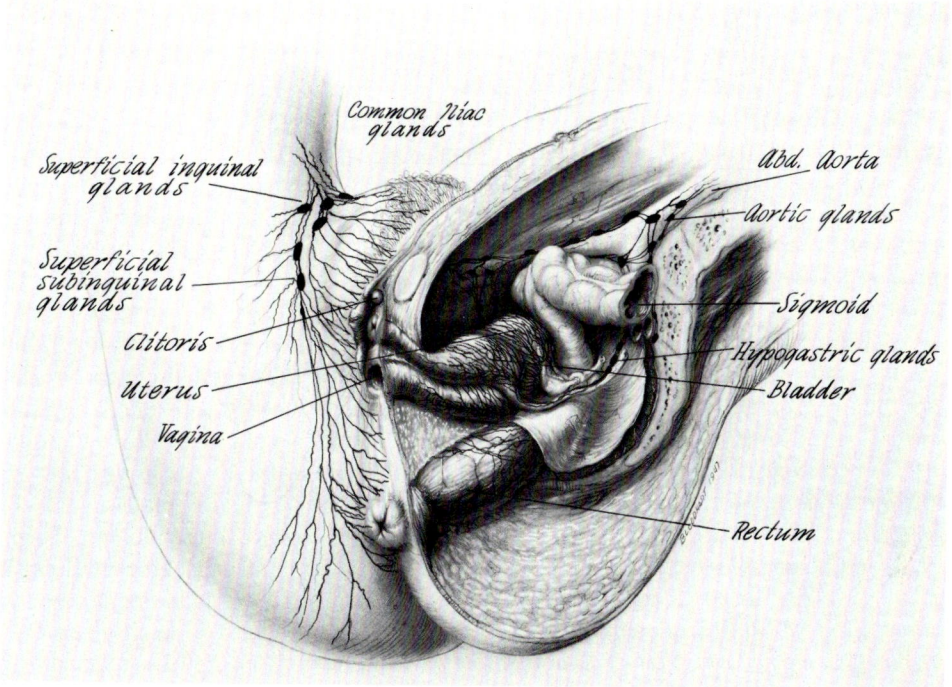

Fig. 7-4 Lymphatic drainage of the vulva. (Courtesy of E. Henriksen, M.D., Clinical Professor of Ob/Gyn, University of Southern California School of Medicine.)

tumors to involve hematogenous transport. The incidence of positive lymph nodes in the surgical series reported varies from approximately 30 to 60%. In most of these series both inguinal and pelvic lymphadnectomies were performed (Table 7-2). Correlation of the incidence of node metastasis with tumor size shows a general tendency for larger tumors to have a greater frequency of node involvement. Collins et al (1963), for example, found positive nodes in 20% of vulvar lesions smaller than 3 cm and in 71% of larger tumors. The frequency of positive nodes also correlates well with the presence or absence of palpable nodes in the inguinal area. Positive nodes are therefore more commonly found in patients with palpable inguinal lymph node enlargement.

TABLE 7-2 INCIDENCE OF POSITIVE NODES

Author	No. Cases	% positive Groin and Pelvic Nodes	% positive Pelvic Nodes
Taussig (1938)	65	46.2	7.7
Cherry and Glucksman (1955)	95	44.2	—
Green et al (1958)	238	58.8	—
Stening and Elliot (1959)	50	40.0	12.0
Way (1960)	143	42.0	16.1
Macafee (1962)	82	40.2	—
Collins et al (1963)	71	31.0	8.5
Rutledge et al (1970)	101	47.6	11.1

Staging Classification

Table 7-3 shows the classification of vulva carcinoma by stages

Along with other authors, we have in previous paragraphs stressed the importance of surgical attack on this disease. In so doing, we have implied that radiotherapy is inappropriate. Here, in contrast with other forms of gynecologic cancer, radiotherapy is at a distinct disadvantage because this relatively radioresistant neoplasm occurs in a very radiosensitive area. Whereas squamous cell carcinomas of the cervix and the vagina are just as radioresistant per se, the normal tissues of these areas can tolerate a large amount of irradiation.

For vulvar malignancy, the radiotherapeutic index is most unfavorable. Some radiobiologists have explained this by stating that the vulvar area has a disporportionately large number of end arteries to be exposed to radiation necrosis. Certainly radiation produces a diffuse vasculitis, and such a concept is possible. In addition, this disease usually occurs in elderly individuals in whom the processes of atherosclerosis and arteriosclerosis have compromised the blood supply sufficiently to create a favorable background for radiation injury. This situation and the absence of adequate collateral circulation render this region particularly vulnerable. Thus the peculiar characteristics of the vulvar skin are such that cancericidal dosages of ionizing radiation cannot be administered without producing undesirable side effects, which take the form of acute vulvitis, severe pain, and often radiation necrosis with infection and sloughing.

Surgical attack is the primary and accepted modality of therapy for this lesion.

TABLE 7-3 STAGING (CLINICAL) FIGO

Stage I	T1	N0	M0	All lesions confined to the
	T1	N1	M0	vulva, with a maximum diameter of 2 cm or less and no suspicious groin nodes.
Stage II	T2	N0	M0	All lesions confined to the
	T2	N1	M0	vulva, with a diameter greater than 2 cm and no suspicious groin nodes.
Stage III	T3	N0	M0	Lesions extending beyond the
	T3	N1	M0	vulva but without grossly positive groin nodes.
	T3	N2	M0	Lesions of any size confined
	T1	N3	M0	to the vulva and having
	T2	N3	M0	suspicious or grossly positive
	T1	N2	M0	groin nodes.
	T2	N2	M0	
Stage IV	T3	N3	M0	Lesions extending beyond the
	T4	N3	M0	vulva with grossly positive nodes.
	T4	N0	M0	Lesions involving mucosa of
	T4	N1	M0	rectum, bladder, or uretha, or
	T4	N2	M0	involving bone.
	M1A			All cases with distant or
	M1B			palpable deep pelvic metastases.

Important points relevant to the sugical radicality concern (1) removal of the mons veneris, (2) excision of a sufficiently wide margin around the tumor, (3) dissection to an adequate depth with removal of all tissues superficial to the urogenital diaphragm, and (4) resection of neighboring structures such as the urethra, the anus, or even bone if the tumor has reached these sites.

The extent of the vulvectomy can be logically supported by recalling the course of the collecting lymphatic channels and the frequency with which multifocal lesions are found in this disease. Dissection should be carried laterally to at least the genital-crural fold, and the necessity for inclusion of the mons will be apparent on this basis. Skin excision may be extended into both inguinal areas forming the "horns" on the specimen. The amount of skin that should be excised is increased in cases in which the inguinal nodes have palpable tumor. Palpable nodes in the inguinal area suggest more strongly that the skin of the area may be involved with tumor, and in these instances larger strips of skin from the inguinal areas should be removed with the specimen.

The rationale for considering the use of a combination of local surgery followed by radiation of the regional nodes has some merit. However, the results (Table 7-4) do not show that combined treatment is any better than simple vulvectomy. Granted that these procedures are usually performed on patients who are far advanced or have serious medical complications, the 5 year survival rates are approximately only 30% for both partial treatment plans.

Modern surgical treatment of carcinoma of the vulva was pioneered by the work of Taussig (1938, 1940) and Way (1960, 1966). Under the influence of Taussig, Mr. Stanley Way was stimulated to embark on his extensive and fruitful clinical experiment with this disease in the late 1940's. With a team approach and a consistent treatment plan, he treated 146 patients with carcinoma of the vulva. The 5 year survival rate for all stages was 74%. His fantastic success with this surgical approach stimulated our present therapy. Way insists on an extremely wide excision, a view that is not upheld in this country by many. His recommended skin incision begins at the mons and is directed downward and lateral to the crural fold, extending into the gracilis region to a point lateral to the anus. It then curves upward and inward to reach the perineum at a point immediately above the external sphincter, where the two opposing incisions meet. Only rarely can the skin edges be approximated; thus healing occurs by granulation and secondary intention if, indeed, a skin graft is not used.

TABLE 7-4 5 YEAR SURVIVAL RATES (%) FOR VULVAR CARCINOMA BY TREATMENT REGIMEN

Series	Radiotherapy Alone	Vulvectomy Alone	Vulvectomy and Radiotherapy	Radical Vulvectomy and Lymphadenectomy
Smith and Pollack (1947)	16.7	47.6	5.6	52.6
Huber (1953)	19.2	39.4		36.4
Taussig (1940)	4.8	8.3		58.5
Lunin (1949)	20.0	25.0		100
Brandstetter and Krataeluvill (1961)	10.3	17.6		58.3

Operation

Our policy for radical vulvectomy is such that the distal limits of the operation include the mons veneris, with resection along the course of the labial-crural folds, crossing the perineum above the anus (Fig. 7-5). The inner incision line follows the hymenal ring, leaving minimal margins of mucosa about the urethral meatus. Great individualization of these resection lines is necessary because of variable locations and sites of the primary disease. The deep fascia limits the depth of the vulvar incision, which is usually carried down to the urogenital diaphragm. On occasions, excision of the urogenital diaphragm and dissection of the ischiorectal fossa and paravaginal spaces may be necessary if the disease has extended to these areas.

The ingunal lymphadenectomy is ordinarily done with the vulvectomy as a one stage procedure and usually antecedes the vulvectomy. Strips of skin from each groin area are excised. The skin of the anterior thigh is then undermined with a plane just anterior to Scarpa's Fascia. Undercutting easily allows access to the point at which the sartorius muscle crosses the adductor magnus to form the inferior limits of the femoral triangle. Removal of the nodes containing fibrofatty tissue as one specimen is completed on each side. Excision is started by incising the fascia lata along the lateral border of the sartorius muscle, reflecting the fascia medially, while protecting the femoral nerve and deep divisions of the femoral artery. The contents of the femoral triangle are removed, leaving the stripped vein and artery to be covered by the transplanted sartorius muscle. The subcutaneous fibrofatty tissue along Poupart's ligament extending up to the lower abdomen is included in the specimen to assure total removal of the superficial nodes as well as the lymphatic vessels. Cloquet's node within the femoral canal can usually be found and submitted for frozen section analysis during the operation. It has been stated that Cloquet's node is the most representative node of the inguinal dissection. If this node or any other groin node is positive, immediate dissection of the pelvic lymph nodes is carried out.

If the external iliac, hypogastric, and obturator nodes are to be dissected, the

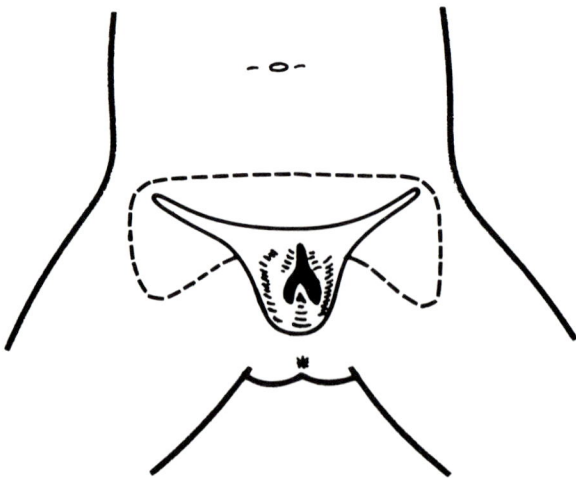

Fig. 7-5 Incision for radical vulvectomy with ileofemoral and possibly pelvic lymphadenectomy. Amount of skin removed from groin area depends on presence and extent of lymph node involvement. (From DiSaia, P.J. et al, Calif. Med. 118:13, No. 6, 1973.)

retroperitoneal spaces are reached through an incision above and parallel to Poupart's ligament. The fibers of the external oblique muscle are separated, and the internal oblique and transversalis muscles are divided. Fibrofatty tissue containing lymphatics and lymph nodes about the external iliac vessels, the obturator nerve, and along the superior border of the internal iliac vessels are removed, often as a single specimen. Rarely does the dissection extend above the level of the common iliac artery bifurcation.

Results

The survival rates in this disease depend on the analysis of the results by absolute survival versus modified life-table methods. It may be stated that the 5 year absolute survival rate for all cases treated by radical vulvectomy with lymphadenectomy ranges between 60 and 70%. In the series from M. D. Anderson Hospital, the 5 year survival rate for 139 patients treated for cure was 83% when modified by the life-table methods. Because of the age group commonly affected by vulvar cancer, intercurrent disease often plays a large role in the calculation of 5 year survivals. In the series from M. D. Anderson Hospital 53 patients with negative inguinal nodes were followed for 5 years or more, and none of them developed recurrence. Thirty patients had positive nodes, and 13 or 39% survived free of disease. Throughout the literature the 5 year survival rate for patients with positive nodes (Table 7-5) varies from 12 to 38% for 5 years.

The inguinal and pelvic lymphadenectomy has undergone considerable alteration as a standard component of the surgical attack. Most authors agree that the radical vulvectomy should be accompanied by inguinal lymphadenectomy. The only exception to this statement is the belief of Morris (1967) and others that a unilateral inguinal lymphadenectomy may be indicated for small lesions localized to one side of the vulva. The rationale for this therapeutic approach derives from the fact that the contralateral inguinal nodes are almost never positive when the ipsilateral inguinal nodes are negative. Morris advocates analysis of the ipsilateral inguinal nodes before the bilateral dissection and avoidance of a contralateral inguinal lymphadenectomy when the ipsilateral inguinal nodes are negative for tumor. It must be added, however, that this view is not popularly held.

Whether the pelvic nodes should or should not be removed has been discussed extensively in the literature in the past several decades. The lymphatics of the labia do not drain directly to the deep pelvic nodes, but drain via the femoral nodes. However, other organs of the vulva, such as the clitoris and urethral meatus, do partially drain to

TABLE 7-5 SURVIVAL RATES FOR PATIENTS WITH POSTIVE PELVIC NODES

Series	Number of Patients	5 Year Survival Rate (%)
Green et al (1958)	16	12.5
Way (1957)	9	22.2
Way (1960)	8	37.5
Merrill and Ross (1961)	3	33.3
Collins et al (1963)	6	16.7
	42	21.4

the pelvic nodes. We have thus adopted the policy of performing the pelvic lymphadenectomy under the following circumstances:

1. If the inguinal lymph nodes are positive.
2. If the clitoris is involved with the lesion.
3. If mucous membrane of the urethra, vagina or anus is involved.

In addition, because of the correlation between the incidence of positive pelvic nodes and a large primary lesion, we often perform a pelvic lymphadenectomy if the primary lesion is greater than 3 cm at its widest point. Deep pelvic lymphadenectomy probably should also be performed when melanoma, sarcoma or adenocarcinoma is present.

Recurrences may be local or distant. The distant recurrences usually appear with in the first year or two after treatment. They usually take the form of disease in the lymph nodes beginning with the high pelvic and paraaortic chain. In addition, pulmonary metastases are not uncommon. The local recurrences tend to occur within the first 3 years. The frequency of local recurrences may be minimized by examination of the surgical margin by frozen section at the time of surgery. Certainly the area of vaginal mucosa closest to the primary lesion should be examined at the time of surgery by frozen section for a tumor-free margin.

The treatment of recurrences is a frustrating problem. Local excision has been the mainstay of treatment, but interstitial irradiation is often useful as a palliative procedure for local control. Recurrences above the pelvis are rarely treated, but radiotherapy and chemotherapy may have some value.

7-3 MELANOMA OF THE VULVA

Melanoma of the vulva, although a rare malignancy, is the second most common cancer occurring in this region. The tumor affects women predominantly in the peri- and postmenopausal age groups; the average at diagnosis is 57. The growth may arise from a preexisting junctional nevus or the junctional component of a compound nevus, or it may originate *de novo*. The patient usually becomes aware of the malignancy because of pruritis, enlargement of a mole, bleeding, or discovery of the tumor itself.

Most melanomas are elevated, pigmented, frequently ulcerated growths usually surrounded by an inflammatory margin. Differential diagnosis includes benign nevus, furuncle, pigmented basal cell carcinoma, and epidermoid inclusion cyst. The amelanotic variety may simulate epidermoid carcinoma. Prognosis is related to size of the lesion, depth of dermal invasion, extension to the urethra or vagina, and presence or absence of regional lymph node metastasis and distant metastasis. More than 80% of vulvar melanomas arise from the labia minora and clitoris. Treatment consists of en bloc groin lymphadenectomy and radical vulvectomy. The pelvic nodes should also be dissected. If the lesion involves the urethra or vigina, exenteration may be necessary. The 5 year survival rate for lesions confined to the vulva is 80%.

Some authorities recommend the removal of any pigmented nevus of the vulva prophylactically, as it is several times more likely to be of the junctional variety. The obstetrician-gynecologist has a unique opportunity to screen women for these pigmented lesions of the vulva.

7-4 SARCOMA OF THE VULVA

Primary sarcoma of the vulva is certainly an unusual malignancy; only about 150 cases have been reported in the world literature. An exact listing is made difficult, however, by the confusion in the early reports between sarcoma and other morphologically similar lesions such as melanoma. Lundwall (1961) in his study of vulvar malignancy reviewed his own series and those of other authors. He found 12 cases of definite sarcoma among 1120 patients with vulvar cancer for an incidence of 1.1%.

The location of these lesions seems to follow the same pattern as that of squamous cell carcinoma of the vulva. In a series of 12 patients reported by DiSaia et al (1971), 6 had lesions on the labium majus, 3 on the labium minus, and 3 on the perineum and clitoral areas. The age incidence is agreed to be between 30 and 50 years. The median age in the group reported in most series is between 35 and 38 years. In most cases, the presenting symptom is local discomfort. Lesions of the labia minora often result in pain during coitus, while those of the labia majora are more ofter associated with irritation from undergarments. The average patient has symptoms from 3-12 months before her initial visit to a physician. Pain with defecation is a complaint in patients with lesions of the perianal area.

The pathologic diagnosis has considerable bearing on the prognosis for the patient. Rhabdomyosarcoma appears to be a rapidly growing lesion that metastasizes early, and the patient's fate is decided shortly after treatment. Leiomyosarcoma, on the other hand, is a slow growing, indolent disease with late local and distant recurrences. Radical vulvectomy with inguinal and pelvic lymphadenectomy appears to be the treatment of choice. Patients in whom the sarcoma is of the well differentiated variety appear to show better survival rates. In the series reported by DiSaia et al, 7 of the 12 patients underwent lymphadenectomy; 4 were without evidence of disease 18-88 months after surgery and 2 were found to have distant metastasis without local disease 22 and 39 months after treatment. The patient who had a lymphadenectomy with a positive node has now survived for 5 years. Should her case eventuate in a long-term cure, it would be difficult to argue against inguinal node dissection, especially in a patient such as her with a small lesion. In general, however, patients with poorly differentiated sarcomas, especially of the rhabdomyosarcoma variety, were doomed to distant metastasis and a short survival. On the other hand, patients with well differentiated lesions, especially of the leiomyosarcoma variety, often had prolonged survivals, even though occasionally complicated by multiple local recurrances. A patient with a well differentiated leiomyosarcoma of the vulva had four local recurrences, which were treated surgically; the patient eventually succumbed to her disease 16 years after the primary procedure was carried out.

7-5 ADENOCARCINOMA OF THE VULVA

Adenocarcinoma of the vulva is one of the rarest of gynecologic malignant lesions. When it does occur, it usually arises from Bartholin's gland. Women with Bartholin's adenocarcinoma average nearly a decade younger than women with epidermoid cancer of the vulva but the symptoms are quite similar. A history of Bartholin gland inflammatory disease during the reproductive years may be obtained, and all too often the cancers themselves are mistaken for abscesses, with the error leading to efforts at surgical drainage and delay in diagnosis. It is important to recognize that uncomplicated inflammatory disease of Bartholin's gland is uncommon after the fourth decade and does not occur in the postmenopausal years. Biopsy specimens must be taken from all such lesions in these age groups to exclude neoplastic disease.

Bartholin gland adenocarcinoma tends to be more advanced at diagnosis than epidermoid vulvar cancer. This is probably owing to its location deep to the skin in proximity to the vagina, perineal body, anal canal and pubic ramus. The region is vascular and its lymphatics may drain directly to the pelvic wall as well as the groin. Because of these considerations the minimal treatment for adenocarcinoma of Bartholin's gland should be radical vulvectomy and bilateral ilio-inguinal (groin and pelvic) lymphadenectomy. Extending the operation to remove portions of vagina, levator, ischial-rectal fat, and even more radical modifications may be required, depending upon the growth pattern of the individual tumor.

Survival data from the literature are of little value because of the small numbers of cases. Patients with clinically suspicious nodes have an especially bad prognosis.

In the category of adenocarcinoma of Bartholin's gland there is a special group that encompasses the so-called adenoid cystic carcinoma. This lesion histologically is similar to the corresponding tumor of the major salivary glands. It tends to remain localized, seldom giving rise to widespread metastasis. Lymphatic spread does occur and lymphadenectomy should be included in the surgical treatment.

REFERENCES

Barclay, D. L., Collins, C. G., and Macey, H. B.: Cancer of the Bartholin gland. *Obstet. Gynecol.* 24:329, 1964.

Beohm, F., and Morris, J.: Paget's disease and aprocrine gland carcinoma of the vulva. *Obstet. Gynecol.* 38:185, 1971.

Brandstetter, F., and Krataeluvill, A.: Ergebnisse der Therapie beim Vulva Karzinom. *Krebsaryt* 16:16, 1961.

Chamlian, D. L., and Taylor, H. B.: Primary carcinoma of Bartholin's gland. *Obstet. Gynecol.* 39:489, 1972.

Cherry, C. P., and Glucksman, A.: Lymphatic embolism and lymph node metastasis in cancer of the vulva and uterine cervix. *Cancer* 8:564, 1955.

Collins, C. G., et al: Cancer involving the vulva. *Am. J. Obstet. Gynecol.* 87:762, 1963.

DiSaia, P. J., Morrow, C. P., Townsend, D. E.: Cancer of the vulva. *Calif. Med.* 118:13, 1973

DiSaia, P. J., Rutledge, F. N., and Smith, J. P.: Sarcoma of the vulva. *Obstet. Gynecol.* 38:180, 1971.

Green, T. H., Ulfelder, H., and Meigs, J. V.: Epidermoid carcinoma of the vulva. *Am. J. Obstet. Gynecol.* 75:834, 1958.

Huber, H.: Das primare Carcinom der Vulva. *Strahlentherapie* 29:61, 1953.

Langfelt-Anderson, B: Cancer of the vulva. *Acta Radiol.* 51:369, 1959.

Lundwall, F.: Cancer of the vulva: A clinical review. *Acta Radiol (Suppl.)* 208:1, 1961.

Lunin, A. B.: Carcinoma of the vulva. *Am. J. Obstet. Gynecol.* 57:742, 1949.

Macafee, C. H. G.: Some aspects of vulvar cancer. *J. Obstet. Gynaecol. Brit. Commonw.* 69:177, 1962.

McKelvey, L., in Pack, G. T., and Ariel, I. M., Eds: *Treatment of Cancer and Allied Diseases. VI. Tumors of the Female Genitalia.* Hoeber Medical Division, Harper & Row, New York, 1962, Chapter. 4, pp. 69-88.

Merrill, J. A., and Ross, W. L.: Cancer of the vulva. *Cancer* **14**:13, 1961.

Morris, John M.: Personal Communication (1967).

Morrow, C. P. & Rutledge, F. N. Melanoma of the vulva. *Obstet. Gynecol.* **39**:745, 1972.

Parry-Jones, E.: Lymphatics of the vulva. *J. Obstet. Gynaecol. Brit. Commonw.* **70**:751, 1963.

Rutledge, F. N. and Sinclair, M.: Treatment of intraepithelial carcinoma of the vulva by skin excision and graft. *Am. J. Obstet. Gynecol.* **102**:806, 1968.

Rutledge, F. N., Smith, J. P., and Franklin, E. W.: Carcinoma of the vulva. *Am. J. Obstet. Gynecol.* **106**:1117-1130, 1970.

Smith, F. R., and Pollack, R. S.: Carcinoma of the vulva. *Surg. Gynecol. Obstet.* **84**:78, 1947.

Stening, M., and Elliott, P.: Primary carcinoma of the vulva with special reference to "leukoplakia" *J. Obstet. Gynaecol. Brit. Emp.* **66**:897, 1959.

Taussig, F. J.: A study of the lymph glands in cancer of the cervix and cancer of the vulva. *Am. J. Obstet. Gynecol.* **36**:819, 1938.

Taussig, F. J.: Cancer of the vulva: An analysis of 155 cases. *Am. J. Obstet. Gynecol.* **40**:764, 1940.

Way, S.: Results of a planned attack on carcinoma of the vulva. *Brit. Med. J.* **2**:780, 1954.

Way, S.: Carcinoma of the vulva. In Meigs, J. V. and Sturgis, S. H. (eds.): Progress in Gynecology. Vol. 3 Grune & Stratton, Inc., New York, 1957.

Way, S.: Carcinoma of the vulva. *Am. J. Obstet. Gynecol.* **79**:692, 1960.

Way, S. and Hennigan, M.: The late results of extended radical vulvectomy for carcinoma of the vulva. *J. Obstet. Gynaecol. Brit. Commonw.* **73**:594, 1966.

Woodruff, J. D., et al: The contemporary challenge of carcinoma *in situ* of the vulva. *Am. J. Obstet. Gynecol.* **115**:677, 1973.

CHAPTER EIGHT

Gestational Trophoblastic Disease

The growth disturbances of the human trophoblast manifest a wide range of biologic behavior. Three distinct clinical–pathologic forms are recognized: hydatidiform (hydatid) mole,* invasive mole (chorioadenoma destruens), and choriocarcinoma. The term chorionepithelioma has sometimes been used to designate both invasive mole and choriocarcinoma. Because of the extraordinary success of chemotherapy in the management of invasive mole and choriocarcinoma, a histopathologic diagnosis has limited clinical relevance at the present time. A more functional, therapeutically oriented classification of trophoblastic disease has been developed by the Union Internationale Contre le Cancer (Table 8-1).

As a maternal neoplastic disease, the gestational trophoblastic tumors are unique insofar as they are derived from fetal tissue. They also exhibit a number of other unusual features that makes them of special interest. Both invasive mole and choriocarcinoma are capable of elaborating steroid and protein hormones. The production of human chorionic gonadotropin (hCG) is a hallmark of these tumors. Both neoplasms are known to undergo spontaneous regression, although such an occurrence with choriocarcinoma is rare. Of all the malignant diseases, choriocarcinoma is the greatest imitator of other pathologic conditions because of its proclivity for hematogenous spread and the production of focal hemorrhagic lesions. Although a "benign" neoplasm, invasive mole is locally invasive and produces distant metastases, features usually confined to malignant tumors. Finally, choriocarcinoma has the distinction of being the only disseminated solid tumor that can be regularly cured by chemotherapy alone. A review of the clinical aspects of gestational trophoblastic disease is presented in this chapter. For a more detailed exposition of the subject, the interested reader is referred to the excellent monographs by Bagshawe (1969), Park (1971), and Hertig (1968), as well as the original papers in the bibliography.

---

*From L. *hydatid = watery vesicle + moles = a mass.*

230

TABLE 8-1   CLASSIFICATION OF
TROPHOBLASTIC NEOPLASIA, UICC, 1965

A. GESTATIONAL
(B. NONGESTATIONAL)

I. Clinical diagnosis
   1. Nonmetastatic
   2. Metastatic
     a. Local (pelvic)
     b. Extrapelvic (specify location)
   3. Other required information
     a. Evidence
       (i) Morphologic
       (ii) Nonmorphologic
     b. Antecedent Pregnancy (specify duration)
       (i) Normal (ii) Abortal
       (iii) Molar
     c. Previous treatment
       (i) Untreated
       (ii) Treated (specify)
II. Morphologic Diagnosis
   1. Hydatidiform mole
     a. Noninvasive
     b. Invasive
   2. Choriocarcinoma
   3. Uncertain
   4. Other required information
     a. Diagnostic basis (specify)
       (i)   C = Curettage
       (ii) U = Excised uterus
       (iii) N = Necropsy
       (iv) O = Other
     b. Date of diagnosis (with respect to date of onset of treatment)
     c. Subsequent change in morphologic diagnosis. Specify diagnostic basis as in II.4a.

8-1   NORMAL TROPHOBLAST

The initial mitotic cleavage of the zygote produces daughter cells of unequal size. It is believed that the larger cell gives rise to the trophoblast, while the smaller develops into the embryonic plate. Not only the cyto- and syncytiotrophoblast, but also the blood vessels and supporting tissues of the placenta, originate from the multipotential, primitive trophoblastic cells. The trophoblast comprises a major portion of the blastocyst at the time of implantation, which takes place 5–8 days after fertilization. It is essential to this process that the trophoblast has the capability of invading the endometrium. The physical-chemical means by which this is accomplished are unknown, but proteolytic enzymes do not seem to be involved. In the process of placentation the trophoblastic tissue invades the whole thickness of the endometrium or decidua within approximately 6 weeks. Some syncytiotrophoblastic cells normally penetrate the myometrium. Rarely, villi extend into the myometrium, producing the condition referred to as placenta accreta.

An even greater enigma of placentation is the ability of the fetal allograft (F_1 hybrid) to establish itself successfully in the maternal tissue without eliciting an immune response. It is known definitely that the trophoblast is of fetal origin and that the uterus is not an immunologically privileged site. Nor can the immunologic tolerance be explained on the basis of antigenic immaturity of the early trophoblast since transplantation antigens have been demonstrated. At the present time the most plausible explanation for this phenomenon is the presence of a nonantigenic barrier at the maternal-fetal (placental) interface. Electron microscopic studies suggest that every syncytiotrophoblastic cell is enveloped by a layer of mucoprotein, mainly sialomucinous in character, which prevents the fetal tissue from being recognized as foreign by the maternal lymphocytes. Recent studies have also demonstrated that hCG has an immunosuppresive quality. The role that this plays in the maternal immunologic tolerance of the fetus is unknown, however.

The great propensity of the human trophoblast for vascular invasion is undoubtedly essential to the establishment of the hemochorial placenta. Since the epithelial coverings of the placental villi are continuously bathed by maternal blood, it is not surprising that trophoblastic cells are commonly deported to the lungs, particularly during the latter weeks of pregnancy and parturition. The deportation of trophoblast is not known to be either beneficial or harmful to the mother.

The duration of viability of the fetal trophoblast is self-limited, but the mechanism by which this is accomplished is unknown. Hormonal and immunologic controls have been postulated, but not substantiated. The maximum life span of normal trophoblast under optimal conditions seems to be only slightly longer than the duration of gestation. This inherent limitation of survival and invasiveness of normal trophoblast sharply distinguishes it from malignant tissue.

8-2 HYDATIDIFORM MOLE

The hydatidiform mole is an abnormal conceptus characterized grossly by vesicular swelling of the placental villi and the absence of an intact fetus or embryo (Fig. 8-1). Microscopically there is an hyperplasia or benign neoplastic proliferation of the trophoblastic epithelium (Fig. 8-2). Although the diagnosis of hydatid mole is usually obvious on gross examination, histologically hydropic degeneration of the villi of an early aborted conceptus may resemble the villi of an hydatid mole. The diagnosis of molar pregnancy should be reserved for conceptuses demonstrating a proliferation of the cyto- and syncytiotrophoblast. Occasionally an abortus will have grossly hydropic villi but no trophoblastic hyperplasia, the so-called transitional mole. When the pathologic findings are equivocal, the management should be the same as for an hydatid mole.

The incidence of molar pregnancy varies from 1 in 125 deliveries in Taiwan to 1 in 2000 deliveries in the United States. The occurrence of hydatid mole is significantly more frequent in the over 40 and under 20 maternal age groups. The risk of developing a second mole is 4–5 times greater than that of the initial molar pregnancy. Somewhat paradoxical is the finding that repeated molar pregnancies are less likely to be complicated by malignant sequelae than the initial mole. The fertility and reproductive performance of patients having hydatid moles is evidently unimpaired unless chemotherapy is required. Patients who receive drugs have an increased rate of spontaneous abortions and placenta accreta, but their pregnancies and offspring are otherwise normal.

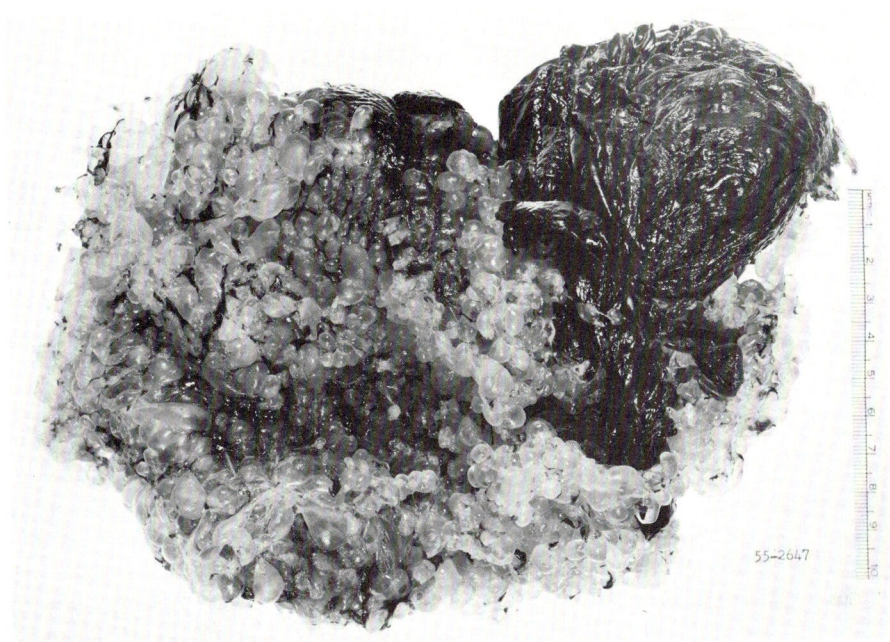

Fig. 8-1 Gross appearance of hydatid mole. The pathognomonic vesicles result from fluid accumulation within the placental villi.

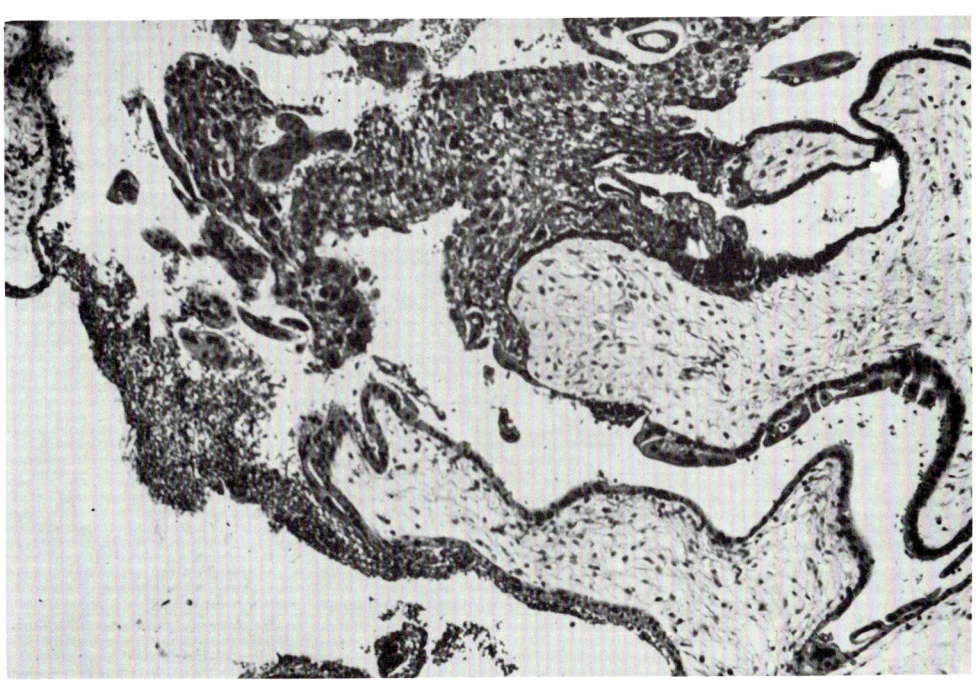

Fig. 8-2 Photomicrograph of hydatid mole. The villi are avascular and edematous. An area of trophoblastic hyperplasia is present.

233

The frequent occurrence of trophoblastic disease in the Orient has supported a nutritional etiology, perhaps involving a deficiency of folic acid. Other conjectures regarding causality include consanguinity, racial susceptability, fetal-maternal histocompatibility, and infectious agents. Bagshawe (1969) has reported that women who have blood type A married to men with blood type O have the greatest risk of developing choriocarcinoma. Chromosomal triploidy is a common finding in abortuses but is unusual in hydatid mole. It is of interest that 80% of hydatid moles are sex chromatin positive, although studies with choriocarcinoma indicate an even sex distribution. The predominantly female chromatin pattern in moles has led to the speculation that they may be derived from polar bodies rather than normal ova.

Diagnosis

Hydatid mole is recognized clinically only 50% of the time before expulsion of the pathognomonic vesicles. The diagnosis should be suspected in any woman with bleeding in the first half of pregnancy, hyperemesis gravidarum, or toxemia before 24 weeks' gestation (Table 8-2). The suspicion may be reinforced by finding on physical examination a uterus large for the estimated length of gestation, the absence of fetal heart tones, or the presence of bilateral ovarian masses compatible with theca-lutein cysts.

When the diagnosis of hydatid mole is entertained, a determination of the urinary hCG excretion may be helpful. If measurements are made after 100 days of amenorrhea, values greater than 500,000 IU/24 hours are usual with hydatid moles, in contrast to normal pregnancy values of less than 100,000 IU. However, lower than normal pregnancy values may be associated with hydatid mole, and values greater than 500,000 IU may be associated with a multiple gestation. Consequently, the hCG assay cannot be depended on absolutely to make a diagnosis of hydatid mole, although it frequently adds strong supportive evidence.

A firm diagnosis of hydatid mole before the spontaneous expulsion of vesicles can be made by means of transabdominal amniocentesis or B-mode ultrasonography. The latter is not universally available, but its simplicity and reliability make it the diagnostic method of choice. It is nonoperative and may be performed repeatedly without apparent harm to

---

TABLE 8-2   DIAGNOSIS OF HYDATID MOLE

Clinical data
  Bleeding in first half of pregnancy
  Lower abdominal pain
  Toxemia before 24 weeks of gestation
  Hyperemesis gravidarium
  Uterus large for dates (only 50% of cases)
  Absent fetal heart tones and fetal parts
  Theca-lutein cysts (about 30% of cases)
Diagnostic studies
  Urinary hCG > 500,000 IU/24 hours
  Ultrasound
  Amniocentesis and amniography

---

the fetus or mother. This study should be carried out in any patient who has bleeding in the first half of pregnancy to facilitate the earlier diagnosis of hydatid mole and other abnormalities of early gestation. The characteristic findings of molar pregnancy on B-scan are demonstrated in Fig. 8-3. Because of its almost universal availability, amniocentesis combined with amniography is the diagnostic test most widely used to confirm the presence of hydatid mole. If amniotic fluid is withdrawn after introducing the needle, a diagnosis of normal pregnancy is presumed and dye is not injected. A small risk of inducing premature labor accompanies the use of the radiopaque material, and the probability of obtaining additional useful information in this circumstance is too remote to warrant its use. (Rarely a mole may coexist with a normal, separate fetus. When this condition is suspected, an ultrasound scan should be obtained.) If no amniotic fluid is withdrawn, radiopaque dye is injected, after which radiographs of the abdomen are taken. The typical honeycomb appearance produced by the dispersion of the dye around the distended hydatid vesicles is shown in Fig. 8-4. Amniography, like sonography, is reasonably safe and accurate, but, of course, false interpretations of either study can be made.

Numerous biochemical serum and urine measurements can be expected to be at variance in normal pregnancy and hydatid mole, but none has an established role in the differential diagnosis of these two conditions. Such substances include human placental lactogen, total estrogens, estriol, estetrol, pregnanediol, neutrophil alkaline phosphatase, leucine aminopeptidase, and oxytocinase.

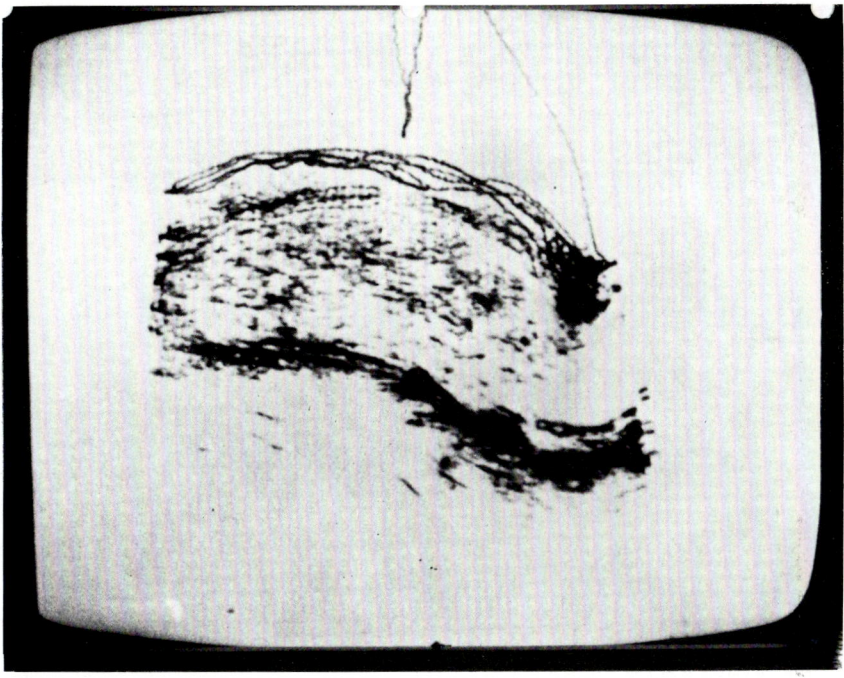

Fig. 8-3 Ultrasonic scan, longitudinal sectional 1 cm to the left of the umbilicus. The patient's pelvis is to the right. The vertical line at the top center marks the umbilicus. The characteristic multiple intrauterine echoes are evident.

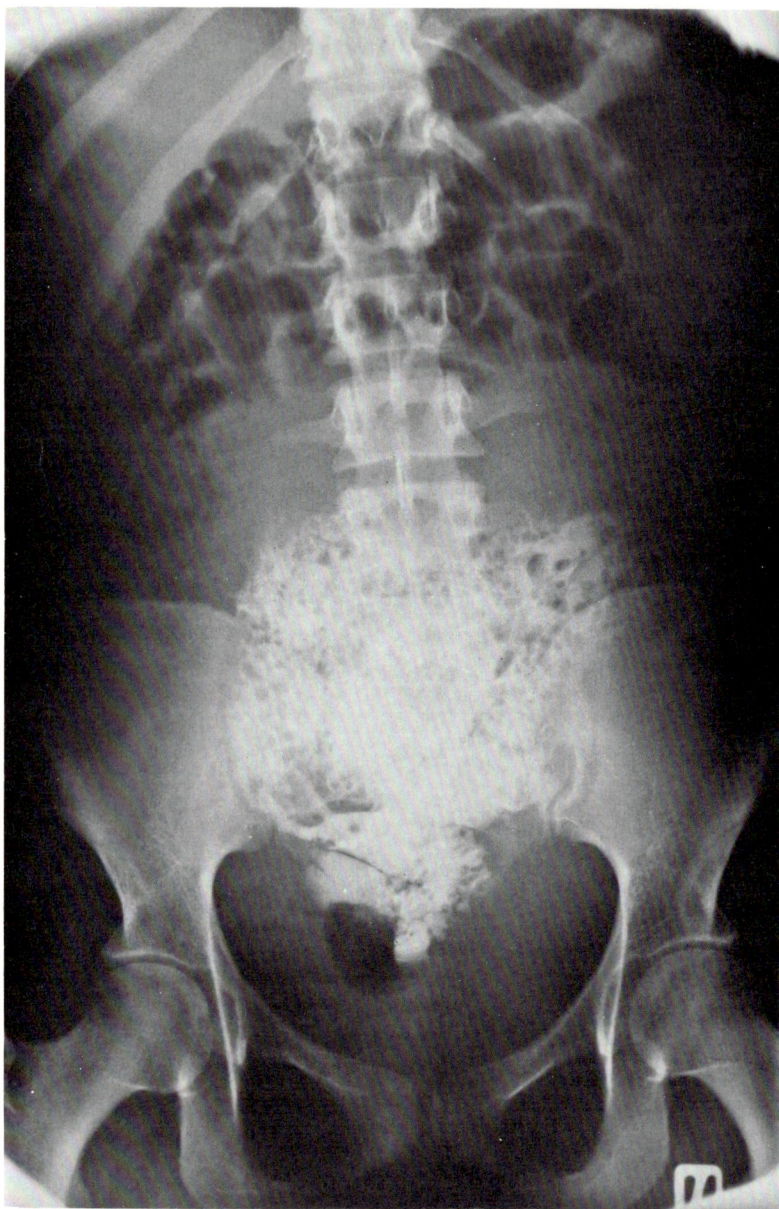

Fig. 8-4 Classic radiographic honeycomb or moth-eaten appearance of hydatid mole obtained after intrauterine injection of water-soluble radiopaque dye.

Complications

Although the outcome of molar pregnancy is generally uneventful, medical complications are potentially both numerous and serious. Anemia from chronic blood loss, toxemia, hyperthyroidism, high output cardiac failure, and abortion with hemorrhage and sepsis are constant threats and become increasingly menacing as the duration of the pregnancy advances. In the interests of avoiding these complications, early diagnosis and prompt evacuation are advisable.

Evacuation

As soon as the diagnosis is confirmed, termination of a molar pregnancy should be carried out with no more delay than is necessary to evaluate the patient adequately and prepare her for therapeutic intervention. Suction curettage is the preferred method of evacuation. After suction evacuation, a sharp curettage is performed to complete the removal of the molar tissue. The curettings are submitted as separate specimens for pathologic examination. Hysterotomy, pitocin induction, and the intraamniotic injection of hypertonic solutions (saline, glucose, urea) are not acceptable alternatives. Hydatid mole is seldom diagnosed in the first trimester of pregnancy, when emptying the uterus by means of conventional curettage would be a safe procedure. Termination of a molar pregnancy by primary hysterectomy is a reasonable option in the management of patients who are good surgical candidates and who desire sterilization. Parenthetically, these individuals still should be followed with gonadotropin titers, although the likelihood of metastatic trophoblastic disease developing is remote.

A little publicized but potentially lethal complication of molar pregnancy is trophoblastic pulmonary embolization at the time of evacuation. Undoubtedly, some embolization occurs in most patients, but occasionally it is massive and produces a major systemic disorder characterized by dyspnea, cyanosis, hypotension, and tachycardia. Deaths have been reported. Such extreme examples of trophoblastic embolization are related to uterine contractions and may be observed whether labor is spontaneous or pitocin induced. Evacuation by suction curettage before the onset of labor may prevent this complication.

Unilateral or bilateral enlargement of the ovaries due to multiple theca-lutein cysts is clinically detectable in approximately 30% of patients with hydatid moles (Figs. 8-5a and 8-5b). Such extreme hyperplasia is believed to result from the high levels of hCG, but it appears that some pituitary hFSH is required in addition. Occasionally theca-lutein hyperplasia does not develop until after the mole is evacuated; it is then related possibly to an increase in pituitary gonadotropin release.

None of the clinical or laboratory features of hydatid mole is associated with an increased probability of malignant sequelae, nor are there any pathologic features that will provide a dependable clue to the behavior of the trophoblast in the individual case. Hertig (1968) has devised a grading system based on the histologic and cytologic characteristics of molar tissue. Initially, there were six groups but he reduced these to three grades: apparently benign, potentially malignant, and apparently malignant. The histologic criteria for the grading system are based on the degrees of trophoblastic hyperplasia and anaplasia. With advancing grade there is an increased risk of developing neoplastic complications. Patients with Grade 3 moles carry a 50% chance of having invasive mole or choriocarcinoma, compared with a 15% chance for Grade 2. Although such a grading system has some predictive capacity it is too inexact to be of much clinical value. It must be emphasized that Hertig's grading system is based on the examination of tissue obtained by sharp curettage of the uterus after evacuation of the mole. These curettings are frequently of a more advanced grade than the molar tissue.

8-3 INVASIVE MOLE

Invasion of the myometrium by molar villi produces a condition designated as invasive mole. This form of mole reportedly comprises 15% of all molar pregnancies, although

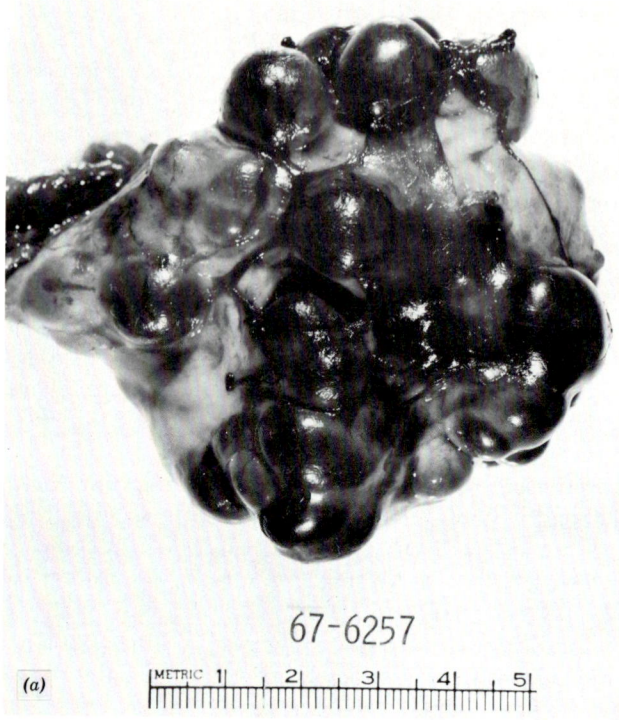

67-6257

(a)

Fig. 8-5a Ovarian theca-lutein hyperplasia associated with hydatid mole. Gross appearance of intact ovary.

Llewellyn-Jones (1967) found only 5 in 71 molar hysterectomy specimens. Histological-ly, invasive mole is characterized by hydropic villi and proliferating trophoblastic epithelium invading the uterine muscle. Associated are hemorrhage and tissue necrosis. The neoplasm may penetrate the full thickness of the uterine wall and extend into the broad ligament or pelvic cavity. Severe vaginal or intraperitoneal hemorrhage may occur. Invasive mole is capable of producing metastases, most commonly to the vagina and lungs, although rare instances of secondary lesions in the brain and spinal cord have been documented. Invasive mole has all the features of a malignant tumor with the exception that its duration of viability is self-limited. If no hemorrhagic complications occur, the tumor can be expected to involute spontaneously without serious trouble developing. Invasive mole can seldom be diagnosed without excising the uterus. Even with a proven invasive mole, however, metastases probably represent choriocarcinoma. Although invasive mole behaves more aggressively than noninvasive mole, it is no more likely to be complicated by choriocarcinoma.

8-4 CHORIOCARCINOMA

Choriocarcinoma follows hydatid mole in approximatley 3% of cases. It is a highly malignant tumor with a predisposition to hematogenous spread. The organs involved by metastasis are, in decreasing order of frequency, the lung, lower genital tract (cervix, vagina, vulva), brain, liver, kidney, and gastrointestinal tract. Although instances of

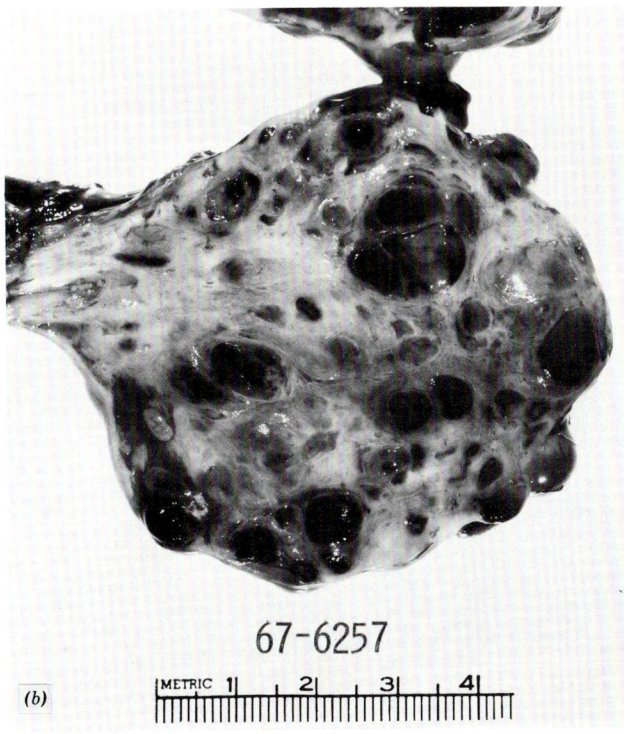

(b)

Fig. 8-5*b*   Cut section of same ovary, showing edematous stroma and multiple theca-lutein cysts.

spontaneous regression have been well documented, this rarely occurs. Choriocarcinoma is a great imitator of other disease processes. Because of its gonadotropin excretion, amenorrhea may develop, simulating an early pregnancy. Usually vaginal bleeding occurs, and a threatened abortion or ectopic pregnancy is suggested. Some cases present with intraperitoneal hemorrhage secondary to a ruptured liver, ruptured theca-lutein cyst, or bleeding ovarian metastasis (Fig. 8-6). Patients with pulmonary spread may present with cough, hemoptysis, pleuritic pain, dyspnea, "asthma," or evidence of respiratory failure. A variety of lesions may be seen on the chest radiograph (Figs. 8-7 to 8-9). Gastrointestinal involvement is accompanied by chronic blood loss and melena or by massive gastrointestinal hemorrhage. Spinal and intracranial metastases are often manifested by focal neurologic signs resulting from spontaneous bleeding. The clinical picture usually suggests a brain tumor or vascular accident. A clinical syndrome with right upper quadrant pain and jaundice resembling cholecystitis is sometimes seen with extensive liver metastases. Rarely patients have presented with hematuria from renal involvement.

Approximately 50% of all cases of gestational choriocarcinoma follow hydatidiform mole. In the others the antecedent pregnancies are evenly divided between abortions (including ectopic pregnancies) and normal pregnancies. Choriocarcinoma follows a term gestation about once in 40,000 cases. Considering the 3% risk of developing choriocarcinoma after hydatid mole, it is apparent that molar pregnancy increases the risk of choriocarcinoma about 1000-fold. Trophoblastic disease following a normal pregnancy is always choriocarcinoma and never a mole or invasive mole.

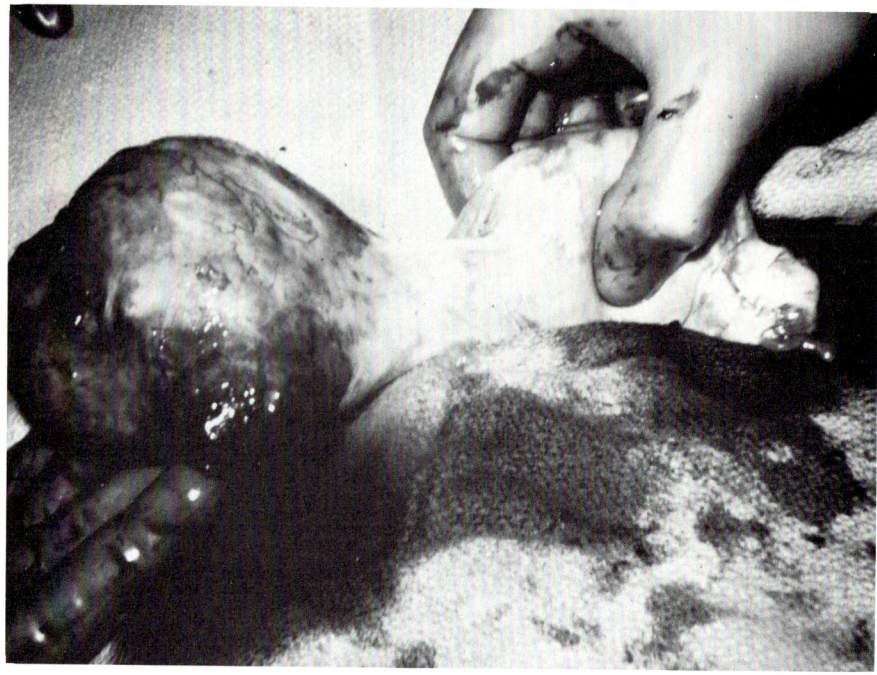

Fig. 8-6 Gestational choriocarcinoma metastatic to the ovary found at laparotomy. On the right is the uterine fundus. The patient presented with a hemoperitoneum 1 year after delivery of an hydatid mole. She had been followed for 3 months only, at which time a routine pregnancy test was negative. Brain and lung metastases were also present.

Choriocarcinoma that follows normal term pregnancy is usually manifested by delayed postpartum bleeding, a rather common complication of normal pregnancy. Because delayed postpartum bleeding is rarely due to choriocarcimina, the diagnosis is seldom suspected. Uterine curettage is often performed for postpartum bleeding, but even when choriocarcimoma is present a tissue diagnosis from the curettings is unusual. In the case of postpartum bleeding or, indeed, any atypical postpartum illness it is appropriate to obtain routinely a pregnancy test to screen for choriocarcinoma. Unfortunately, the diagnosis is not usually made until the patient develops symptoms from metastases.

8-5 MANAGEMENT OF GESTATIONAL TROPHOBLASTIC DISEASE

Human Chorionic Gonadotropin Assay

An adequate assay for hCG is indispensable to the diagnosis, treatment, and follow-up of trophoblastic disease. In common with pituitary lactogenic hormone (hLH) and follicle stimulating hormone (hFSH), hCG is a glycoprotein composed of two polypeptide chains or subunits designated alpha and beta. The alpha subunits of hCG, hLH, and hFSH are identical; their function is concerned with the rate of combination of the molecule with the target cell receptor site. However, the beta chain of each hormone is chemically different; it determines the biological activity of the molecule. Usually hCG is considered

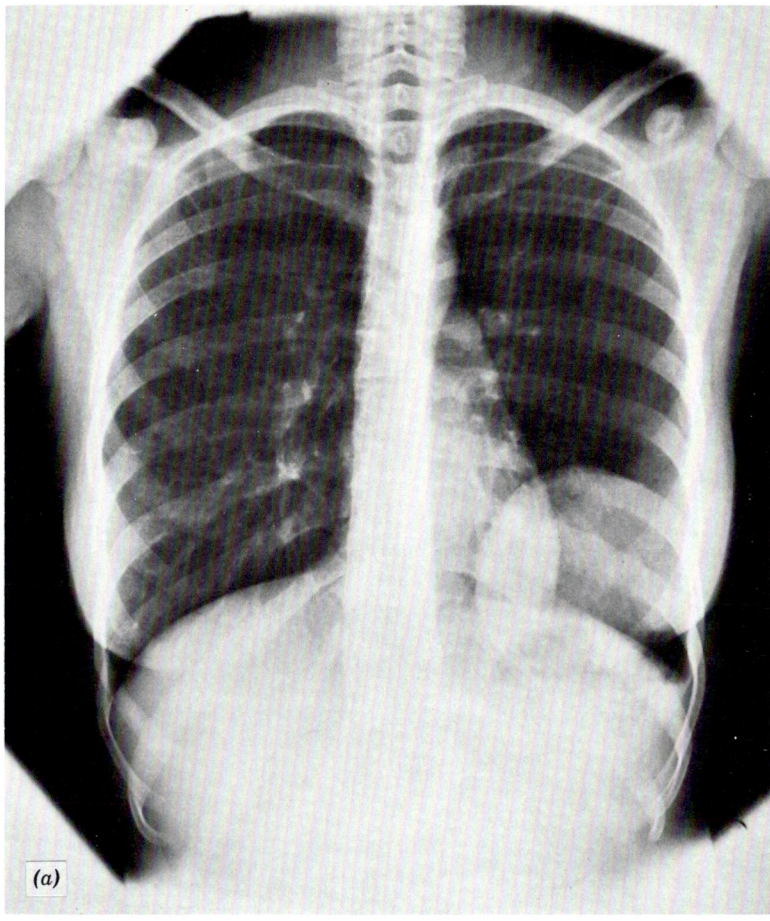

Fig. 8-7a Chest radiographs demonstrating a single, large, sharply circumscribed metastasis in the left posterior lung field. The lesion was still present, although much smaller, 1 year after remission induction. Posterior-anterior radiograph.

a product unique to trophoblastic tissue, whether of fetal or of teratomatous origin, although recently it has been demonstrated that nontrophoblastic malignancies often produce low levels of hCG (Braunstein et al, 1973). It is uncertain whether hCG is secreted by the cytotrophoblast, syntrophoblast, both, or some intermediary cell.

The first laboratory tests for detecting hCG in serum or urine utilized small animals and were dependent on the biologic activity of the molecule. With the exception of the mouse and rat uterine weight assay and the rat ventral prostate assay, none of them was sufficiently sensitive or quantifiable to monitor trophoblastic disease (Table 8-3). The uterine weight assay measuring total gonadoptropins (hCG, hLH, and hFSH) is time consuming and expensive. Nevertheless, its sensitivity and reliability made it the standard assay for trophoblastic disease supervision until the successful application of immunoassay methods to the measurement of hCG. Immunoassay has been widely adapted to pregnancy testing as a commercial enterprise. Immunologic pregnancy tests are quantal in

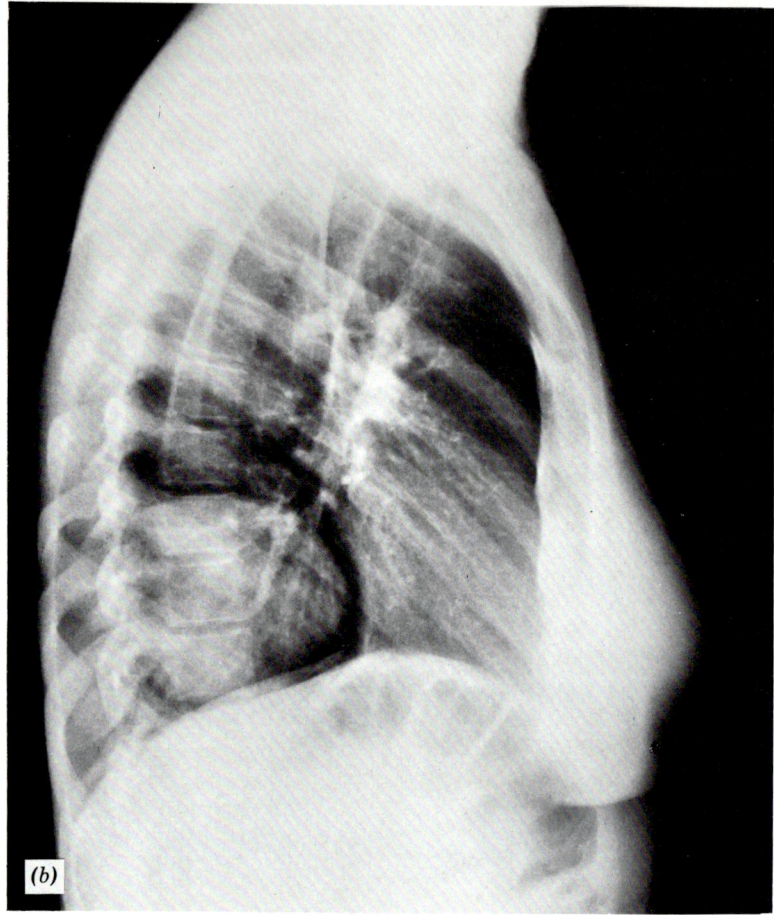

Fig. 8-7b   Lateral radiograph. Same patient as figure 8-7a.

design, giving a positive reaction for any concentration of hCG above a preset lower limit, usually in the range of 1000-3000 IU/L. Some commercial tests are available for quantitative measurements of gonadotropin in the concentration range above their minimum sensitivity.

Recently, radioimmunoassay (RIA) has been applied to the measurement of hCG in serum and urine. This method, described in Fig. 8-10, has a sensitivity of 1 IU/L. For the assay an antibody is made against the intact hCG molecule, which cross-reacts with pituitary hLH because of the common alpha subunit. Although the nonpregnant woman should have no hCG in her serum or urine, since the assay measures hLH in addition to hCG the "normal" range of values for hCG is that for hLH. During the reproductive years, hLH levels from 5 to 25 IU/L are considered normal except during the preovulatory phase of the menstrual cycle, when the hLH surge may produce values in excess of 100 IU/L. In the castrated or postmenopausal woman hLH levels exceeding 200 IU/L may be achieved. In 1972 Vaitukaitis et al reported a RIA that specifically measures

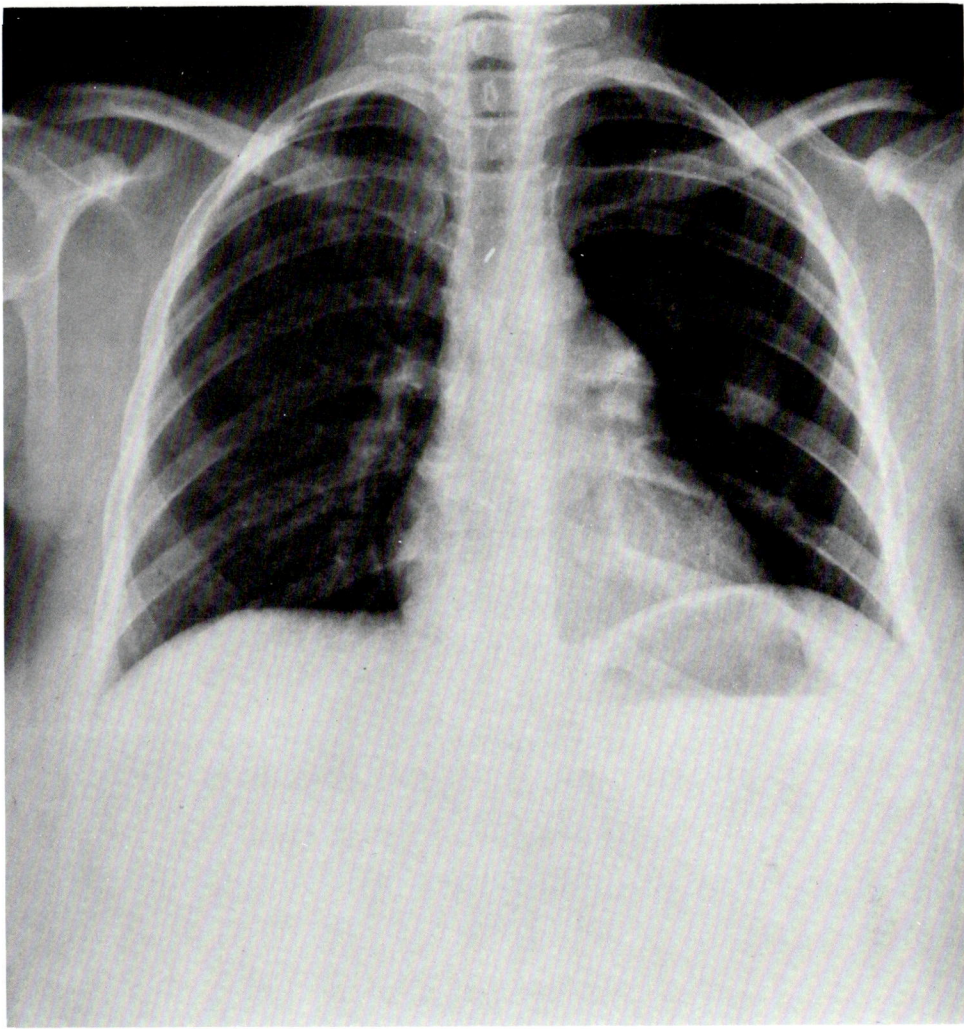

Fig. 8-8 Solitary metastasis in left mid-lung field which is smaller and less distinct than the lesion in **Fig. 8-7.** This lesion proved refractory to chemotherapy.

hCG in the presence of hLH by utilizing an antibody generated against the beta subunit of hCG. The sensitivity of the assay is adequate to distinguish hCG from follicular or luteal phase levels of hLH and is thus ideal for the diagnosis, treatment, and follow-up of trophoblastic disease when gonadotropin levels fall to the normal hLH range.

Postmole Surveillance

A program for monitoring patients after delivery of a hydatid mole is outlined in Table 8-4. A chest x-ray and pelvic examination are performed as part of the initial evaluation to identify metastases and establish a baseline for future reference. Uterine curettage is unnecessary after the initial evacuation procedure. Urine or serum hCG values are obtained at weekly intervals until three consecutive measurements are normal. The

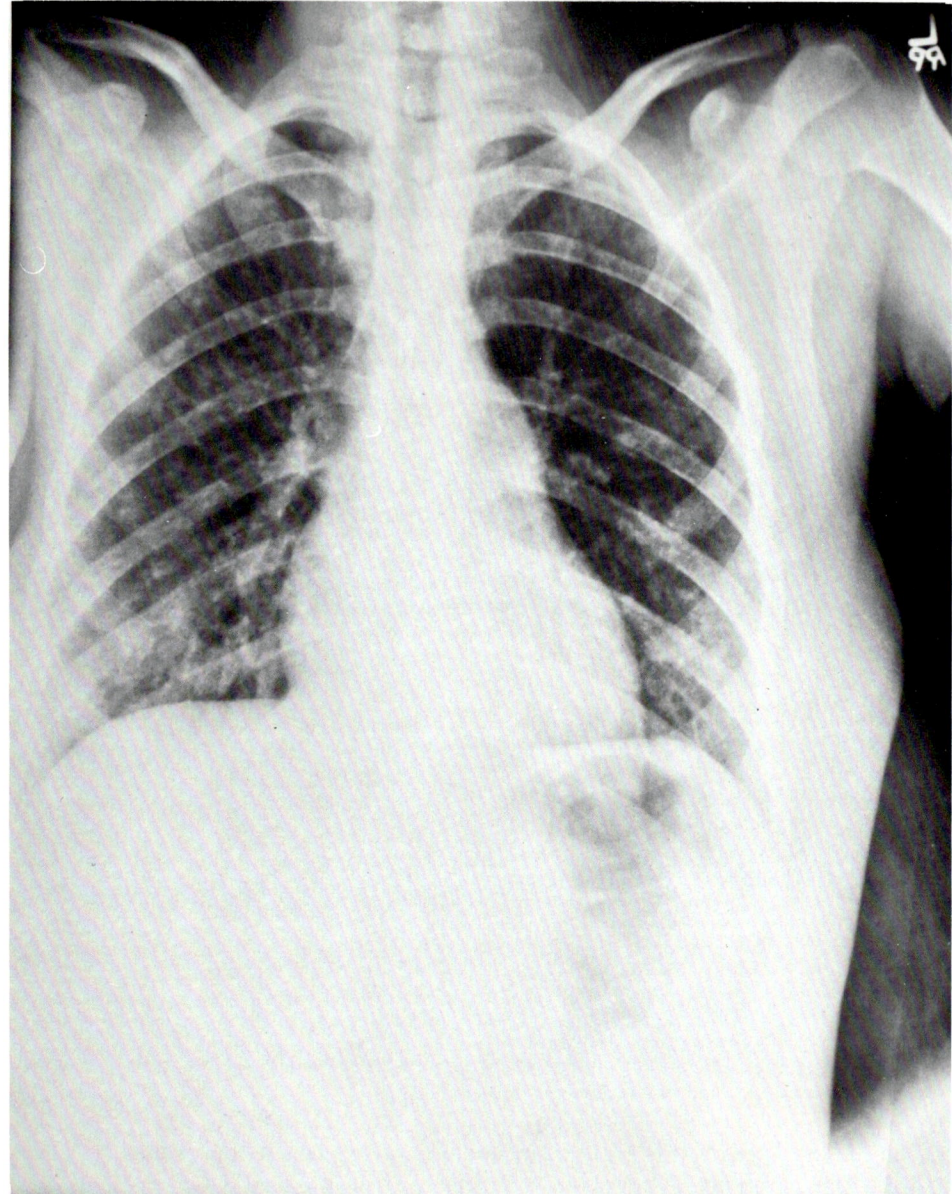

Fig. 8-9 Bilateral diffuse pulmonary metastasis from gestational choriocarcinoma. This patient presented with a complete spinal cord block secondary to an extradural metastasis.

patient is then considered to be in remission, after which hCG values are obtained at monthly intervals for 6 months and bimonthly for 6 months. Since the hCG produced by neoplastic trophoblast is indistinguishable biologically and immunologically from pregnancy hCG, it is important that pregnancy be avoided during the postmole follow-up period to avoid confusion regarding the etiology of rising levels of hCG. The use of combination oral contraceptives is recommended since they not only accomplish the goal of preventing pregnancy but also suppress the midcycle hLH peak.

TABLE 8-3 SENSITIVITY OF VARIOUS PREGNANCY TESTS AND hCG ASSAY METHODS

Name		Approximate Sensitivity[a] (IU^{b} hCG/L)	Test Time
1. Pregnancy tests			
Biologic			
Ascheim-Zondek	Immature female mouse	3000	4—5 days
Freidman	Immature female rabbit	3000	1—2 days
Galli-Mainini	Male toad (Bufo arenarum)	2500	1—3 hours
Hogben	Female toad (Xenopus laevis)	2500	18 hours
Ovarian hyperemia	Immature female rat	250	16—24 hours
Immunologic			
Latex agglutination—slide		700-1000	2 minutes
Latex agglutination inhibition—slide		2000-5000	2 minutes
Hemagglutination inhibition—tube		500-2000	2 hours
2. hCG assays			
Biologic			
Uterine weight	Mouse	100	3—4 days
Uterine weight	Rat	100	4—5 days
Ventral prostate	Rat	100	4—5 days
Ovarian hyperemia	Rat	400	16-24 hours
Ovarian weight	Rat	400	4—5 days
Spermiation	Toad or frog	4000	2—5 hours
Immunologic			
Hemagglutination inhibition—tube		500-1000	2 hours
Radioimmunoassay		1-10	3—5 days

[a]Minimal detectable amount of hCG in unconcentrated urine.

[b]1 International Unit of hCG is defined as the amount of hormone that will double the rat ovarian weight.

Pregnancy tests are woefully inadequate for postmolar surveillance. Of those commercially available, the most sensitive detects concentrations of hCG no lower than 500 IU/L and most are less sensitive. In addition, while the pregnancy test remains positive it gives no indication whether the hCG concentration is falling, has leveled off, or is rising. The commercial quantitative immunoassays may be used to measure the hCG levels after molar pregnancy until the titer drops below their sensitivity, after which it is imperative that the hCG measurements be continued with a more sensitive assay (RIA or uterine weight assay). The involution of theca-lutein cysts accompanying molar pregnancy may be slow and should not be interpreted as evidence of active disease. Provided that the hCG returns to normal levels, the cysts always regress.

The studies of Delfs (1959), Brewer et al (1971), and more recently Bagshawe et al (1973) and Goldstein (1974) provide a firm basis for the interpretation of postmolar gonadotropin values relative to the diagnosis of progressive trophoblastic disease and the need for therapeutic intervention. Brewer et al reported that by 60 days after molar evacuation approximately 70% of their patients achieved a normal hLH-hCG level, that is,

RADIOIMMUNOASSAY FOR hCG

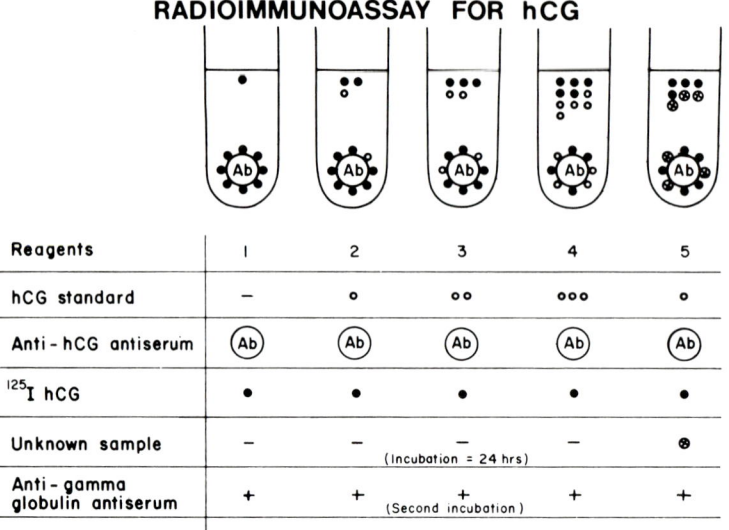

Reagents	1	2	3	4	5
hCG standard	–	o	o o	o o o	o
Anti – hCG antiserum	(Ab)	(Ab)	(Ab)	(Ab)	(Ab)
^{125}I hCG	•	•	•	•	•
Unknown sample	–	–	– (Incubation = 24 hrs)	–	⊗
Anti – gamma globulin antiserum	+	+	+ (Second incubation)	+	+

Fig. 8-10 Radiolabeled hCG is incubated with excess anti-hCG antibody. Unlabeled hCG (standard or unknown) displaces the radioactive hCG. The bound radioactivity will then be lower than in the *control* in reverse relation to the amount of unlabeled hCG added. The anti-hCG antibody is precipitated (second incubation), and the radioactivity in the precipitate counted. The amount of hCG in the unknown (tube 5) is read from a curve constructed from the measurement of radioactivity in the standard dilution series (tubes 1-4).

less than 25 IU/L. An additional 15% demonstrated a continuous drop in their titers, although the values were still higher than normal. The remaining 15% of the group at 60 days postmole had elevated titers, either plateaued or rising. In an earlier study Brewer et al (1968) found that nearly half of these patients had histologic evidence of choriocarcinoma; the rest had invasive mole. It is this group of patients that is selected for treatment.

The indications for initiating therapy during the postmolar follow-up period are given in Table 8-5. Of course, treatment should be instituted whenever there is a tissue diagnosis of choriocarcinoma or invasive mole, but this is seldom possible on the basis of uterine curettings. The presence of metastasis is sufficient cause for initiating chemotherapy at any point in time relative to the antecedent pregnancy. Although invasive mole can be associated with pulmonary and vaginal secondary lesions, metastases are far more likely to be the result of choriocarcinoma, and delaying treatment with the expectation that the metastatic lesions may regress spontaneously is not in the best interests of the patient.

TABLE 8-4 POSTMOLE SURVEILLANCE PROGRAM

1. Chest x-ray
2. Pelvic examination q 2 weeks until hCG normal, then monthly
3. Oral estrogen-progestin contraceptives X 12 months
4. Quantitative hCG determinations
    a. Weekly until 3 consecutive normal values (< 25 IU/L) obtained
    b. Monthly X 6 months
    c. Every 2 months X 6 months

TABLE 8-5 INDICATIONS FOR INITIATING
TREATMENT DURING POSTMOLE FOLLOW-UP

1. Tissue diagnosis of choriocarcinoma or invasive mole
2. hCG values rising or plateaued
3. hCG value elevated at 8 weeks postevacuation
4. Presence of metastasis
5. Elevation of hCG value after reaching normal

Usually therapy for progressive trophoblastic disease after the delivery of a hydatid mole is instituted because of an abnormal regression curve. A steadily falling hCG level portends a favorable outcome, and treatment is unnecessary unless the value exceeds 500 IU at 8 weeks postdelivery. If a significant rise in the hCG measurement occurs or if it remains constant for a period of 2 weeks treatment is indicated.

At the time that a decision is made to initiate therapy for progressive trophoblastic disease a complete evaluation of the patient is made (Table 8-6). Abnormal vaginal bleeding and lactation are common in patients with active trophoblastic disease. If there is much tumor in the uterus, bleeding may be profuse. The majority of patients have an enlarged uterus; ovarian enlargement due to theca-lutein hyperplasia is also common. Special attention is paid to the lower genital tract for evidence of metastasis. Biopsy of metastatic lesions should be avoided since major hemorrhage may ensue, particularly if the visible nodule is continuous with a pelvic metastasis. A chest x-ray, intravenous urogram, liver scan, and brain scan are performed in search of metastatic disease. Baseline blood counts and renal and liver function studies are obtained since these values must be monitored during chemotherapy. An endometrial curettage is unnecessary in evaluating these patients, however, because the selection of treatment is not predicated on the tissue diagnosis.

Nonmetastatic Trophoblastic Disease

Methotrexate and actinomycin D have demonstrated clear cut superiority to all other cytotoxic agents in the treatment of trophoblastic neoplasia. The recommended dosage and schedule for these agents are listed in Table 8-7. The therapeutic efficacy of these two drugs is apparently equivalent, but actinomycin D is favored by some authors

TABLE 8-6 WORK-UP FOR
TROPHOBLASTIC DISEASE

1. History, physical and neurological examination
2. Chest x-ray
3. Liver and brain scans
4. Intravenous urogram
5. hCG determinations
6. Complete blood count, platelet count
7. BUN[a], creatinine, SGOT[b] SGPT[c]

  a. blood urea nitrogen
  b. serum glutamic oxalo-acetic transaminase
  c. serum glutamic pyruvic transaminase

TABLE 8-7   SINGLE AGENT CHEMOTHERAPY FOR NONMETASTATIC
TROPHOBLASTIC DISEASE

---

1. Actinomycin D: 10-12 μg/kg/day IV X 5 days (maximum single dose: 0.5 mg)

    or

    Methotrexate: 0.4 mg/kg/day IM or IV X 5 days (maximum single dose: 30 mg)
2. Repeat cycle after minimum gap of 7 days if: Granulocytes > 1500/mm^3; Platelets > 100,000/mm^3; Stomatitis and gastrointestinal toxicity recovered; SGOT, SGPT, and BUN normal (methotrexate only)
3. Continue chemotherapy cycles until:
    a.   One course past normal hCG level
    b.   hCG values reach plateau or begin rising
4. Weekly hCG values and peripheral blood counts
5. Before each treatment cycle, SGOT, SGPT, BUN, and pelvic examination
6. Monthly titers for 6 months, every 2 months X 6 months, then every 6 months.
7. Continue oral contraceptives for 1 year after remission induction

---

because its use is attended by less systemic toxicity. Methotrexate is not recommended in the presence of parenchymal liver disease and is contraindicated when renal function is impaired. Each treatment cycle is repeated as soon as the normal tissues (bone marrow, gastrointestinal tract) have recovered, with a minimum 7 day gap between the last day of one course and the first day of the succeeding course. While the patients are under treatment, weekly gonadotropin values and peripheral blood counts are obtained. Before each course of therapy a pelvic examination and liver and renal function studies should be done. Provided that the gonadotropin levels continue to fall under therapy, additional chest x-rays are not necessary. Chemotherapy is continued until three consecutive weekly titers are normal.* A minimum of one course of drug therapy should be given after the first normal hCG determination. On the average, three to four courses of single drug therapy are required. The number of treatment cycles necessary to induce remission is proportional to the magnitude of the hCG concentration at the initiation of therapy. After remission has been induced and the treatment completed, hCG assays are obtained monthly for 6 months, every 2 months for the subsequent 6 months, and every 6 months thereafter. It is recommended that the patient take combination oral contraceptives for gonadotropin suppression and prevention of pregnancy during the first follow-up year.

Occasionally a patient with nonmetastatic trophoblastic disease will demonstrate resistance to single agent therapy, invariably after an initial response. Resistance is more likely to occur with choriocarcinoma than invasive mole, and, as a rule, the resistant focus is deep in the myometrium. These patients are more likely to have higher titers at initiation of therapy and a longer interval since the antecedent pregnancy than patients who do not demonstrate drug resistance. If the hCG values fail to drop significantly during two consecutive treatment courses, a change to actinomycin D or methotrexate, depending on which was the initial drug, is frequently successful in eradicating the disease. If the patient is not desirous of further childbearing, hysterectomy is indicated (Table 8-8) when the tumor manifests drug resistance. Before operation, the patient is reevaluated for metastatic disease. A pelvic arteriogram is obtained to demonstrate disease in the uterus (Fig. 8-11). Occasionally the arteriogram will be negative because the tumor is confined to the endometrium. An endometrial curettage will be positive in such cases. For the woman who is strongly motivated to retain her reproductive capability and whose uterine disease is not eradicated by changing drugs, a bilateral hypogastric artery infusion using methotrexate or actinomycin D can be performed (Hammond and Parker, 1970).

*The beta assay is employed to confirm remission hCG values and follow-up treated patients.

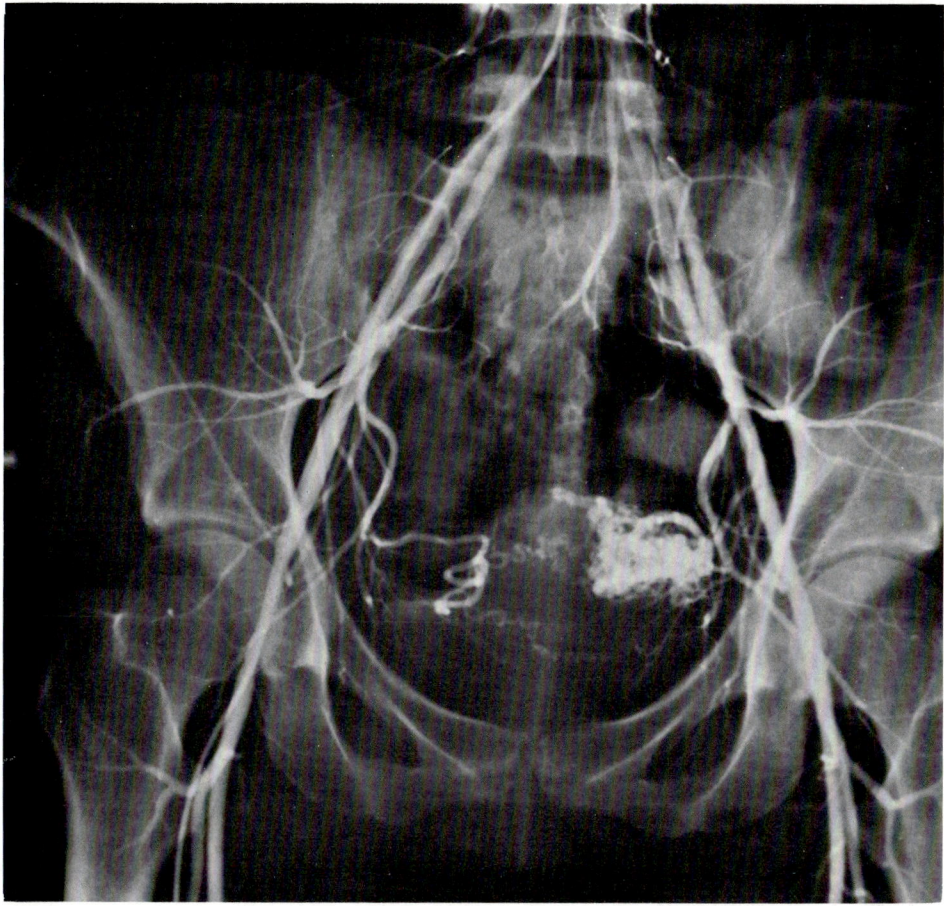

Fig. 8-11 Pelvic arteriogram showing features characteristic of trophoblastic desease within the myometrium. The left uterine artery is enlarged, and there is early filling of the ipsilateral veins due to arteriovenous shunting. In this case hysterectomy was performed because of drug resistance, and a small focus of choriocarcinoma was found deep in the myometrium near the left cornu. The patient has remained in remission for 1 year.

Smith (1973) has achieved excellent results using alternate courses of methotrexate and actinomycin D for nonmetastatic and metastatic trophoblastic disease. This regimen avoids the cumulative toxicity of methotrexate and may reduce the incidence of resistance developing to conventional single agent therapy.

The prognosis in this group of patients is exceptionally good; a nearly 100% cure rate can be anticipated. Hammond and Parker reported only 1 death among 47 patients with nonmetastatic trophoblastic disease following hydatid mole.

TABLE 8-8   INDICATION FOR HYSTERECTOMY IN TROPHOBLASTIC DISEASE

1. Primary management of hydatid mole—good operative candidate who requests sterilization
2. Primary management of nonmetastatic trophoblastic disease—good operative candidate who requests sterilization
3. Uterine disease resistant to chemotherapy

Metastatic Trophoblastic Disease

Patients with metastatic trophoblastic disease are subdivided into good and poor prognosis categories according to criteria established by Ross et al (1965) at the National Institutes of Health (Table 8-9). Patients with a good prognosis are managed in the same manner as those with nonmetastatic disease. A remission rate of nearly 100% can be expected. However, in the NIH experience, when individuals with demonstrable metastases had a urinary output of hCG greater than 100,000 IU/24 hours at the initiation of treatment or had delivered more than 4 months previously, a remission rate of only 40% was achieved with single agent therapy (Ross et al, 1965). In addition, patients with brain or liver metastasis have a poor prognosis regardless of titer or duration of disease at the onset of therapy.

Because of the limited success of single agent therapy in managing the poor prognosis group, new approaches to treatment were investigated. Hammond et al (1973) reported 7 complete remissions among 10 patients with poor prognosis metastatic trophoblastic disease, using a modified regimen of Li's triple therapy as the initial treatment (Table 8-10). However, among 7 individuals who were treated with combination chemotherapy after failure on single agent therapy remission was achieved in only 1 case. The addition of 2000 rads whole organ irradiation given in 2 weeks simultaneously with the initiation of triple drug therapy when brain or liver metastases are present has improved the prognosis in this high risk group; a complete remission rate of approximately 50% can be anticipated. It is not certain whether the irradiation exerts its beneficial effect by destroying the tumor in combination with the drug therapy or whether it serves to prevent a fatal hemorrhage, which would preclude the administration of drugs long enough to eradicate the disease. Toxicity is much less predictable with combination drug therapy than with single agents, and the threat of serious complications is significantly increased. Nevertheless, it is of critical importance to avoid severe toxicity that delays treatment, permitting significant regrowth of the tumor. Chemotherapy is continued until three consecutive weekly gonadotropin values are normal and the patient has had two courses of drug therapy after the first normal determination.   A principle in the management of trophoblastic disease is that the drug therapy is administered utilizing the gonadotropin measurements as the sole guide to tumor response and activity. Radiographically, lung lesions may remain for months after complete destruction of all viable trophoblastic tissue. In such cases chemotherapy is discontinued after remission has been achieved, as determined by hCG studies irrespective of the x-ray findings.

No chemotherapeutic regimen has established efficacy in the treatment of patients demonstrating resistance to triple drug therapy. Surgical excision of resistant foci outside the uterus has proved to be unsuccessful with few exceptions. Regional arterial infusion has been applied to liver metastasis. In selecting drugs for treatment of trophoblastic disease resistant to triple drug therapy, consideration should be given to agents that have

TABLE 8-9   POOR PROGNOSIS METASTATIC TROPHOBLASTIC DISEASE

1.   Metastatic disease with urinary hCG excretion > 100,000 IU/24 hours
2.   Metastatic disease with duration of disease > 4 months (interval since antecedent pregnancy)
3.   Brain or liver metastasis (regardless of disease duration or level of hCG)
4.   Metastatic disease resistant to single agent chemotherapy

TABLE 8-10 COMINATION CHEMOTHERAPY FOR POOR PROGNOSIS METASTATIC TROPHOBLASTIC DISEASE

1. Actinomycin D: 8-10 μg/kg/d IV (maximum 0.5 mg) X 5 days
    Methotrexate: 0.3 mg/kg/d IV or IM (maximum 15 mg) X 5 days
    Chlorambucil[α] 0.2 mg/kg/day PO (maximum 12 mg) X 5 days
2. Repeat cycle after minimum gap of 9 days
    if bone marrow and gastrointestinal toxicity
    recovered
3. Continue cycles until two courses given
    after first normal hCG value
4. Remission: three consecutive weekly hCG values
    normal (less than 25 IU/L)
5. hCG determination monthly X 12 months, every 2 months
    X 6 months then every 6 months
6. Monitor closely for toxicity
7. Pregnancy prophylaxis

[α]Or cyclophosphamide: 3-5 mg/kg/d IV (maximum 250 mg)

demonstrated activity against this malignancy: 6-mercaptopurine, 6-diazo-5-oxo-L-norleucine (DON), vincristine, and vinblastine.

8-6 PROPHYLACTIC CHEMOTHERAPY

The routine administration of methotrexate or actinomycin D during or immediately after the evacuation of hydatid mole has received attention as a potential means of eliminating postmolar neoplastic sequelae. Because of the relatively low incidence of postmolar choriocarcinoma and invasive mole, and the almost 100% cure rate when adequate follow-up and treatment are implemented, the use of prophylactic chemotherapy needs to be free of significant complications and uniformly successful to be justifiable. Goldstein (1972) has reported the best results with this approach to the management of hydatid mole. Employing actinomycin D and evacuating the mole during a 5 day treatment course reduced but did not eliminate the incidence of neoplastic sequelae. No serious drug effects were encountered. In view of this experience, prophylactic chemotheray seems suitable only for patients who cannot be followed after evacuation. Similarly, the concept of "covering" patients with systemic chemotherapy while they undergo surgery (uterine curettage, hysterectomy) for trophoblastic disease would seem to be applicable only when drug therapy is otherwise indicated.

REFERENCES

Aguero, O., and Zighelboim, I.: Fetography and molegraphy. *Surg. Gynecol Obstet.* **130**:649, 1970.

Attwood, H.D., and Park, W.W.: Embolism to the lungs by trophoblast. *J. Obstet. Gynaecol Brit. Commonw.* **68**:611, 1961.

Bagshawe, K. D.: *Choriocarcinoma: The Clinical Biology of the Trophoblast and Its Tumours.* Williams and Wilkins, Baltimore, 1969.

Bagshawe, K. D., Wilson, H., Dublon, P., Smith, A., Baldwin, M., and Kardana, A.: Follow-up after hydatidiform mole: Studies using radioimmunoassay for urinary human chorionic gonadotrophin (HCG). *J. Obstet. Gynaecol. Brit. Commonw.* **80**:461, 1973.

Borell, U., Fernstrom, I., Moberger, G., and Ohlson, L.: *The Diagnosis of Hydatidiform Mole, Malignant Hydatidiform Mole and Choriocarcinoma with Special Reference to the Diagnostic Value of Pelvic Arteriography.* Charles C Thomas, Springfield, Ill., 1966.

Brace, K. C.: The role of irradiation in the treatment of metastatic trophoblastic disease. *Radiology* **91**:540, 1968.

Braunstein, G. D., Vaitukaitis, J. L., Carbone, P. P., and Ross, G. T.: Ectopic production of human chorionic gonadotrophin by neoplasms. *Ann. Int. Med.* **78**:39, 1973.

Brewer, J. I., Eckman, T.R., Dolkart, R. E., Torok, E. E., and Webster, A.: Gestational trophoblastic disease. *Am. J. Obstet. Gynecol.* **109**:335, 1971.

Brewer, J. I., Smith, R. T., and Pratt, G. B.: Choriocarcinoma. *Am. J. Obstet. Gynecol.* **85**:841, 1963.

Brewer, J. I., Torok, E. E., Webster, A., and Dolkart, R. E.: Hydatidiform mole. *Am. J. Obstet. Gynecol.* **101**:557, 1968.

Choriocarcinoma, UICC Monograph Series, Vol 3, J. F. Holland and M. M. Hreshchyshyn, Eds. Springer-Verlang, New York; *Berlin Heidelberg,* 1967.

Delfs, E.: Chorionic gonadotrophin determinations in patients with hydatidiform mole and choriocarcinoma. *Ann. N.Y. Acad. Sci.* **80**:125, 1959.

Goldstein, D. P.: The chemotherapy of gestational trophoblastic disease. *J. Am. Med. Assoc.* **220**:209, 1972.

Goldstein, D. P.: Prevention of gestational trophoblastic disease by use of actinomycin D in molar pregnancies. *J. Obstet. Gynecol.* **43**:475, 1974.

Goldstein, D. P., Aono, T., Taymor, M. L., Jochelson, K., Todd, R., and Hines, E.: Radioimmunoassay of serum chorionic gonadotropin activity in normal pregnancy. *Am. J. Obstet. Gynecol.* **102**:110, 1968.

Goldstein, D. P., Winig, P., and Shirley, R. L.: Actinomycin D as initial therapy of gestational trophoblastic disease. *Obstet. Gynecol.* **39**:341, 1972.

Gottesfeld, K. R., Taylor, E. S., Thompson, H. E., and Homes, J. H.: Diagnosis of hydatidiform mole by ultrasound. *J. Obstet. Gynecol.* **30**:163, 1967.

Hammond, C. B., Borchert, L. G., Tyrey, L., Creasman, W. T., and Parker, R. T.: Treatment of metastatic trophoblastic disease: Good and poor prognosis. *Am. J. Obstet. Gynecol.* **115**:451, 1973.

Hammond, C. G., Hertz, R., Ross, G.T., Lipsett, M.'B., and Odell, W.D.: Primary chemotherapy for nonmetastatic gestational trophoblastic neoplasms. *Am. J. Obstet. Gynecol.* **98**:71, 1967.

Hammond, C. B., and Parker, R. T.: Diagnosis and treatment of trophoblastic disease. *Obstet. Gynecol.* **35**:132, 1970.

Hendrickse, J. P. de V., Willis, A. J. P., and Evans, K. T.: Acute dyspnoea with trophoblastic tumours. *J. Obstet. Gynecol. Brit. Commonw.* **72**:376, 1965.

Hertig, A. T.: *Human Trophoblast.* Charles C Thomas, Springfield, Ill., 1968.

Hertz, R.: Gestational trophoblastic neoplasia. *Hosp. Prac.,* January, p. 157, 1972.

Kaye, M. D., and Jones, W. R.: Effect of human chorionic gonadotropin on *in vitro* lymphocyte transformation. *Am. J. Obstet. Gynecol.* **109**:1029, 1971.

Kerber, I. J., Inclan, A. P., Fowler, E. A., Davis, K., and Fish, S. A.: Immunologic tests for pregnancy. *Obstet. & Gynecol.* **36**:37, 1970.

Kolstad, P., Hoeg, K., and Norman, N.: Malignant trophoblastic neoplasia. *Acta Obstet. Gynecol. Scand.* **51**:275, 1972.

Kolstad, P., and Liverud, K.: Pelvic arteriography in malignant trophoblastic neoplasia. *Am. J. Obstet. Gynecol.* **105**:175, 1969.

Lewis, J. L.: High risk pregnancy: Hydatidiform mole and choriocarcinoma. *J. Reprod. Med.* **7**:57, 1971.

Lewis, J. L.: Chemotherapy of gestational choriocarcinoma. *Cancer.* **30**:1517, 1972.

Li, M. C.: Trophoblastic disease: Natural history, diagnosis, and treatment. *Ann. Int. Med.* **74**:102, 1971.

Llewellyn-Jones, D.: Management of benign trophoblastic tumors. *Am. J. Obstet. Gynecol.* **99**:589, 1967.

Park, W. W.: *Choriocarcinoma: A Study of Its Pathology.* F. A. Davis, Philadelphia, 1971.

Physiology and pathology of trophoblastic tumors *in vivo* and *in vitro.* Ann. N.Y. Acad. Sci. **172**:277, 1971. Steinetz, B. G. ed.

Ross, G. T., Goldstein, D. P., Hertz, R., Lipsett, M. B., and Odell, W. D.: Sequential use of methotrexate and actinomycin D in the treatment of metastatic choriocarcinoma and related trophoblastic diseases in women. *Am. J. Obstet. Gynecol.* **93**:223, 1965.

Smith, J. P.: Trophoblastic disease: Diagnosis and management. *In Endocrine and Nonendocrine Hormone-Producing Tumors*, a Collection of Papers presented at the Sixteenth Annual Clinical Conference on Cancer, 1971, at the University of Texas, M. D. Anderson Hospital and Tumor Institute, at Houston. Yearbook Medical Publishers, Chicago, 1973.

Trophoblastic disease. *Clin. Obstet. Gynecol.:* **10**, No. 2, 1967.

Vaitukaitis, J. L., Braunstein, G. D., and Ross, G. T.: A radioimmunoassay which specifically measures human chorionic gonadotropin in the presence of human luteinizing hormone. *Am. J. Obstet. Gynecol.* **113**:751, 1972.

Van Thiel, D. H., Grodin, J. M., Ross, G. T., and Lipsett, M. B.: Partial placenta accreta in pregnancies following chemotherapy for gestational trophoblastic neoplasms. *Am. J. Obstet. Gynecol.* **112**:54, 1972.

CHAPTER NINE

Cancer
of the Fallopian Tube

Although the fallopian tube is an organ commonly involved in nonneoplastic tumor formation such as tubal pregnancy, pyosalpinx, and hydrosalpinx, it is rarely the primary site of true neoplasia. Benign tumors occur but are reported with less frequency than are malignant tumors. Of the reported benign tumors the most common are cystic teratomas, which are histopathologically the same as ovarian dermoid cysts. Solid teratoma, neurilemmomas, and adenomatoid tumors have also been reported in the fallopian tube. Most of the teratomas were symptomatic and palpable on pelvic examination.

INCIDENCE

Primary carcinoma of the fallopian tube accounts for only 0.1-0.5% of all gynecologic malignancies. It is interesting to speculate why the various sections of the müllerian tract should have such different susceptibilities to cancer. Cancer of the tube is rarest of all; more frequent is cancer of the endometrium and still more prevalent is cancer of the cervix. Cancer of the fallopian tube is, for the most part, an adenocarcinoma, although rare neoplasms of many varieties have been reported (e.g., sarcoma, endothelioma, lymphosarcoma, carcinosarcoma, and mixed tumors). In all, approximately 800 cases have been reported in the world literature. No official staging has been established; however, the spread, treatment, and prognosis of the disease are similar to those of serous carcinoma of the ovary, and it seems reasonable to adapt the staging system for ovarian carcinoma to tubal carcinoma (Table 9-1).

Chronic salpingitis of a tuberculous (less than 5%) and nontuberculous nature has been implicated in the genesis of this disease. On statistical grounds, however, this is unlikely since pelvic inflammatory disease is seen so frequently and carcinoma of the tube is rare. However, a history of infertility is common (more than 40% nulliparous). Some reports have indicated that the presence of occluded fimbria improves the prognosis, presumably because it prevents spillage of tumor within the peritoneal cavity.

The average age of patients with tubal carcinoma is about 55 years with the great

TABLE 9-1 SUGGESTED STAGING OF FALLOPIAN TUBE CARCINOMA

Stage 0	Carcinoma *in situ.*
Stage Ia	One tube involved—no serosa.
Stage Ib	Both tubes involved—no serosa.
Stage Ic	One or both tubes involved with ascites or positive peritoneal fluid cytology.
Stage IIa	Involvement of tubal serosa.
Stage IIb	Involvement of ovaries, uterus, or pelvic wall.
Stage III	Extension of tumor beyond the pelvis but limited to abdominal cavity.
Stage IV	Extension outside the abdominal cavity

majority occurring between 45 and 60 years of age. The youngest patient reported was 18 years old, and the oldest was aged 80.

SYMPTOMS AND DIAGNOSIS

The clinical triad of pain, vaginal discharge, and adnexal mass is suggestive of tubal carcinoma (present in two thirds of patients). Vaginal cytology is reported to be of no value in detecting this disease, but cases have been reported with a positive Papanicolaou smear. Bilaterality has been reported in about 20% of the cases. Tubal carcinoma should be suspected in any patient with postmenopausal bleeding not explained by physical examination or endometrial curettage. It is also suggested in the patient with a clinical history and findings suggestive of PID in a postmenopausal state. Although some authors have recommended histologic grading of these tumors, such a system has little prognostic value except for the poorly differentiated, nonpapillary solid tumors.

Vaginal discharge is frequently associated with this disease. This is of special significance in the postmenopausal group. At times the discharge is clear yellow or amber and has been mistaken as symptomatic of urinary tract fistula because of the persistence and profuseness. A sporadic watery discharge like hydrops tubae profluens associated with hydrosalpinx is also seen in some patients. Another important symptom is cramplike abdominal pain. Hysterosalpingography has not proved to be of value in diagnosis nor has laparoscopy, largely because the latter cannot distinguish between inflammatory disease and tubal carcinoma. Preoperative diagnosis is made in less than 5% of the cases; as a matter of fact, many coexistent lesions are found because myomas of the uterus, ovarian cysts, and pelvic inflammatory disease frequently provide the physical signs for which operation is performed. There is no significant correlation in the coincidence of myoma uteri and ovarian enlargements with this tubal disease. In one case reported by Mitchell and Mohler (1945) a carcinoma was discovered accidentally in the portion of a tube that had been resected as part of a sterilization operation during a cesarean section.

When curettage does not reveal a neoplasm, the persistence of vaginal bleeding in a postmenopausal woman should always raise the suspicion of tubal carcinoma. An abnormal Pap smear with negative findings at curettage should also suggest the possibility of tubal carcinoma.

SURVIVAL

Schiller and Silverberg (1971) studied 76 patients and reported a gross 5 year survival rate of 91% in patients with intramucosal lesions, 53% with tubal involvement reaching the serosa, and 25% or less in all more advanced tumors. It is obvious that survival in any series will depend to a great extent on the stage of the cases within that series. About 50% of the patients in whom the disease is limited to the tube at the time of primary operation can be expected to survive for 5 years, whereas only occasional reports of those with more advanced disease surviving for 5 years are recorded.

TREATMENT

Treatment of choice for fallopian cancer is total abdominal hysterectomy and bilateral salpingo-oophorectomy. If no residual tumor is present after surgery, consideration should be given to pelvic and abdominal irradiation. However, the effectiveness of irradiation therapy has not been established by a controlled study in the literature. Tubal carcinoma is known to respond to progestins, 5-fluorouracil, alkeran, and cytoxan, and undoubtedly patients who have unresectable bulky disease should be treated with chemotherapy. Of 27 cases from the Mayo Clinic reported by Hanton et al (1966), 7 patients received some form of chemotherapy: 5, systemic alkylating agents and 2, 5-FU; none of these agents caused any significant tumor regression. Boronow (1973) recently reported a patient with metastatic poorly differentiated adenocarcinoma to lungs and skin who underwent a complete objective response maintained over 13 months with the institution of alkeran therapy. At the present time the drugs of choice at our institution are an alkylating agent such as alkeran in combination with a progestin. The use of a progestin is theoretical, based on the similar müllerian origins of the endosalpinx and the endometrium, as well as the proven response of the latter to progestin chemotherapy. All patients should have adjunctive therapy after surgery, even if there is no known residual disease.

REFERENCES

Boronow, R. C.: Chemotherapy for disseminated tubal cancer. *Obstet. Gynecol.* 42:62-66, 1973.

Boutselis, J., and Thompson, J.: Clinical aspects of primary carcinoma of the fallopian tube. *Am. J. Obstet. Gynecol.* 111:98, 1971.

Dodson M., et al: Clinical aspects of fallopian tube carcinoma. *Obstet. Gynecol.* 36:935, 1970.

Erez, S., et al: Clinical staging of carcinoma of the uterine tube. *Obstet. Gynecol.* 30:547, 1967.

Hanton, E. M., et al: Primary carcinoma of the fallopian tube. *Am. J. Obstet. Gynecol.* 94:832, 1966.

Hertig, A. T., and Gore, H.: *Tumors of the Female Sex Organs*, Part 3: Tumors of the Ovary and Fallopian Tube. In *Atlas of Tumor Pathology*, Sect. 9, Fasc. 33. Armed Forces Institute of Pathology, Washington, D.C., 1961.

Hurlbutt, F. R., and Nelson, H. B.: Primary carcinoma of the uterine tube. *Obstet. Gynecol.* 21:730, 1963.

Kneale, B. L. G., and Attwood, H. O.: Primary carcinoma of the fallopian tube. *Am. J. Obstet. Gynecol.* 94:840, 1966.

Mazzarella, P., Okagaki, T., and Richart, R. M.: Teratoma of the uterine tube—a case report and review of the literature. *Obstet. Gynecol.* 39:381, 1972.

Mitchell, R. M. and Mohler, R. W.: Primary carcinoma of the fallopian tube. *Am. J. Obstet. Gynecol.* 50:283, 1945.

Momtazee, S., and Kempson, R. L.: Primary adenocarcinoma of the fallopian tube. *Obstet. Gynecol.* 32:649, 1968.

Okagaki, T., and Richart R. M.: Neurilemmoma of the fallopian tube. *Am. J. Obstet. Gynecol.* 106:929, 1970.

Pauerstein, C. J., Woodruff, J. D., and Quinton, S. W.: Developmental patterns in adenomatoid lesions of the fallopian tube. *Am. J. Obstet. Gynecol.* **100**:1000-1007, 1968.

Schiller, H., and Silverberg, S.: Staging and prognosis in primary carcinoma of the fallopian tube. *Cancer* **28**, 389, 1971.

Steile, S. J.: Carcinoma of the fallopian tube. *Proc. Roy. Soc. Med.* **60**:884, 1967.

Turunen, A.: Diagnosis and treatment of primary tubal carcinoma. *FIGO* 7:294, 1969.

CHAPTER TEN

Chemotherapy

10-1 RATIONAL BASIS FOR CANCER CHEMOTHERAPY

The most significant advance in the treatment of cancer during the past 15 years has been the unequivocal demonstration that certain disseminated malignancies can be cured by chemotherapy alone. The concept of curing human tumors with drugs is thousands of years old, but until the past quarter century such an accomplishment seemed to be more a fanciful wish than a legitimate endeavor of orthodox medical science. Cancer chemotherapy had an ironic and serendipitous beginning in World War I when Krumbhaar reported that victims of mustard gas poisoning developed severe leukopenia and lymphopenia. This observation led to the treatment of human leukemia with nitrogen mustard in the early 1940s. Initially, drug regimens were necessarily empiric, and the constant threat of serious complications coupled with evanescent tumor responses encouraged widespread skepticism. Although therapists dreamed of cures, they administered drugs expecting, at the most, temporary palliation. Numerous derivatives of nitrogen mustard were synthesized in an effort to increase the tumoricidal effect, reduce the toxicity, and expand the spectrum of sensitive malignancies. An intense search for more active compounds was initiated. The sex steroids estrogen and testosterone, naturally occurring growth regulators of certain normal tissues, were discovered to have an inhibitory effect on breast and prostate cancer. The antifolics aminopterin and amethopterin (methotrexate) were the first of numerous antimetabolites enjoined in the drug warfare against malignant neoplastic disease.

Information derived from molecular biology and cell kinetics is recruited continuously to optimize drug dosages and schedules. As a result clinical chemotherapy is progressing rapidly from an entirely empiric practice to one of the most scientifically sophisticated subspecialties in modern medicine. The substantive nature of this progress is demonstrated by the two human malignancies now curable by chemotherapy alone: gestational choriocarcinoma and Burkitt's lymphoma. Complete remissions of several months to years have also been achieved in childhood leukemia, lymphoma, Wilm's tumor, and metastatic carcinoma of the ovary, uterus, and breast with drug therapy alone or in combination with radiation and surgery.

258

Knowledge of the scientific basis of cancer chemotherapy is indispensable to the development of improved treatment protocols and the optimal use of antineoplastic drugs. A brief review of the relevant cellular biology, cell cycle kinetics, and the characteristics of tissue growth, including the relationship of these factors to drug action, dosage, and schedule, is presented here.

Molecular Biology

The cell is the fundamental unit of living tissue, normal or neoplastic. Its metabolic and biologic activities are controlled and directed by the genetic data incorporated into nuclear deoxyribonucleic acid (DNA). The elucidation of the genetic code and the mechanism by which it governs the synthesis of nucleic acids and protein ranks as one of man's greatest intellectual achievements. Deoxyribonucleic acid with its protein coating composes the substance of nuclear chromatin. During cell division the chromatin reorganizes to form the familiar paired chromosomes of metaphase. The protein coating stabilizes the DNA macromolecule and assists in regulating its activities. The DNA molecule consists of two strands wound in a double helix. Each strand or chain is a polymer of nucleotide subunits composed of deoxyribose, a purine or pyrimidine base, and a phosphate group. The two chains are joined by chemical bonds between specific base pairs. The pyrimidines cytosine and thymine always bind to the purines guanine and adenine, respectively.

The basic dogma of modern biology is expressed in the equation:

$$\text{DNA} \xrightarrow{\text{Transcription}} \text{RNA} \left(\begin{array}{c} \text{Transfer} \\ \text{Messenger} \\ \text{Ribosomal} \end{array} \right) \xrightarrow{\text{Translation}} \text{Protein}$$

Replication

At the time of cell division, DNA replication is accomplished by a progressive uncoiling of the double helix and the addition of complementary purine and pyrimidine bases to each strand under the direction of DNA polymerase. The end product is duplicate molecules of double stranded DNA, each composed of one old and one new chain. An additional function of DNA is the determination of cell structure and function through its control of protein synthesis. The information stored in the sequential purine and pyrimidine code is transcribed to ribonucleic acid (RNA). Deoxyribonucleic acid serves as a template for RNA, which is synthesized with the aid of RNA polymerase and is composed of a single strand of polymerized nucleotides which differ from DNA in that they contain ribose rather than deoxyribose and uracil instead of thymine. Three RNA species of varying sizes and functions exist; they have been designated as messenger (mRNA), ribosomal (rRNA), and transfer (tRNA) ribonucleic acid. Messenger RNA enters the cytoplasm, where it assembles the ribosomes (composed of rRNA) of the endoplasmic reticulum in preparation for protein synthesis. The synthesis of protein, a polymer of amino acids, is controlled by the sequence of bases in the mRNA. Each tRNA unit contains three nitrogenous bases, the sequence of which is specific for one amino acid. It escorts the amino acid to the polyribosomal structure, where it is inserted into an appropriately coded segment of the mRNA template under the guidance of the associated ribosomal RNA. In this manner the amino acid sequence characteristic for the coded protein is an exact expression of the DNA blueprint.

Antineoplastic drugs are nonspecific and exert their cytocidal effect by interfering with the replication of DNA or the transcription of its information to RNA (Fig. 10-1). These agents may act by combining with functional units of the DNA macromolecule or by disrupting the synthesis of its purine and pyrimidine precursors. Since the precursors in normal and malignant tissue are qualitatively identical, the effectiveness of chemotherapy is dependent on differences in metabolic demands, reflecting the greater replicative activity of the tumor cells. Although nucleotides can be synthesized from preformed dietary bases, the major pathway involves *de novo* synthesis from amino acid precursors (Fig. 10-2). Analogs of essential purine and pyrimidine metabolites prevent *de novo* synthesis of the normal subunits by tying up enzymes. As fraudulant monomers they may be incorporated into DNA and RNA, where they prevent the normal expression of the involved functional units. Although cell death can result from interference with RNA synthesis, a more common effect is deterring cells from entering the S phase, thus protecting them from lethal injury. The only reaction essential to DNA synthesis that is not involved in RNA synthesis is the conversion of deoxyribotide uracil monophosphate (dUMP) to deoxythymidine monophosphate (dTMP). Thymidine is present in DNA but not in RNA. The last step in the synthesis of dTMP is the methylation of dUMP at the 5 position. This methyl group is donated by a tetrahydrofolic acid derivative, and the reaction is catalyzed by the enzyme thymidylate synthetase. Both methotrexate and 5-fluorouracil act by inhibiting the synthesis of dTMP. Whether induced by chemical agents, therapeutic radiations, or ultraviolet light, DNA injuries are not necessarily permanent. If the injury is not lethal, repair enzymes can excise the damaged DNA segment and insert a normal part. Cancer cells are believed to have defective repair enzyme systems and therefore may be more susceptible to lethal injury than normal cells.

Growth Kinetics

Simply stated, cancer is a problem of uncontrolled proliferation. Its deviant behavior is best understood in the context of normal growth. There are three categories of normal adult tissues, based on the growth kinetics involved in maintaining a balance between parenchymal cell production and loss. The *expanding* tissues are composed of differentiated cells which normally survive the lifetime of the organism and do not

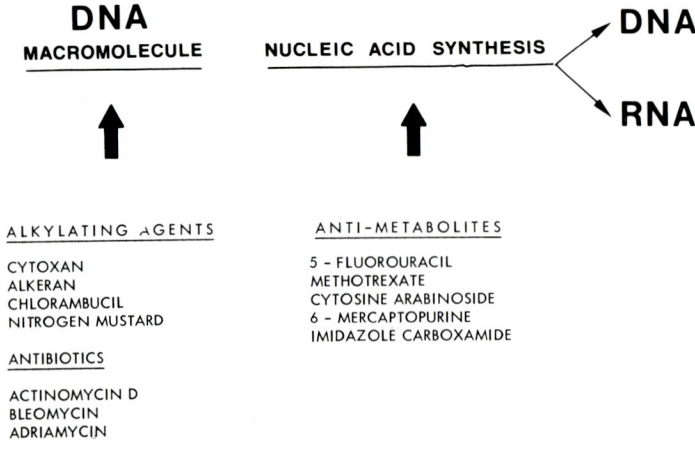

Fig. 10-1 Sites of action of chemotherapeutic agents.

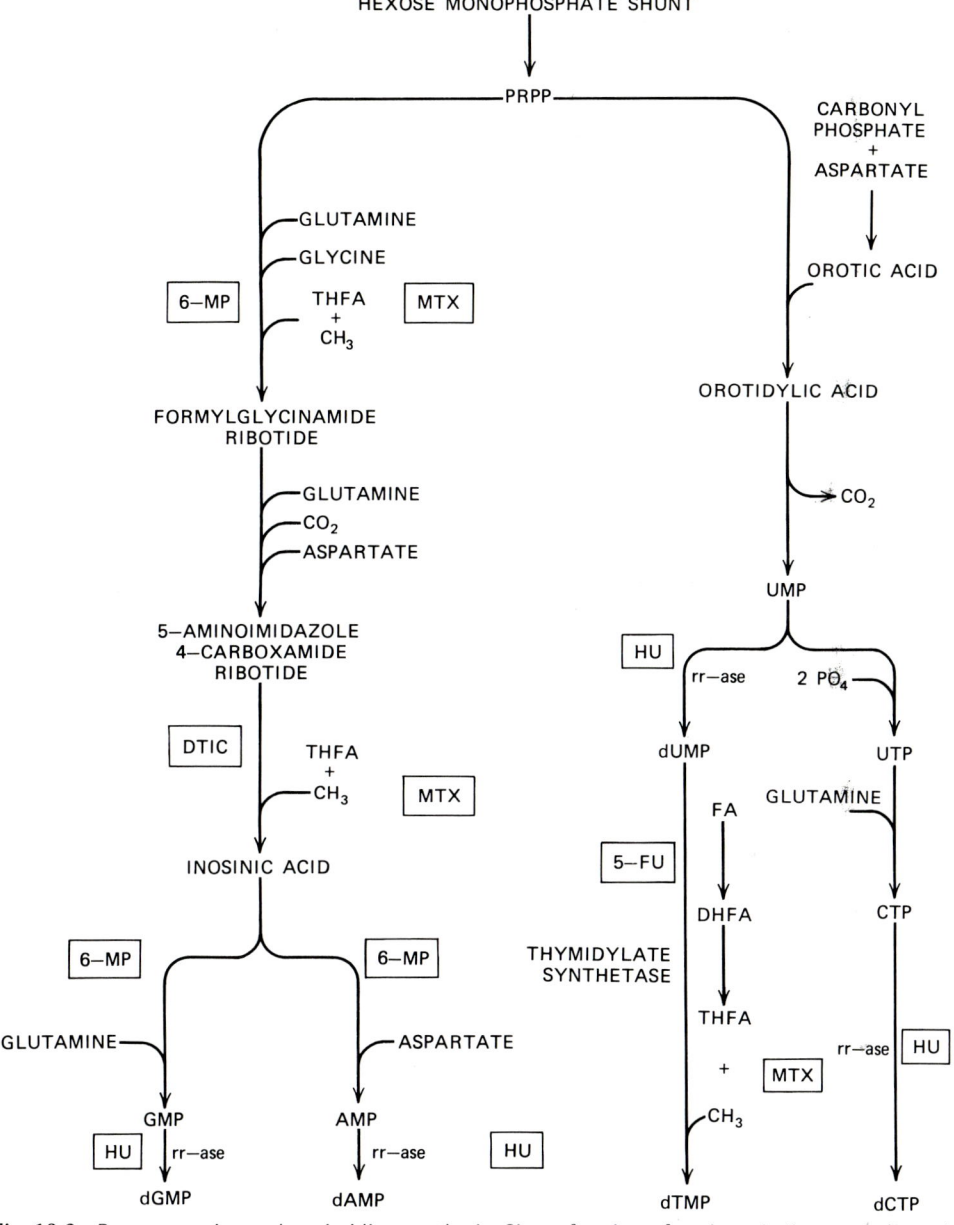

Fig. 10-2 *De novo* purine and pyrimidine synthesis. Sites of action of antimetabolites are indicated. AMP = adenosine monophosphate; CTP = cytidine triphosphate; DHFA = dihydrofolic acid; DTIC = dimethyltriazenoimidzole carboxamide; dTMP = deoxythymidine monophosphate; FA = folic acid; 5-FU = 5-fluorouracil; GMP = guanosine monophosphate; HU = hydroxyurea; MTX = methotrexate; 6-MP = 6-mercaptopurine; PRPP = phosphoribosyl pyrophosphate; rr-ase = ribonucleotide reductase enzyme system; THFA = tetrahydrofolic acid; UMP = uridine monophosphate.

require replacement. In the event of accidental loss, however, the cells of the expanding tissues, which retain the capacity to replicate, are able to replace the lost cells. The liver, kidney, and endocrine glands are examples of expanding tissues. The cells of nerve and striated muscle tissue are highly differentiated and have lost permanently the capacity to divide, even in the event of accidental loss. These tissues are designated as *static*. The third type of tissue, *renewing*, contains differentiated cells with a relatively short life span, requiring constant renewal from a stem cell or clonogenic subpopulation. The stem cell production of new differentiated cells is in equilibrium with the continuous loss of differentiated cells. The bone marrow, gastrointestinal mucosa, epidermis, and hair follicle are examples of renewing tissues.

The cell population of malignant tumors resembles the renewing type of tissue (Fig. 10-3). Essential to the survival of any malignant tumor is a subpopulation of cells capable of sustained reproduction. These clonogenic or stem cells may be actively proliferating, or they may occupy the temporarily nondividing compartment (G_0). A third compartment in the tumor cell population is composed of permanently nondividing cells, which have lost their ability to replicate because of differentiation, hormone effect, immune host defenses, or injury resulting from crowding and ischemia. The recruitable G_0 cells form a reserve from which the proliferating compartment may be replenished. From the therapist's viewpoint, the permanently nondividing cells are nonviable since, having lost the ability to replicate, they are doomed to die. These cells do comprise mass, however, and occupy volume that may hinder accurate evaluation of tumor response. Stem cells in the proliferating compartment are most vulnerable to injury by cytotoxic drugs, whereas resting stem cells are partially or completely insensitive to these agents. Thus the relative proportions of these two compartments, that is, the growth fraction, will have a crucial bearing on the responsiveness to chemotherapy. The blood cells and gastrointestinal mucosa as renewing tissues are the normal tissues most susceptible to injury from antineoplastic drugs because of their large proliferating compartments. However, the stem cells in these tissues protect them from total destruction since they have the ability to repopulate the tissue after the drug effect is over. On the other hand, the static and expanding tissues are protected from injury because all their cells are arrested in G_1.

Normally a cellular "brake" prevents overgrowth of any one cell type for the benefit of the community of cells. Under such special circumstances as wound healing and liver regeneration, the brake is released and then reset at a time that is optimal for the well being of the organism. Cancer tissue has lost this genetically determined brake. As depicted in Fig. 10-4, the initial growth of both normal and malignant tissues is exponential and would soon result in host death. However, normal tissue growth reaches

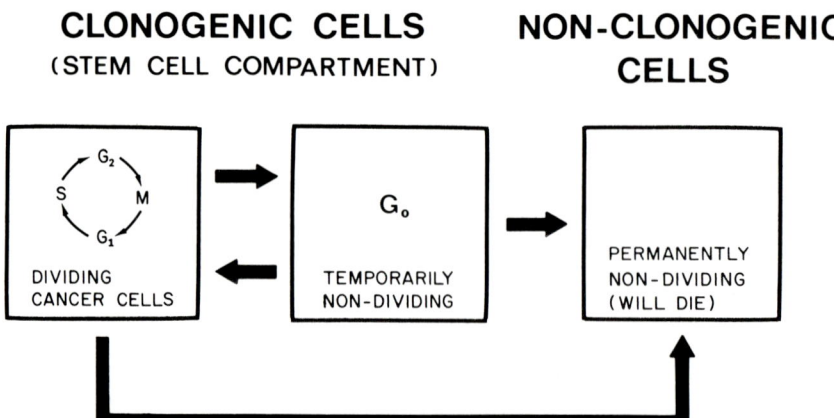

Fig. 10-3 Cell compartments in tumor mass. Modified from De Vita, 1971.

LETHAL NUMBER OF CELLS

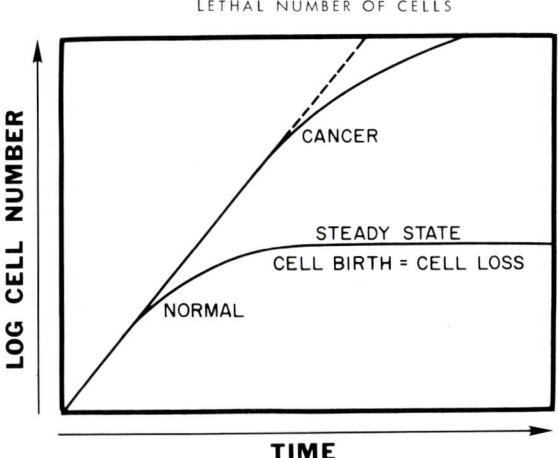

Fig. 10-4 Comparison of normal and malignant growth. Modified from De Vita, 1971.

a steady state after achieving a critical mass that is optimal for host survival. The kinetics of the steady state depend on whether the tissue is of the expanding, static, or renewing type. The last class of tissue may actually replicate faster than most cancers, but the balance between cell birth and cell loss is maintained. In contrast to normal tissue, cancer continues to grow, although not exponentially, until host death intervenes. As the tumor volume increases, the doubling time lengthens probably because of crowding and poor vascularization. There is an increased cell loss through central necrosis and also decreased production as cells move from the proliferating pool into the resting compartment because of hypoxia and nutrient shortages. The cells occupying the ischemic zones of solid tumors are probably inaccessible to therapeutic levels of systemically administered drugs.

The Cell Cycle

For many years two morphologically distinct intervals in the life cycle of the cell have been recognized: mitosis, with its classical subdivisions prophase, metaphase, anaphase, and telophase; and the interval between successive mitoses, which is designated as interphase. Tritiated thymidine pulse labeling of DNA has made it possible to identify three metabolically and functionally distinct subdivisions of interphase (see Fig. 10-5).

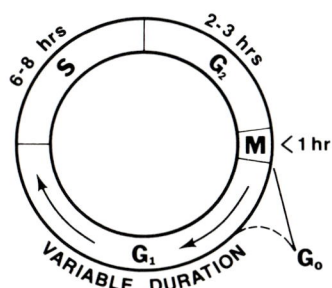

Fig. 10-5 The cell cycle.

After mitosis an interval of variable duration precedes the initiation of DNA synthesis. This G_1 phase is characterized by a diploid DNA content and an absence of DNA synthesis (actually a small amount of DNA synthesis for repair purposes occurs). During G_1, RNA and protein synthesis take place at a normal rate until immediately before the onset of the S phase, when a burst of RNA synthesis occurs. The cell then enters the S phase of the replicative cycle, during which time the entire nuclear DNA complement is duplicated. It lasts 6-8 hours on the average in mammalian cells. After the S phase the second postmitotic gap, G_2, appears. It is characterized by an absence of DNA synthesis and a tetraploid DNA content; RNA and protein synthesis proceed in preparation for cell division. During the M phase little RNA and protein are synthesized. A duplicate set of chromosomal DNA is inherited by each daughter cell, restoring the normal diploid condition. The interval between successive mitoses, the cell generation time, varies according to the length of G_1 since S, G_2, and M are relatively constant for any cell type. Although G_1 has a minimal time interval, it has no fixed maximum limit (see Fig. 10-6). As the G_1 phase becomes more prolonged, the cell is considered to enter a resting or temporarily nondividing state designated as G_0. The metabolic characteristics of the various phases of the generation cycle have a profound influence on the susceptibility of the cell to drug injury.

The elegant studies of Bruce (1966) on AKR mouse lymphoma have provided a classification of chemotherapeutic agents (Fig. 10-7) based on the relative dose-survival curves for normal hemopoietic and lymphoma colony forming (stem) cells. The fraction of surviving colony forming cells after 24 hours of drug exposure *in vivo* was determined by the spleen colony assay. Agents in Class I (ionizing radiation and nitrogen mustard) are lethal to cells in all phases of the cell cycle, and resting cells are as sensitive as proliferating cells. These are considered nonspecific agents. Class II drugs are phase specific, exerting their lethal effects exclusively or primarily during one phase of the cell cycle, usually S or M. Proliferating cells are killed whereas resting cells are spared.

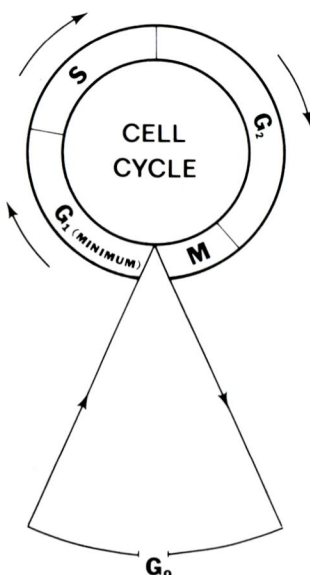

Fig. 10-6 Relationship of G_1 and G_0 phases.

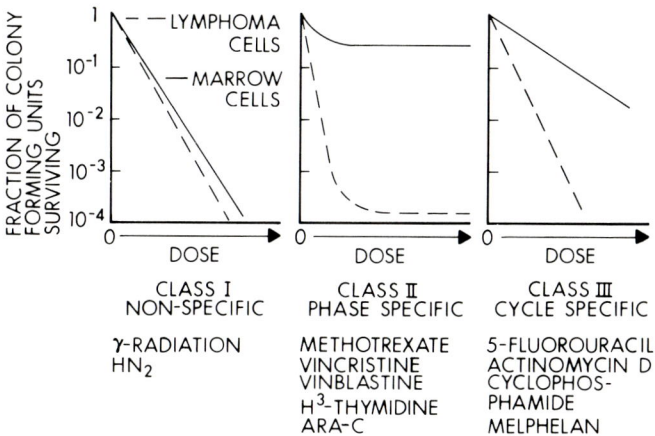

Fig. 10-7 Dose-survival curves of normal hemopoietic and AKR mouse lymphoma stem cells for various cytotoxic agents. (After Bruce 1966.)

Dissociation of the lymphoma and marrow curves reflects the relative number of stem cells in each tissue. Class III drugs are designated as cycle specific and are capable of damaging both resting and cycling cells, although the latter are much more sensitive. Again the dissociation of the dose-survival curves reflects the larger fraction of stem cells in the marrow than in the lymphoma cell population.

The L-1210 Mouse Leukemia Model

Much of the experimental foundation for clinical chemotherapy has been derived from the studies of Skipper et al (1964) on L-1210 mouse leukemia. One of the features that makes it suitable as a laboratory model is that its tumor cell population can be quantified. Several principles have been established from the study of this model which serve as guidelines to clinical chemotherapy:

1. Host survival is inversely related to the number of cells remaining after treatment or present when drug therapy is initiated (inoculum);
2. A single tumor cell is capable of multiplying and killing the host;
3. The tumor effect is dose related within the limits of drug toxicity, and the dose-response curve is steep;
4. A given dose of an effective drug kills a constant fraction of cells and not a constant number, regardless of the number of cells present (fractional kill hypothesis);
5. Tumor growth has the same slope after the drug effect is over as it did before treatment.

These principles, derived from a nonsolid animal tumor, must be applied with great circumspection to human solid tumors. Their validity is probably limited to the very early growth of solid tumors and rapidly proliferating malignancies such as choriocarcinoma, since the growth characteristics in these circumstances closely resemble those of nonsolid tumors. Nevertheless, these are concepts of fundamental importance, and the fractional kill hypothesis in particular needs emphasis by exposition.

One gram of tumor contains approximately 10^9 cells, but seldom is even the most superficially located tumor diagnosed with such a small cell population. The minimum palpable subcutaneous disease is approximately 6×10^7 cells (60 mg). Most patients with visceral tumors are estimated to have 10^{10}-10^{11} tumor cells (10-100g) at the time of diagnosis. The tumor cell volume producing host death is about 10^{12} cells, only 1-2 orders of magnitude less than the total number of cells in the human adult. As demonstrated in Table 10-1, a 90% reduction of a 10^{10} (10 billion) tumor cell population from a single course of drug therapy will produce a complete clinical remission. The reduction of a palpable 10 g mass to a nonpalpable 1 g mass makes the patient apparently tumor free. Since each course of drug therapy will kill the same fraction of cells and not the same number, to eradicate the last surviving cell at least 10 additional courses of drug therapy are required (so-called exponential iceberg). In dealing with visceral solid tumors the residual tumor burden may be vastly in excess of 1 billion cells without any clinical evidence of disease. The influence of the fractional kill mechanism of drug therapy and the volume of tumor at the onset of therapy on outcome is illustrated in Fig. 10-8. The patient on the left with 10^{11} cells gets a good response for several courses of therapy and the tumor volume is reduced 4 decades, but resistance develops and the patient is lost. On the right the initiation of therapy at a time when subclinical disease is present (10^4 cells) produces a cure. The larger the initial tumor volume and the smaller the fractional kill, the more likely is resistance to develop. (It is of some interest that normal tissues do not develop resistance to antitumor drugs). The results of therapy in sensitive tumors, therefore, will be directly proportional to the number of cells present when treatment is begun. Since the response is dose related, more aggressive treatment should improve the response rate provided that toxicity remains in an acceptable range. The effect of successive doses of drug will depend on the fractional kill and the number of existing cells. Since the number of cells present at the initiation of a cycle of therapy is dependent on the number of cells surviving the preceding treatment and the tumor cell production between treatment cycles, it is imperative that this interval not be determined by chance but be reduced to a strict minimum, that is, the time required for restoration and recovery of normal tissues. Obviously cell destruction must exceed interval production for chemotherapy to be successful.

TABLE 10-1 TUMOR DEPOPULATION RELATED TO SUCCESSIVE DRUG
CYCLES ASSUMING A 90% FRACTIONAL KILL IN A MODEL SYSTEM

Drug Treatment No.	Tumor Weight (g)	Number of Tumor Cells	Number of Tumor Cells Killed	Number of Tumor Cells Surviving	
1	10.0	10,000,000,000 (10^{10})	9,000,000,000	1,000,000,000	Clinical
2	1.0	1,000,000,000 (10^9)	900,000,000	100,000,000	Disease
		Complete Clinical Remission			
3	0.1	100,000,000 (10^8)	90,000,000	10,000,000	Subclinical
4	0.01	10,000,000 (10^7)	9,000,000	1,000,000	Disease
5	0.001	1,000,000 (10^6)	900,000	100,000	
6	0.0001	100,000 (10^5)	90,000	10,000	
7	0.00001	10,000 (10^4)	9,000	1,000	
8	0.000001	1,000 (10^3)	900	100	
9	0.0000001	100 (10^2)	90	10	
10	0.00000001	10 (10^1)	9	1	
11	0.000000001	1 (10^0)	1	0	

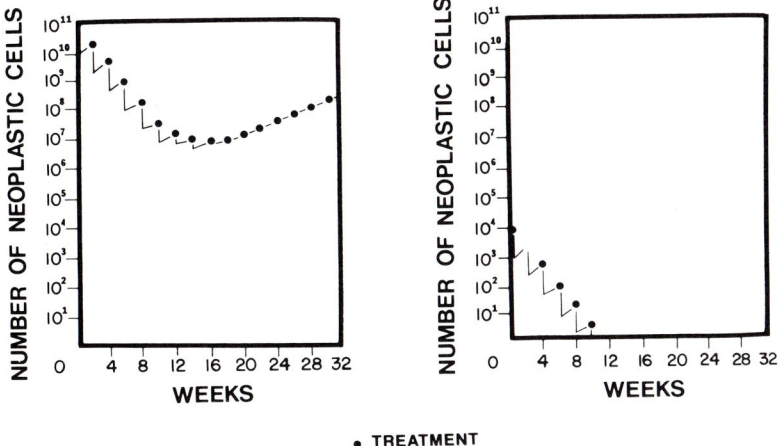

• TREATMENT

Fig. 10-8   Role of inoculum size in treatment outcome. (Luce 1967.)

Principles of Clinical Chemotherapy

The dose and the schedule of drugs have a vital influence on the therapeutic index. The steep dose-response curve for most drugs indicates that the highest tolerable dose (i.e., the dose producing an acceptable degree of reversible toxicity) should be used in the treatment of sensitive tumors. The aim is to achieve a maximum cell kill with a minimum toxicity. A twofold increase in dose may produce a tenfold increase in the fractional kill. In addition to drug dose, optimal therapy must take into consideration the length of time that a therapeutic concentration of drug is maintained. Maximal effectiveness of some oncolytic drugs is primarily dependent on peak tissue concentration, while that of others depends on the duration of exposure. In general, the phase specific drugs (Fig. 10-9) are optimally administered in 5 day courses (approximately two average cell generation times), during which time a therapeutic concentration is maintained. Since proliferating cells do not progress through the generation cycle in a synchronized fashion, prolonged exposure permits a higher fraction of the proliferating cells to pass through a vulnerable phase of their life cycle. In contrast, the cycle specific drugs are optimally administered as

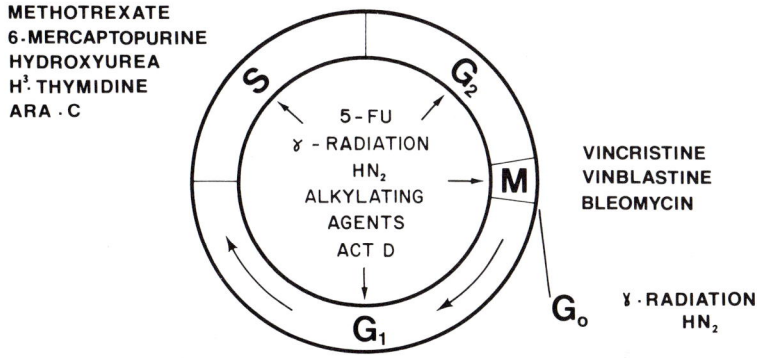

Fig. 10-9   Drug activity related to phases of cell cycle.

an intravenous bolus, utilizing the highest tolerable dose, and repeated after the normal target tissues have recovered.

High dose, intermittent therapy has been the most successful schedule against tumors with a large growth fraction. Some myelosuppression and immunosuppression are acceptable since recovery occurs between treatment cycles. Immunosuppression, which is more pronounced when drugs are given continuously, is a side effect of most cytotoxic drugs, but cyclophosphamide, 6-mercaptopurine, and prednisone are particularly toxic to the immune system. Suppression of the host's natural immune defenses is an important aspect of chemotherapy and must not be overlooked. Slow growing tumors have a large component of permanently nondividing cells and a small growth fraction. Theoretically, drugs active against cells in G_0 and administered on a continuous basis should produce the best results in these tumors. However, immuno- and myelotoxicity must be negligible, or chronic therapy is not likely to be feasible. No currently available drug meets all of these criteria.

Antitumor drugs have been combined either concurrently or sequentially in an effort to increase their effectiveness. It seems logical that drugs having different limiting toxicities and different modes of action might increase the fractional kill without a parallel rise in damage to normal tissues, including immunocompetent cells. In addition, the likelihood of resistance developing should be reduced. Tumors are composed of numerous cell clones which vary in their sensitivity to drugs. The use of multiple agents should lessen the possibility of the tumor being repopulated by a resistant clone. Sequential, concomitant, or complementary blockade of metabolic pathways should avoid the problem of drug resistance secondary to the utilization of alternate pathways or the emergence of a protective random mutation. As a rule, drugs selected for polychemotherapy must be effective as single agents if any improved results are to be expected. Unfortunately, the toxicities of most antitumor drugs are similar, and selecting drugs with no overlapping side effects is not usually possible. Nevertheless, combination chemotherapy has proved superior to single agent therapy in the management of leukemia, lymphoma, and some rapidly proliferating solid tumors. Drug combinations have not been used extensively in the slow growing, solid tumors because the risk of serious toxicity does not always seem to be justified by the small chance of substantial tumor control.

In summary, successful drug therapy requires the administration of an effective agent, utilizing an optimal dose and schedule. The tumor usually must have a high growth fracton and not inhabit the pharmacologic sanctuaries (central nervous system, ovary, ischemic zones). The tumor volume must be small or the fractional kill large to avoid the emergence of a resistant clone or the development of tolerance in previously sensitive clones. The recovery of normal tissue from drug injury must precede regeneration of tumor to pretreatment levels.

Adjuvant Therapy

Surgery and ionizing radiation have probably been maximally exploited as independent modalities for the control and cure of regional malignant disease. Their complementary use has provided improved treatment results in the management of some malignant tumors. The employment of cytotoxic agents as adjuvants to regional surgical and radiation therapy is a logical step since chemotherapy, including hormone therapy and immunotherapy, provides the only means of systemic treatment for disseminated disease. Increased survival with this multidisciplinary strategy has already been realized for, at least, Wilm's tumor. The malignant neoplasms most suited to adjuvant chemotherapy are those that have significant cure rates from surgery or radiation therapy and also demonstrate a significant response to chemotherapy. Among the gynecologic malignancies, ovarian, tubal, and endometrial carcinoma would seem to be well qualified. The best results with chemotherapy as a surgical adjuvant are probably achieved after surgery rather than before. In this cooperative effort surgery and radiation therapy would have as their primary role the reduction of the tumor burden, ideally to a subclinical or occult level. Such a reduction of the necrotic and ischemic zones of bulky tumors minimizes the cell population inaccessible to therapeutic drug levels. Increased proliferative activity of the residual cell population probably follows tumor depopulation, enhancing the likelihood of eradicating the disease with antineoplastic agents. It must be kept in mind that high doses of radiation produce vascular damage, leading to the formation of ischemic sanctuaries for potentially sensitive cells. Adjuvant drug therapy can be used intraoperatively to prevent the spread of cancer during surgery. Rarely the administration of an antineoplastic agent will make an inoperable tumor resectable.

The status of immunotherapy in gynecologic cancer is reviewed in Chapter 13. It is distinctly possible that chemotherapy need not destroy all the residual cancer cells. The host immune defenses stimulated by nonspecific immunotherapy may be capable of destroying 10^5 tumor cells.

The intraarterial infusion of drugs has been utilized to increase the concentration of drug delivered to the tumor without raising the systemic toxicity. This is most suitable for tumors with a long doubling time and has been used frequently in combination with x-ray therapy. The concept is to have drugs available in the tissues to react with the free radicals produced by the ionizing radiation. Continuous exposure of a tumor to cycle and phase specific agents provides the opportunity for resistant resting cells within the tumor bed to enter the drug sensitive proliferative cycle.

10-2 CHEMOTHERAPEUTIC AGENTS IN GYNECOLOGIC MALIGNANCIES

I. Alkylating agents
    A. Nitrogen mustard compounds
        Mustargen (mechlorethamine)
        Leukeran (chlorambucil)
        Cytoxan (endoxan, cyclophosphamide)
        Alkeran (L-sarcolysin, melphalan)
    B. Ethylenimines
        Thiotepa (triethylenethiophosphoramide)
    C. Alkyl sulfonates
        Busulfan (myeleran)
II. Antimetabolites
    A. Folic acid analogs
        Methotrexate (amethopterin)
    B. Pyrimidine analogs
        Fluorouracil (5-FU)
        Cytosar (cytosine arabinoside)

        C.   Purine analogs
               Purinethol (6-mercaptopurine)
               Imidazole carboxamide
III.   Antibiotics
               Cosmegen (actinomycin D)
               Blenoxane (bleomycin)
               Adriamycin
IV.   Vinca alkaloids (periwinkle drugs)
               Velban (vinblastine)
               Oncovin (vincristine sulfate)
 V.   Progestins
               Provera (medroxyprogesterone acetate)
               Delalutin (hydroxyprogesterone caproate)
               Megace (megestrol acetate)
VI.   Miscellaneous
               Hydrea (hydroxyurea)

Alkylating Agents

This group of compounds originated with "sulfur mustard" (bis-2-chlorethyl sulfide), a poisonous liquid with a vesicant action used in World War I. From it were derived bis-β-chloroethylamine and its N-methyl derivative, the parent compounds of the so-called nitrogen mustards. The alkylating agents are the single most useful group of cancer chemotherapeutic agents, although, despite an enormous amount of basic investigative effort, their mechanism of action as antineoplastic agents is not clear. They are very reactive, electrophilic compounds that readily combine with numerous biologically important sites, for example, amino, phosphate, sulfhydryl, hydroxyl, imidazole and carboxyl groups. Two generally accepted explanations concerning the manner in which these drugs inhibit rapidly proliferating cells are the cross-linking and the cyclo-alkylating hypotheses. Each of these concepts attempts to explain a predominant requirement for activity of these compounds: bifunctionality (i.e., the presence of two or more alkylating groups). Cross-linking implies interaction between the bifunctional compounds and the reactive groups of a macromolecule (e.g., DNA) at two nucleophilic sites, forming a bridge that prevents replication or otherwise alters the biologic properties of the chromosomes, thereby crippling the cell. In addition, these linkages may form large circular chains also injurious to the cell. The specific locus of such an attack has not been determined. Some investigators favor the phosphate groups of the polynucleotides, whereas others consider the nitrogen atoms of the purine and pyrimidine bases to be more likely targets.

    Three main types of alkylating agents currently in clinical use are (a) the nitrogen mustards; (b) the ethylenimines; and (c) the alkyl sulfonates. In the first group, there are four drugs that are in general clinical use: mechlorethamine, chlorambucil, cyclophosphamide, and alkeran (melphalan).

    Mechlorethamine, commonly called nitrogen mustard or HN_2, is commercially available as Mustargen (Merk and Company). The earliest successes with mechlorethamine were in lymphomas, and it is still widely used for treating Hodgkin's disease. It must be dissolved immediately before administration in order to avoid rapid hydrolytic inactivation. The

Nitrogen Mustards

Mechlorethamine (Nitrogen Mustard, HN$_2$, Mustargen)

$$Cl-CH_2-CH_2$$
$$N-CH_3$$
$$Cl-CH_2-CH_2$$

Methyl bis (β-chloroethyl) amine. Basic substance to all nitrogen mustards.

usual intravenous dose is 0.4 mg/kg. In almost all instances nausea and vomiting accompany its administration. The injections should be delivered into the tubing of an intravenous infusion because this highly reactive compound has a vesicant action upon contact with subcutaneous tissues or exposed surfaces and may produce local necrosis, contractures, or thrombophlebitis. The rapid local administration of sodium thiosulfate immediately after accidental extravasation may prevent these toxic effects by inactivation of the reactive groups. Depression of the bone marrow is the most serious toxic manifestation of nitrogen mustard, and treatment is generally not repeated until 4-6 weeks after therapy in order to assure adequate time for recovery.

Because of the effectiveness of other alkylating agents in the treatment of ovarian cancer, nitrogen mustard is uncommonly used in modern gynecologic oncology. Probably its most useful application is in the treatment of pleural effusion and occasionally ascites unresponsive to systemic chemotherapy. Fifteen milligrams of drug mixed with 20 cc of saline is administered into the pleural cavity after thoracentesis. In a similar manner, 20 mg of nitrogen mustard is mixed with 50 cc of saline for intraperitioneal installation after paracentesis. Its effect on persistent ascites is not as dramatic as its effect on pleural effusion.

Chlorambucil (Leukeran)

$$HO-\overset{\overset{\displaystyle O}{\|}}{C}(CH_2)_3$$

with benzene ring, N substituent groups CH_2CH_2Cl and CH_2CH_2Cl

4$-$($p-$[Bis($\beta-$chloroethyl)amino] phenyl)butyric acid

Chlorambucil has had widespread application in the treatment of adenocarcinoma of the ovary. It has also been used in conjunction with methotrexate and actinomycin D for choriocarcinoma and ovarian germ cell tumors. Chlorambucil is generally given in doses of 0.1-0.2 mg/kg/d (6-12 mg/day in the average patient). Often 3-6 weeks elapse before improvement occurs. The maintenance dose frequently must be reduced to approximately 2-4 mg/day in order to keep the white count above 3000 and the platelet count above 75,000. Myelotoxicity may develop slowly, but it is possible to induce marked hypoplasia of the bone marrow with prolonged high doses. Ocassionally patients have gastrointestinal effects, such as nausea and vomiting.

Cytoxan (Endoxan, Cyclophosphamide)

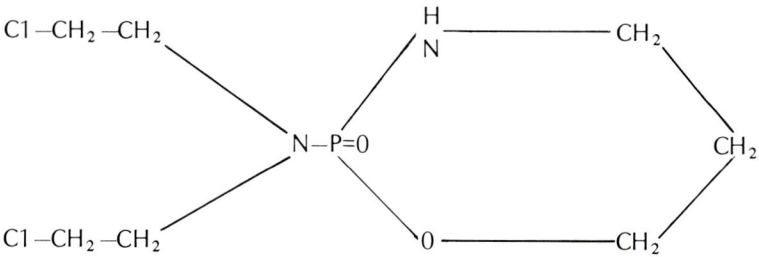

2−[Bis(β−chloroethyl)amino]−2H−1,3,2−oxazaphosphorinane 2−oxide

More literature has appeared on cyclophosphamide than on any other alkylating agent. Cyclophosphamide is unique among the alkylating agents in its ability to produce remissions in a wide spectrum of diseases, including childhood acute leukemia, highly malignant sarcomas of children, Ewing's sarcoma, and multiple myeloma. In the treatment of gynecologic malignancies it has demonstrated considerable activity in uterine sarcomas, ovarian carcinomas, germ cell tumors of the ovary, cervical carcinoma, and recurrent endometrial carcinoma. Frequently it is used in combination with other antineoplastic agents. Cytoxan is inactive *in vivo* until it is converted by the liver to a cytotoxic metabolite.

Cytoxan is administered in a number of dosage regimens. It can be given orally in a dose of 2.5 mg/kg/d. This dose is increased by 50 mg increments each month until chronic leukopenia (WBC ≅ 3000) results. Intravenous dose schedules are numerous, including (a) 1-2 mg/M^2 IV push once every 3−6 weeks; (b) 10−15 mg/kg IV once weekly; and (c) 8mg/kg/d IV push daily for 5 days repeated every 4−6 weeks. When cytoxan is used in combination with other myelosuppressive drugs, a proportionate reduction in dosage is necessary.

Reports of the toxic effects of cyclophosphamide have indicated some interesting manifestations of selectivity. Although leukopenia is regularly seen at higher dosage levels, a significant degree of thrombocytopenia is much less common. The apparent resistance of the megakaryocytes to this agent is even more evident when the hematologic effects of cyclophosphamide are compared to those caused by nitrogen mustard. Another manifestation of the difference in tissue specificity of this drug and other alkylating agents is the frequent occurrence of alopecia; this cosmetically troublesome effect usually is reversible upon discontinuation of cyclophosphamide therapy.

Many patients experience nausea and vomiting during the intravenous administration of the drug, especially when the dose is above 4 mg/kg. These symptoms may appear up to 6 hours after administration of the drug and may last for approximately 24 hours. The breakdown products of cyclophosphamide are excreted in the urine. These substances are very irritating to bladder mucosa, causing hemorrhagic cystitis in some cases. A high urine volume reduces the concentration of these irritating substances and the likelihood of this complication developing. Hemorrhagic cystitis necessitates discontinuation of cytoxan therapy. The hemorrhage may be so severe that urinary diversion is necessary to achieve satisfactory hemostasis.

Melphalan (Alkeran, L-Sarcolysin)

p—Bis(β—chloroethyl)aminophenylalanine

Alkeran is one of the most popular drugs for the treatment of adenocarcinoma of the ovary because of its minimal side effects, high activity, and ease of administration. This drug has also been used in the treatment of cervical and tubal adenocarcinoma in conjunction with progestins. The standard dose regimen is 0.2 mg/kg/d in divided doses for 5 days, repeated every 4 weeks if the WBC is greater than 3000 and the platelet count exceeds 150,000. The drug is usually given 3 times a day with meals in order to avoid a mild degree of gastric irritation. In patients who must receive the drug intravenously, the dose is 1 mg/kg IV push. It is repeated every 3 weeks if the platelets exceed 150,000 and the WBC is greater than 3000.

The toxicity of melphalan is almost purely to bone marrow, and the white blood cells, platelets, or red cells may be affected. The dosage necessary to produce toxicity varies greatly from patient to patient. Patients with uremia may be more susceptible to melphalan toxicity and should receive a smaller initial dose. Although neutropenia is commonly seen during the first several courses of alkeran chemotherapy, it is often suppression of the megakaryocytes that prohibits routine administration of the drug after several months of use. Only an occasional patient complains of thinning of the hair.

Ethylenimines

Triethylenemelamine (TEM) was the first ethylenimine synthesized by industrial chemists for use in improving the finish of rayon fabrics. Because of the presence of ethylenimine groups in its structure, the cytotoxic and pharmacalogic actions were studied by various investigators. The analog triethylenethiophosphoramide (thiotepa) was introduced clinically in 1963.

Thiotepa

$$CH_2-N-P-N-CH_2$$

Triethylenethiophosphoramide

Several authors have reported on the use of thiotepa in the treatment of ovarian cancer with very acceptable remission rates. In recent years, however, it has found less favor than some of the alkylating agents mentioned above. Though thiotepa may be administered orally, it is usually given intravenously or intramuscularly in doses of 10 mg daily for 5 days, followed by maintenance levels of 5-20 mg/week. It was formerly quite common for this drug to be administered as a single intracavitary injection of 10-50 mg in an effort to control peritoneal or pleural neoplastic effusions, but this practice can no longer be recommended since its effects are less predictable than those of the intravenous route. Undesirable effects of thiotepa, like the other ethylenimine derivatives, are depression of the bone marrow and, occasionally, nausea and vomiting.

Alkyl Sulfonates

Busulfan (Myleran)

$$CH_2-CH_2-O-SO_2-CH_3$$
$$CH_2-CH_2-O-SO_2-CH_3$$

1,4–Dimethanesulfonoxybutane

This drug is listed only in the interest of completeness. It is effective primarily in the treatment of chronic granulocytic leukemia, and it has not been used successfully against gynecologic malignancies.

Antimetabolites

Folic Acid Analogs

In order for cells to proliferate, the synthesis of DNA, RNA, and certain coenzymes is essential. A number of analogs of nucleic acid precursors (purine and pyrimidine bases and their nucleosides) have been discovered which interfere with the biosynthesis of these essential substances. Such antimetabolites are structurally similar to normal metabolites. Other agents structurally unrelated may act directly on enzymes involved in nucleotide biosynthesis. These substances inhibit the growth of the most rapidly proliferating cells in the body: the bone marrow, the lining of the digestive tract, germinal cells, hair and nails, and the developing fetus. To a varying degree, these agents inhibit the growth of certain neoplastic diseases as well. The antimetabolites most commonly used in gynecologic oncology are methotrexate (amethopterin) and 5-fluorouracil (5-FU). Cytosar (cytosine arabinoside), 6-mercaptopurine, and imidazole carboxamide are employed only rarely.

Methotrexate (Amethopterin)

4—Amino—N^{10}—methylpteroylglutamic acid

Methotrexate (MTX) combines with folic acid reductase, inhibiting the reduction of folic acid to tetrahydrofolic acid (folinic acid). Folinic acid is important in the transfer of single carbon fragments, which are used in many biosynthetic reactions in the body. The striking clinical results obtained by Farber and his coworkers (1949) in the treatment of acute leukemia in children with folic acid antagonists constituted a milestone in the history of chemotherapy by clearly demonstrating that the previously inexorable progression of this disease could be arrested in some cases with an antimetabolite. Among gynecologic neoplasms, methotrexate has achieved unparalleled success in the treatment of malignant trophoblastic disease. Doses between 20 and 30 mg/day intramuscularly or intravenously for 5 days repeated every 2-3 weeks have been productive of dramatic responses and a high cure rate in an otherwise fatal disease (Chapter 8). Intraarterial methotrexate has been used to palliate recurrent squamous cell cancer of the cervix, vagina, and vulva at a dose of 25 mg per artery per day with simultaneous administration of citrovorum factor (6-9 mg IM 4 times a day). Citrovorum (folinic acid) bypasses the metabolic block neutralizing the systemic action of methotrexate, reducing its toxicity.

Methotrexate can be administered orally, being readily absorbed from the alimentary tract, but is usually given as a parenteral solution of the sodium salt. Its route of administration has great bearing on its toxicity. Large doses given as an intravenous bolus may be considerably less toxic than much smaller amounts given in divided doses. Methotrexate can be retained in human tissues for long periods, for example, for weeks in the kidneys and for several months in the liver. The data strongly suggest that methotrexate retained within the cells is bound primarily to folate reductase, which thereby is prevented from functioning. Since from 50 to 90% of each dose of methotrexate normally is excreted rapidly in the urine, impaired renal function is a relative contraindication to its use. Impaired hepatic function also is associated with marked reduction in tolerance for this drug, which should not be administered under this circumstance.

It is important to emphasize that methotrexate is very poorly transported across the blood-brain barrier; hence neoplastic cells that have entered the central nervous system probably are protected from parenterally administered drug.

Methotrexate may produce severe bone marrow depression, ulcerative stomatitis, and at times bleeding from the mucous membrane lesions. Impaired renal function has been induced by this drug in some patients. A very characteristic diffuse drug rash has been seen in a significant number of patients. Gastrointestinal side effects such as anorexia, nausea, and vomiting, as well as diarrhea, are quite common. One of the pronounced manifestations of methotrexate toxicity is the tendency to be cumulative; repeated doses of this drug are more likely to result in serious toxicity. Severe diarrhea or ulcerative stomatitis is an all too frequent complication and requires adjustment of drug dosage in the next treatment course. Partial alopecia is also seen frequently.

Methotrexate in combination with actinomycin D and cytoxan has current use in the treatment of high risk trophoblastic disease and certain germ cell tumors of the ovary. Recurrent squamous carcinoma of the cervix may be palliated with systemic methotrexate alone or in combination with other drugs.

Pyrimidine Analogs

5—Fluorouracil (5-FU)

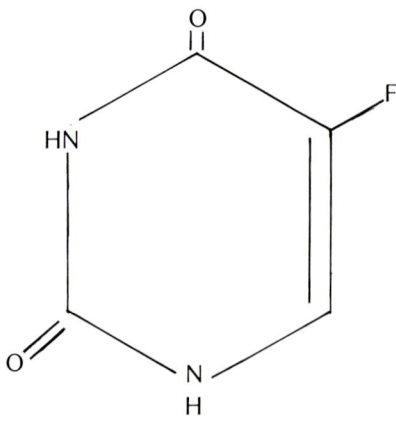

5-Fluorouracil, like uracil, is converted enzymatically to the corresponding ribo-nucleoside and ribonucleotide, and it is thus incorporated into the nucleic acid. In addition, 5-FU ties up thymidylate synthetase, which acts on dUMP to produce dTMP. Thymidine deficiency produced by thymidylate synthetase inhibition, which results in the unavailability of thymidine for cellular replication, is probably the main action of 5-FU.

5-Fluorouracil is usually administered intravenously but also is given orally and intraarterially. Commonly used dose regimens are 15 mg/kg once weekly and 15 mg/kg daily for 5 days, repeated every 4 weeks. In addition, 5-FU has been used as a frequent member of combination chemotherapy regimens at a dose of 5 mg/kg IV each day for 5 days (Act Fu Cy, Table 10-2). Its use intraarterially at a dose of 10 mg/kg/d for 15 days was instituted at the M. D. Anderson Hospital for bulky cervical cancers. This regimen was given concomitantly with irradiation therapy. Gastrointestinal malignancies have been treated by the administration of 5-FU by continuous intravenous infusion over a period of 8 hours, in doses of 1 gm daily (in 1000 ml of 5% dextrose in water) for 5 days. In some institutions this has been followed by the administration of the drug orally for 2-4 weeks. It has been suggested that patients with gut malignancies metastatic to the liver may experience improved palliation from the oral administration of 5-FU on the hypothesis that the portal concentration of drug is higher.

The earliest symptoms of toxicity during the course of 5-FU therapy are anorexia and nausea; these are followed shortly afterwards by stomatitis and diarrhea, which constitute reliable warning signs that a sufficient dose has been administered. Stomatitis may be preceded by a sensation of dryness, followed by erythema and the formation of a white, patchy membrane that develops into a necrotic ulcer. The occurrence of similar lesions in the stoma of colostomies has been observed. The other major toxic effect is myelosuppression. Clinically, this is most frequently manifested as leukopenia, which may begin as early as the 2nd or 3rd day of treatment or as late as the 3rd week. The nadir of the leukopenia is usually between the 9th and 14th day after the first injection of the drug. During this period susceptibility to overwhelming septicemia usually with a gram negative organism, is generally increased, and for this reason patients with infections are poor candidates for therapy. Thrombocytopenia and anemia may complicate the picture; loss of hair occasionally progressing to total alopecia, nail changes, dermatitis, and increased pigmentation and atrophy of the skin may be encountered. Uncommonly cerebellar ataxia is observed.

Cytosine arabinoside requires activation by conversion to the nucleoside triphosphate, which inhibits the important enzyme DNA polymerase. The fact that Ara-C is incorporated into DNA to a small extent may also contribute to its mode of action. The drug has been given experimentally to patients with a variety of neoplastic diseases and has found some application in the treatment of ovarian carcinoma. In all instances it has been used with other drugs in combination chemotherapy, and the doses have been 2 mg/kg/d for 5-10 days, depending on the accompanying antineoplastic agents. Cytosar 50 mg/M^2/d, has been used to treat herpes zoster by IV infusion over 48 hours. The main toxic manifestations of Ara-C are myelosuppression, nausea, vomiting, and stomatitis.

There is still uncertainty as to whether the small amount of 6-mercaptopurine associated with RNA and DNA is incorporated into these macromolecules in the internucleotide linkages; nevertheless, it is now apparent that the important biologic

Cytosar (Cytosine Arabinoside, Ara-C)

1−β−D−Arabinofuranosylcytosine

Purine Analogs

6-Mercaptopurine (6-MP)

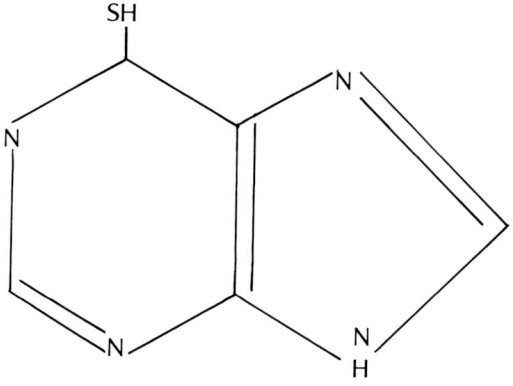

TABLE 10-2 INDICATIONS, DOSE SCHEDULES, AND SIDE EFFECTS
OF THE MOST COMMONLY USED DRUGS IN GYNECOLOGIC ONCOLOGY

Drug	Dose	Indications	Side Effects
Mustargen	15 mg in 20 cc saline given intrapleurally	Malignant pleural effusion	Nausea, pain, fever, bone marrow depression
Cytoxan	1-2 g/M^2 IV once every 3-4 weeks 15 mg/kg IV once weekly 8 mg/kg/day IV X 5 days every 4-6 weeks 2.5 mg/kg/day orally	Ovarian carcinoma, recurrent cervical carcinoma, recurrent endometrial carcinoma	Leukopenia $>$ thrombopenia, nausea, alopecia, hemorrhagic cystitis
Melphelan	0.2 mg/kg/day orally X 5 days every 4 weeks (maximum 12 mg/day) 1.0 mg/kg IV push once every 3 weeks	Ovarian carcinoma, tubal carcinoma, recurrent adenocarcinoma of cervix	Thrombopenia $>$ leukopenia
Thiotepa	10 mg/day IV X 5 days, then once weekly 0.4 mg/kg/day IV X 2 days; in 2 weeks 0.2 mg/kg IV weekly X 4 weeks	Ovarian carcinoma	Thrombopenia $>$ leukopenia
Methotrexate	0.4 mg/kg/day IV or IM X 5 days (maximum 30 mg/day) 0.3 mg/kg/day X 5 days IV or IM as part of MAC	Good risk gestational trophoblastic disease High risk gestational trophoblastic disease, ovarian choriocarcinoma	Bone marrow depression, nausea, vomiting, diarrhea, alopecia, dermatitis, liver and renal failure
5-FU	12-15 mg/kg IV once weekly 12-15 mg/kg/day IV X 5 days every 4 weeks 5 mg/kg/day IV X 5 days as part of Act Fu Cy	Recurrent endometrial carcinoma ovarian germ cell tumors, ovarian carcinoma resistant to alkylating agents	Nausea, stomatitis, ileitis, bone marrow depression, cerebellar ataxia

TABLE 10-2 INDICATIONS, DOSE SCHEDULES, AND SIDE EFFECTS OF THE MOST COMMONLY USED DRUGS IN GYNECOLOGIC ONCOLOGY (cont.)

Drug	Dose	Indications	Side Effects
Actinomycin D	0.01 mg/kg/day IV X 5 days [8-12 μg/kg/day]	Good risk gestational trophoblastic disease	Stomatitis, thrombopenia ⟩ leukopenia, ileitis, diarrhea, nausea, alopecia, dermatitis, local tissue necrosis
	0.01 mg/kg/day X 5 days as part of MAC, VAC, Act Fu Cy	Ovarian germ cell tumors, uterine sarcomas, ovarian carcinoma resistant to alkylating drug	
Bleomycin	15-30 mg/IV or IM weekly (maximum total dose 400 mg)	Recurrent squamous cell carcinoma of cervix, vagina, or vulva	Pulmonary fibrosis, alopecia, fever, skin blisters, stomatitis, kidney injury
Adriamycin	20-30 mg/M² /day IV X 3 days every 3 weeks 60-90 mg/M² IV once every 3 weeks (maximum total dose 450 mg/M²)	Uterine sarcoma, recurrent cervical carcinoma, recurrent endometrial carcinoma	Leukopenia ⟩ thrombopenia, fatal cardiomyopathy, nausea, local tissue necrosis
Vincristine	1.5 mg/M² /week IV as part of VAC	Uterine sarcoma, ovarian germ cell tumors	Neurotoxicity, alopecia, constipation, paralytic ileus

TABLE 10-2 INDICATIONS, DOSE SCHEDULES, AND SIDE EFFECTS
OF THE MOST COMMONLY USED DRUGS IN GYNECOLOGIC ONCOLOGY (cont.)

Drug	Dose	Indications	Side Effects
MAC			
Methotrexate	0.3 mg/kg IM or IV } daily X 5	High risk gestational trophoblastic disease, ovarian choriocarcinoma	Potentially severe bone marrow and gut toxicity, alopecia, nausea, stomatitis, dermatitis
Actinomycin D	0.01 mg/kg IV } every		
Chlorambucil	0.2 mg/kg PO } 2-3 weeks		
	(Cytoxan, 3-5 mg/kg/day IV, may be substituted for chlorambucil)		
Act Fu Cy			
Actinomycin D	0.01 mg/kg } IV daily X 5	Ovarian carcinoma resistant to single agent therapy, malignant germ cell tumors without choriocarcinoma, malignant stromal tumors	Potentially severe bone marrow and gut toxicity, stomatitis, nausea, vomiting, dermatitis
5-FU	5 mg/kg } every		
Cytoxan	5 mg/kg } 4 weeks		
VAC			
Vincristine	1.5 mg/M² IV once weekly X 4-6 weeks, then every 2 weeks	Sarcomas, malignant germ cell tumors	Bone marrow toxicity, neurologic toxicity, constipation, stomatitis, dermatitis, alopecia, ileus
Actinomycin D	0.01 mg/kg } IV daily X 5		
Cytoxan	8 mg/kg } days every 4-6 weeks		
	(when used with XRT, give only vincristine until after XRT is completed)		

actions of the compound necessitate enzymatic conversion to the corresponding ribonucleotide, that is, the thioanalog of inosinic acid. Inosinic acid, a ribonucleotide, is the first purine-containing compound to appear in the pathway of nucleic acid biosynthesis. It is a precursor of both adenylic acid and guanylic acid, which are incorporated into RNA and the corresponding deoxyribonucleotides of DNA. Another major effect of the ribonucleotide of 6-MP is the suppression of *de novo* purine biosynthesis. In gynecologic oncology 6-MP has found its only use in the treatment of trophoblastic disease. Several authors have utilized it alone and in combination with other drugs for metastatic gestational trophoblastic disease. The average daily dose of 6-MP is 2.5 mg/kg. The drug is administered orally as a single dose given at any convenient hour of the day. The usual starting dose range is 150-250 mg/day. The total dose necessary to produce depression of the marrow in the patient with nonhematological malignancies is about 45 mg/kg but ranges from 18 to 106 mg/kg.

The principal toxic effect of this drug is bone marrow suppression, although this, in general, develops more gradually than with folic acid antagonists; thrombocytopenia, granulocytopenia, and anemia may not be encountered even on continued administration of the drug for several weeks. Anorexia, nausea, and vomiting may occur in 25% of adults, but stomatitis and diarrhea are rare.

Imidazole Carboxamide (DTIC)

5—(3,3—Dimethyl—1—triazeno)imidazole—4—carboxamide

Imidazole carboxamide is considered by many investigators to be the most effective single agent for systemic chemotherapy of malignant melanoma, and it is presented in this synopsis for that reason. At the time of the writing of this section, it remains an investigational drug with great promise against this malignancy. Its chief action appears to be as a purine analog which produces a block in the synthesis of purine nucleotide DNA precursors. In addition to its function as an antimetabolite, it appears to have activity, although to a lesser extent, as an alkylating agent.

The usual dosage varies from 70 mg/M^2/d for 10 days, repeated every 4 weeks, to 150 mg/M^2/d for 5 days, repeated every 21 days. The drug has also been administered by intraarterial infusion with an overall response rate of approximately 40%. In these studies the dosage was 250 mg/M^2 for 5 consecutive days, followed by 16 days of rest and then another course of drug. This regimen is continued until toxicity necessitates discontinuation of therapy. DTIC is also used with adriamycin in soft tissue sarcomas.

Antibiotics

Actinomycin D (Cosmegen)

There are specific antibiotics that act at various points on the DNA→ RNA→ protein sequence. Many of the most active antibiotics are inhibitors of RNA synthesis, and the actinomycins, specifically dactinomycin (actinomycin D), are the most potent compounds of this group. In cell cultures, dactinomycin can produce acutely almost complete inhibition of RNA synthesis. Although many of its biological effects resemble those obtained with alkylating agents and x-irradiation, dactinomycin does not produce the chromosome breaks in culture cells typical of radiomimetic agents. All biologically active dactinomycin derivatives contain a quinoidal ring system, a free amino group at position 3 of the the quinoidal ring, and two lactone rings. Each of these structures serves to stabilize the compound and to enhance its ability to exchange hydrogen bonds in binding with DNA. These actinomycins bind to DNA at guanine-containing loci in a manner that raises the energy required for strand separation and displaces the enzyme RNA polymerase. This binding produces a specific block in DNA-dependent RNA synthesis, which causes cell injury and death. The cellular consequences of these subcellular actions are mitotic abnormalities and chromosomal aberrations. The nucleolus becomes smaller and compact. Because of the lack of RNA, particularly mRNA, cell death occurs.

Actinomycin D is highly effective in the treatment of gestational trophoblastic disease. Its activity is equivalent to that of methotrexate, and its toxicity may be less. Certainly in any patient who has hepatic or renal disese the use of actinomycin D in preference to methotrexate is mandatory. Actinomycin D has also demononstrated considerable activity in combination with other drugs in the treatment of epithelial carcinoma of the ovary (Act Fu Cy), sarcomas of the uterus (VAC), and germ cell tumors of the ovary (VAC and MAC). It must be administered intravenously; if given orally, doses equivalent to those tolerated by the intravenous route may cause severe injury to the digestive tract. The local vesicant action prohibits subcutaneous or intramuscular injection. When administered intravenously, it should always be injected into the tubing of a running IV. Infiltration into the subcutaneous tissue will result in slough in a significant number of patients. The usual dose is 0.5 mg 8-12 μg/kg/day IV for 5 days, repeated every 2 weeks, for trophoblastic disease.

Toxic manifestations of actinomycin D are common and may be severe. Nausea and vomiting may begin a few hours after administration and persist throughout the course of therapy. Diarrhea, proctitis, anorexia, glossitis, ulceration of the oral mucous membranes (Fig. 10-10), and depression of the bone marrow with pancytopenia occur from 1 to 7 days after completion of therapy. The last of these often develops rapidly and may first affect the platelets. Alopecia is infrequent, particularly at lower levels of dosage; however, it may be extensive. Severe dermatologic reactions, including an acneiform rash, have been reported with actinomycin D (Fig. 10-11). It frequently produces a local vesicant reaction with erythema in areas exposed to radiation therapy either before, during, or after treatment. Severe enteritis can develop from the simultaneous administration of actinomycin D with abdominal or pelvic irradiation. It is generally not used during abdominal radiation therapy.

Actinomycin D (Cosmegen, dactinomycin)

Bleomycin (Blenoxane)

Bleomycin is the generic name for a group of antibiotics isolated from a strain of *Streptomyces verticillus* in Japan. This new anticancer drug has been reported to have a high order of activity against a wide variety of epithelial cancers, including squamous cell carcinoma, particularly the well-differentiated spindle cell carcinoma, which, in some studies, has been quite resistant to irradiation. This compound is of great interest not only because of its reported clinical activity, but also because of its failure to demonstrate

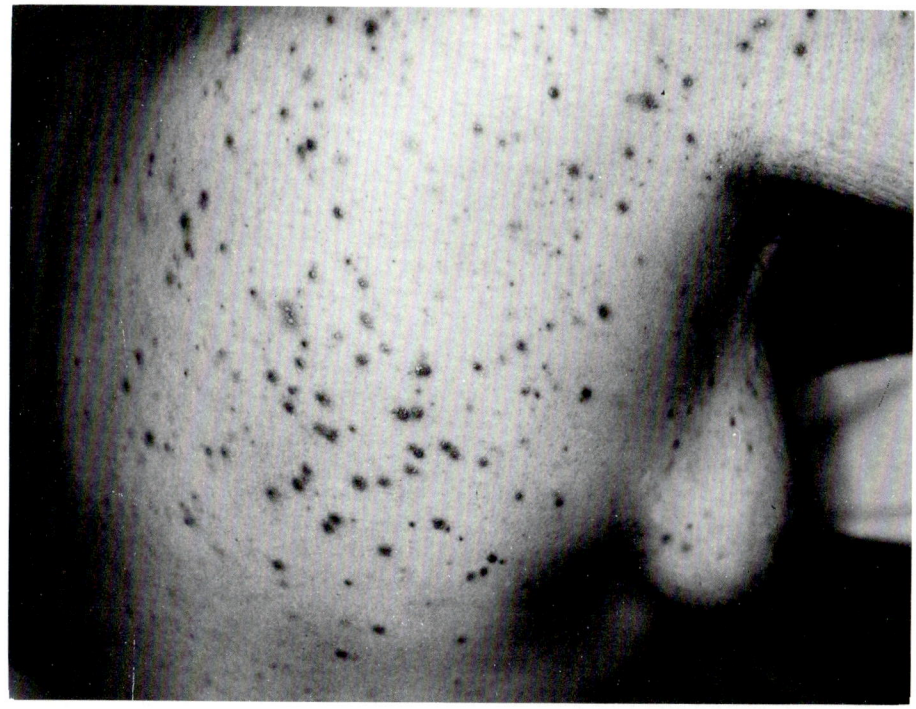

Fig. 10-10 Generalized acneiform eruptions secondary to actinomycin D therapy. The most severe areas occurred on the face and were complicated by secondary infection.

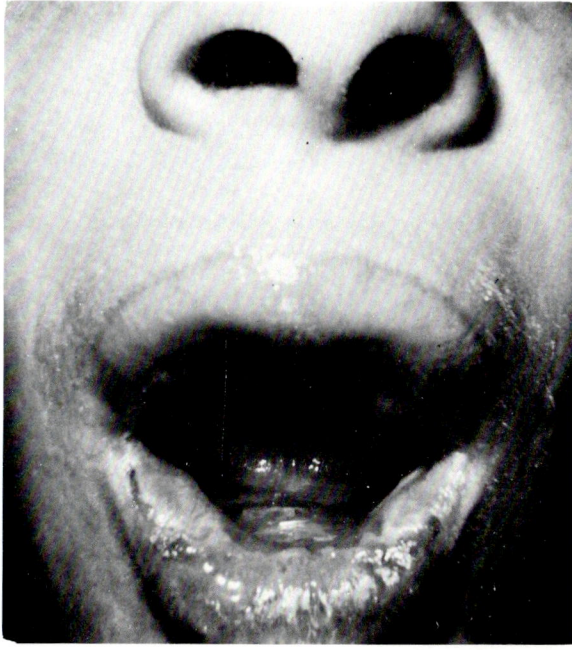

Fig. 10-11 Ulcerative stomatitis involving the mucosal surface of the lower lip. The irregular, thickened border of the ulcer is at the inner lip margin. The patient had received actinomycin D.

significant myeloid toxicity in man. Its dose limiting toxicity is pulmonary. Chemically, the compound consists of at least seven polypeptides that are similar in structure. The main component, bleomycin A_2, is present in at least 50% concentration. Apparently, none of the components has significant antitumor properties when given alone. Bleomycin is capable of splitting single strand DNA, but the exact mechanism of its oncolytic action has not been elucidated. In high concentration it inhibits the synthesis of DNA in HeLa cells and at a much lower concentration causes inhibition of cell division.

In gynecology bleomycin is being used in the treatment of squamous cell carcinoma, recurrent or disseminated, of the cervix, vagina, and vulva. Bleomycin has been largely administered by the intravenous route but it can be given intramuscularly or subcutaneously as well. Local tolerance by the IM route is entirely satisfactory and offers the theoretical advantage of avoiding exposure of the lungs to a large bolus of drug, as occurs in the intravenous route of administration. The most commonly used schedule consists of 15-30 mg administered once weekly to a total cumulative dose of 400 mg. This total cumulative dose limit is recommended since the incidence of pulmonary toxicity greatly increases at higher dose levels. Bleomycin is suitable to intraarterial administration, and infusion of unresectable pelvic carcinoma can be accomplished via catheters placed in the iliac arteries.

From the accumulated human data, no definite bone marrow depression has been demonstrated. However, aggravation of depressed platelet counts from previous chemotherapy has been observed in several patients. The major human toxicities noted with bleomycin are skin, pulmonary, and acute systemic reactions. Skin toxicity includes thickening, reddening, and painful ulceration, particularly over pressure points. Mucosal surface ulcerations, alopecia, and nail changes are also common. All changes are reversible with discontinuation of drug. Pulmonary toxicity is characterized by a peculiar pneumonitis rapidly progressing to pulmonary fibrosis; death may occur. The true incidence of fatal pulmonary complication is approximately 3%. Serial chest x-rays and frequent pulmonary function studies have not been predictive, although they document the deteriorating function once the toxicity begins. Predicting which patients will develop pulmonary fibrosis is not possible. Frequent chest x-rays are indicated, and the drug should be promptly discontinued at the first evidence of pneumonitis. The earliest sign may be basilar rales. In addition to the increasing incidence of pulmonary complications with total dosage exceeding 400 mg, patients over 70 years of age and those with underlying pulmonary disease may be more likely to develop pulmonary toxicity than younger patients.

Acute toxicity reactions include fever after injections in 50% of patients; about 10% develop nausea and vomiting, and (of great importance) a few patients manifest acute allergic reactions, consisting of a shocklike syndrome, pulmonary edema, and a reticular rash. Such anaphylactic reactions have occurred only in patients with lymphoma, and a small test dose is advised under these circumstances.

Adriamycin is an antibiotic structurally related to daunomycin, an antineoplastic drug little used in gynecology. The mechanism of action seems to be interference with nucleic acid synthesis. Adriamycin has shown activity against several gynecologic malignancies, including recurrent cervical and endometrial carcinoma, ovarian carcinoma, and uterine sarcomas. Varying dosage schedules have been used. At the M. D. Anderson Hospital adriamycin has been administered in dosages of 20-30 mg/M^2/d for 3 days, repeated every 3 weeks, or 60-90 mg/M^2 as a single dose, repeated every 3 weeks. The Sloan-Kettering Institute has administered the drug in a dose of 0.5 mg/kg/d for 3

Adriamycin

days, followed by 4 days of rest and then another 3 days of drug. The cycle is repeated until toxicity develops. The maximum cumulative dose should not exceed 450-550 mg/M^2; higher dosages incur a significant incidence of cardiac toxicity. The drug is always administered intravenously.

Adriamycin has yielded consistent toxic side effects. The bone marrow toxicity, at times life threatening, is the dose limiting and the main toxic manifestation of adriamycin. Indeed, in several patients fatal, irreversible bone marrow aplasia has been reported. Leukopenia has been reported in approximately 80% of patients evaluated. The nadir occurs about the 14th day, plus or minus 4 days. The average duration of significant leukopenia is on the order of 7-10 days. Thrombocytopenia occurs much less frequently than leukopenia. Approximately 60% of patients show a drop in platelet count, but this has not been severe. Virtually all patients develop mild to total alopecia.

Stomatitis is reported in approximately 40-60% of patients and is in part a function of dose schedule. The greater the time interval between drug administrations, the lower is the frequency of stomatitis. Typically, the stomatitis begins as a burning sensation and erythema of the oral mucous membrane, which progresses within 1-3 days to frank necrosis and ulceration, especially of the sublingular and lateral tongue margins.

Adriamycin induced cardiac toxicity occurs in a significant number of patients when the total dose exceeds 550 mg/M^2. In a series of patients reported by Gottlieb et al (1972), 20-30% receiving a cumulative dose of adriamycin greater than 550 mg/M^2 developed cardiac toxicity, and most of these died. There is also a cardiac toxicity independent of dose, which is more common in elderly patients and is manifested as EKG abnormalities. This severe dose related complication appears to take the form of myometrial atrophy and "pump failure." It manifests itself as an acute, fulminant congestive heart failure, typically unresponsive to cardiac glycosides and tublular diuretics. Gastrointestinal symptoms, mostly diarrhea, develop in one third to one fifth of the patients. Local thrombophlebitis and necrosis were noted if the drug extravasated, but this complication can be eliminated by injecting the adriamycin into a running IV infusion.

Vinca Alkaloids (Periwinkle drugs)

Unlike the rational design and systematic synthesis that characterized the development of many of the chemotherapeutic agents previously described, the discovery of the vinca alkaloids resulted from empirical observations. The reputed medicinal properties of a species of myrtle, the periwinkle (*Vinca rosea*), and, more specifically, its alleged activity as an oral hypoglycemic agent, prompted an investigation in 1949 of crude fractions obtained from this plant. Working independently with such extracts, Canadian investigators and a group of researchers at the laboratories of Eli Lilly and Company were unable to demonstrate hypoglycemic activity in experimental animals, but consistently observed leukopenia. Subsequent fractionation of these extracts yielded four active alkaloids; two of these, vincristine and vinblastine, have established value in the chemotherapy of neoplastic diseases. These two compounds are complicated dimeric structures and differ only in the oxidation state of a single substitution.

   At the molecular level, they act as mitotic arresting agents by specifically blocking the assembly of the microtubular protein subunits. It has also been observed that vinca alkaloids produce metaphase arrest of human cells in culture, and the possibility exists that their effect resembles that observed with colchicine. Vinblastine produces a greater degree of mitotic inhibition than does colchicine and, at lower concentrations, causes cytologic aberrations that may be related to the damage of spindle development, while a direct effect on the chromosomes appears to be involved at higher doses.

Vinblastine: R = $-CH_3$
Vincristine: R = $-CHO$

Vinblastine (Velban)

This drug has been recommended in the treatment of choriocarcinoma but is less effective than actinomycin D and methotrexate. In some reports vinblastine has been beneficial in patients whose disease has become refractory to methotrexate. The dosages used in these instances were somewhat larger than conventional ones, and the toxic manifestations were proportionally more severe. It is generally recommended that therapy with vinblastine be initiated with a single intravenous injection of 0.1–0.15 mg/kg, after which the response of the patient is observed for 1 week; if the indicated level of leukopenia is not attained, the dose administered weekly may be increased gradually by increments of 0.05 mg/kg until either the desired antitumor effects are noted or the degree of leukopenia precludes further administration of the drug. If the total leukocyte count does not return to 4000/mm^3 within 10-14 days after administration of the drug, the treatment schedule should be adjusted. Doses as high as 0.3-0.4 mg/kg have been used in the treatment of resistant choriocarcinoma, but in almost every instance moderate to severe leukopenia results. In some studies it was necessary to extend the course of therapy for at least 12 weeks to produce a satisfactory result.

The toxic manifestations of vinblastine are related directly to the size of the total dose. After a single intravenous dose, leukopenia (with a nadir that occurs within 4-10 days, followed by recovery within 7-14 days) has been the most important sign of toxicity, as well as the limitation on the size of the dose that can be administered subsequently. Although depression of the platelet count has been noted, this has been considerably less pronounced than the degree of granulocytopenia and usually has not been of serious consequence. Other undesirable effects include, in descending order of frequency, nausea, temporary mental depression, alopecia, vomiting, malaise, parasthesias, phlebitis, temporary loss of deep tendon reflexes, anorexia, and diarrhea. With the exception of nausea and mental depression, the frequency of other toxic manifestations has been less than 10%. Infrequently seen are vesicular stomatitis or dermatitis, headache, convulsions, epistaxis, gastrointestinal bleeding, and ileus. The transient mental depression, which usually occurs on the 2nd or 3rd day after treatment, is of interest since other compounds containing indole derivatives (e.g., reserpine and lysergic acid) have been associated with effects on the central nervous system.

Vincristine (Oncovin)

Vincristine is probably one of the safest of all cancer chemotherapeutic agents; its usefulness, however, is severely decreased by its neurotoxicity. This apparent paradox is explained by the fact that its dose limiting toxicity is rarely, if ever, lethal. In gynecology vincristine has been used in the treatment of squamous carcinoma of the cervix, endometrial sarcomas, sarcoma botryoides, and other rhabdomyosarcomas. It is also useful in the treatment of the highly malignant germ cell tumors of the ovary. An interesting feature is the lack of cross-resistance between vincristine and vinblastine, a remarkable finding in view of their very close structural similarity. Before the advent of adriamycin, vincristine showed the greatest spectrum of clinical activity against human sarcomas. Vincristine has been used in various schedules, nearly always in combination with other drugs. In combination with actinomycin D and cytoxan, a dose of 1.5 mg/M^2/week IV has been employed. The schedule calls for injections for 6 weeks, repeated every 3 months or continued weekly or once every 2 weeks (Table 10-2). The maximum single dose should not exceed 2.5 mg, and the dose should be reduced 50% with neural toxicity. Since this drug is often used concomitantly with radiation therapy in the treatment of sarcomas, myeloid suppression may be seen in instances where it is otherwise relatively uncommon. Vincristine has also been used as a continuous intraarterial infusion at a dose of 0.01-0.02 mg/kg/d, continued until severe neurological toxicity results. When administered by infusion, it must be protected from light exposure.

Neurotoxicity is the most common side effect of vincristine, but there is no general agreement as to the exact site of the neural lesion. Some evidence suggests that the initial site of vincristine toxicity is in the sensory cells of the dorsal ganglia and the anterior horn cells, resulting from impaired neurotubular synthesis and function. The most frequent and troublesome neurotoxicity has been peripheral neuropathy, the earliest signs of which are paresthesias and loss of deep tendon reflexes, usually appearing after a month of therapy. More severe neurotoxicity in the form of neuritic pain, foot drop, wrist drop, and muscular atrophy is not uncommon. A slapping gait as a result of foot drop and muscular weakness has been described. Hoarseness and vocal cord paralysis occasionally occur. Severe constipation, considered a form of neurotoxicity, has been a troublesome and frequent complication of vincristine therapy. The use of a feces wetting agent and a methylcellulose bulk laxative 3 times a day is recommended. High fecal impaction, with no stool in the ampulla, has been considered a manifestation of vincristine induced bowel hypomotility. Ileus, manifested by abdominal cramps and vomiting, also occurs fairly frequently, but diarrhea is much less common. Mild neurotoxicity can be reduced or even eliminated if the dosage is lowered. Hair loss, often total, occurs in almost half of the patients, but regrowth begins when the drug is discontinued or when a lower dose is used for maintenance. Bone marrow toxicity has been seen only with high dose regimens. Vincristine is one of the few cancer chemotherapeutic agents that can be used without hesitation in leukopenic patients.

Progestins

Progestins have played a role in gynecologic oncology primarily in the treatment of metastatic endometrial carcinoma, but they have been used also, with equivocal results, in the treatment of mixed mesodermal sarcoma of the endometrium, stromal cell sarcoma, endocervical adenocarcinoma, adenocarcinoma of the fallopian tube, and carcinoma of the ovary. A considerable amount of literature has been accumulated on the use of injectable medroxyprogesterone acetate (Depo-Provera, Upjohn) and 17—α—hydroxyprogesterone caproate (Delalutin, Squibb). With both agents the results appear to be similar in that 30-40% of patients treated for metastatic endometrial carcinoma will show an objective response. Recently a potent oral progestin, megestrol acetate (Megace, Mead-Johnson), has become available. Preliminary studies indicate it to be as effective as the injectables.

The mechanism of action of progestins on endometrial adenocarcinoma has not been identified. Possible modes include an immunosuppressive effect, a change in endogenous sex steroid support, and a direct action on neoplastic cells. That large doses of synthetic progestins have an immunosuppressive effect has been demonstrated in transplant experiments. The mechanism of this immunologic suppression, however, is not understood. Studies of serum protein electrophoresis in patients receiving large doses of progestins have revealed no change in the pattern. For progestin therapy to be beneficial

Medroxyprogesterone Acetate (Provera)

17—α—Hydroxyprogesterone caproate (Delalutin)

Megestrol Acetate (Megace)

in transplant experiments, a suppression of the cell mediated immune response must be postulated, and this would be contrary to the interest of the host in its immunologic reaction to malignancy. If indeed progestins exert their beneficial effect via their immunosuppressive capabilities, it must be in the direction of suppressing substances such as "blocking antibodies."

Synthetic progestins can also be potent inhibitors of pituitary gonadatropin hormones. The pituitary suppression would seem to be specific for gonadatropins without affecting adrenocorticotropic hormone secretion, although the latter has not been carefully measured. This may conceivably result in an antiantigen effect, which may be of assistance in suppressing the malignancy. Many have felt that the rationale for the use of progestins in the treatment of advanced endometrial carcinoma is closely allied with its antagonism to estrogen. The relationship between carcinoma of the endometrium and prolonged estrogen stimulation of the endometrium seems evident. The suppressive effect of progestins on endometrium, the inhibition of experimental estrogen carcinogenesis, and the regression of induced endometrial carcinoma in animals reinforce the clinical observations that far advance endometrial carcinoma in human beings may remit under the influence of progestin adminstration.

The original premise on which the use of progestins in endometrial adenocarcinoma was based was that a neoplasm which arose from an epithelium sensitive to sex steroids might retain this sensitivity. Since benign but atypical endometrial changes in human females can be reversed by the administration of synthetic progestins, it was only logical to anticipate that endometrial adenocarcinoma could be altered with similar drugs. Histologic changes in the endometrium with progestin therapy include an initial secretory effect on the cytoplasm, followed by destruction of the architecture of the glands with a narrowing of the lumina and a decrease in gland size. The epithelium changes to a flattened cuboidal type with a marked decrease in mitotic activity, and, finally, marked epithelial atrophy results. In adenocarcinoma of the endometrium, these kinds of histopathologic changes can be seen to occur also with progestin therapy, culminating in an arrest of progress and disappearance of evidence of malignancy both in the uterus and at metastatic sites. The inference is that progestin is acting directly at a cellular level and that the effects of this hormone therapy are not mediated by extrinsic mechanisms.

The doses of synthetic progestin utilized by various institutions in the treatment of metastatic adenocarcinoma of the endometrium have varied widely. Depo-Provera is recommended in doses from 500 to 1500 mg/week intramuscularly. There is evidence to suggest that the time from the onset of therapy to response is dependent on the loading dose given. Patients given doses exceeding 1 g/week respond more quickly to progestin therapy than those receiving lesser doses. Even in the face of massive doses of progestin, objective response will often require 6-12 weeks. Megace has been used in dosages of 20-120 mg orally twice a day. The recommended maintenance dose at our institution is 40 mg orally twice a day. The dose of Delalutin has ranged from 250 to 1000 mg 1-3 times a week, with most authors reporting regimens of 1000 mg intramuscularly once or twice weekly.

Only minimal sytemic reactions have been observed in progestin therapy. Patients have developed nodules at the site of injection, and an occasional woman will complain of lethargy. A significant number of patients on progestin therapy develop a sense of well being associated with weight gain. Serious side effects are unknown.

Miscellaneous

Hydroxyurea (Hydrea)

$$NH_2-\overset{\overset{\displaystyle O}{\|}}{C}-NH-OH$$

Hydroxyurea is a simple chemical compound whose structure is that of urea with a hydroxyl group replacing a hydrogen atom in one of the amino groups. Theoretically this drug is promising because of its ability to enhance radiosensitivity. The fluctuation in radiosensitivity with different phases of the cell cycle forms the basis for the use of combined hydroxyurea and radiotherapy. The cycle influence is almost as great as the oxygen effect since radiosensitivity can vary by a factor of 2.5 among the various phases. In most investigations done *in vitro* with culture cell lines, sensitivity to irradiation therapy is at its maximum just before DNA synthesis (late G_1) and is reduced to a minimum during DNA synthesis (S phase). Hydroxyurea has been proposed as a radiosensitizing agent that might improve the control of locally advanced cancer by destroying cells in the radioresistant S phase and synchronizing other cells in the relatively radiosensitive late G_1 phase. In other tissue culture studies it was found that hydroxyurea inhibited the incorporation of thymidine into DNA and suggested that its action was a result of interference with ribonucleotide (diphosphate) reduction. In gynecology hydroxyurea has been used primarily as an adjunct to radiation therapy in patients with large cervical lesions. A cooperative study under the auspices of the Gynecologic Oncology Group is being carried out to evaluate its effectiveness in these patients. The dose employed in this study is 80 mg/kg orally every 3 days during radiation therapy; a maximum single dose of 6000 mg is observed. Others have used a dosage of 20-30 mg orally in divided doses each day. Since the drug may potentiate the effect of irradiation, and since its peak blood level is relatively brief, it is ideally administered 4 hours before and 4 hours after radiation.

Toxicity is mainly hematologic, with the occurrence of leukocyte, platelet, or red cell depression. Reversal is usually rapid with return to normal levels within 10-30 days after discontinuing the drug. With high dose regimens anorexia and vomiting occur occasionally, and skin rash, stomatitis, and alopecia have been reported.

10-3 GENERAL GUIDELINES FOR CHEMOTHERAPY

1. Under most circumstances treatment should not be instituted if:
    White blood cell count is less than 3000.
    Neutrophil count is less than 1200.
    Platelet count is less than 150,000.
2. Blood transfusions should not be given for anemia per se unless the hematocrit is less than 24% and/or the patient is symptomatic.
3. Patients should receive multivitamin preparations with iron.
4. Moderate toxicity should be accompanied by at least 25% reduction in dosage for the next course of drug. When toxicity is severe, the reduction should be 50% (refer to Table 10-3). It is acceptable to reduce the dosage of only the drugs that are responsible for the toxicity. In every case the overall condition of the patient and the virulence of the malignancy in relation to the probability of drug effect must be considered when doses are adjusted.
5. All drugs should be discontinued immediately if signs of toxicity develop during treatment. The nadir of toxicity develops within 1-3 weeks after administration of most drugs; therefore any toxicity during therapy is an ominous sign.
6. Patients should be under treatment for two or three courses of drug before concluding that the regimen is ineffective.
7. Growth of tumor, appearance of serous effusion, or failure to control serous effusion is definite evidence of drug failure and an indication for a change of therapy if an adequate trial has been completed.
8. When known tumor is present, the location should be identified with drawings and the size (cm), the volume (cc), or weight (g) should be indicated at each examination.
9. A patient who is discharged after the administration of multiple drug chemotherapy should alert her physician in the event of a febrile episode or other symptom of significant toxicity.
10. The best indicators of the hemopoietic reserve are the neutrophil and platelet counts. They should be normal and stable before each treatment cycle.
11. Patients who have had prior irradiation (especially pelvic) or chemotherapy, are elderly or debilitated, or have advanced disease should receive no more than one half to two thirds of the normal initial drug dose.
12. Vigorous supportive care is essential to successful chemotherapy. Platelet count depression below $50,000/mm^3$ is associated with an increasing liklihood of spontaneous bleeding, although platelet tranfusions are seldom necessary above $20,000/mm^3$ in the absence of other complications. Granulocytopenia below $1000/mm^3$ is associated with an increased probability of infection, especially in the presence of gut toxicity. Patients with less than $500/mm^3$ should receive prophylactic antibiotics (Keflin: 2 g every 6 hours, and carbenicillin: 5 g every 4 hours) and be placed in reverse isolation.

TABLE 10-3   CHEMOTHERAPY TOXICITY OUTLINE

Hematologic toxicity
1. Leukopenia (normal value: 5-10,000/mm³)

    3000—5000 WBC/mm³   mild
    1000—3000 WBC/mm³   moderate
    〈 1000 WBC/mm³   severe

2. Neutropenia (normal value: 1900-6700/mm³)

    700—1699/mm³   mild
    699—301/mm³   moderate
    〈 300/mm³   severe

3. Thrombopenia (normal value: 150,000—350,000/mm³)

    100,000—150,000/mm³   mild
    50,000—100,000/mm³   moderate
    〈 50,000   severe

Hepatic toxicity
1. SGOT (normal value: 10-40 units)

    43—100 units   mild
    101—500 units   moderate
    〉 500 units   severe

2. BSP (normal value: ≤5% retention at 45 minutes)

    15—20%   mild
    21—30%   moderate
    〉 30%   severe

Gastrointestinal toxicity
1. Nausea, vomiting, diarrhea

    1-2 emeses or stools/day . . . . mild

    3-5 emeses or stools/day . . . . moderate
    Persistant and requires drug treatment

    Antiemetic or antidiarrheal . . . . severe
      agents provide little or no benefit
    May need hospitalization

2. Stomatitis, proctitis

    Superficial ulceration . . . . mild
    No difficulty in eating most foods

    Ulceration with secondary infection . . . . moderate
    Difficulty in eating

    Systemic infection . . . . severe
    Inability to eat any foods

Neurotoxicity

    Paresthesias, no motor loss, constipation . . . . mild

    Paresthesias disturbing to the patient . . . . moderate
    Motor loss of less than 25%
    Constipation requiring vigorous laxation

    Motor loss greater than 25% . . . . severe
    Paresthesias
    Constipation requiring repeated enemas

Febrile response, sepsis (usually accompanied by neutropenia)

    Temperature up to 101°F . . . . mild

    Temperature greater than 101°F . . . . moderate

    Any temperature with shaking, chills, ... severe
      and/or positive blood culture

REFERENCES

Anderson, D. G.: The possible mechanisms of action of progestins on edometrial adenocarcinoma. *Am. J. Obstet. Gynecol.* 113:195, 1972.

Ansfield, F. J.: *Chemotherapy of Malignant Neoplasms*, 2nd Ed. Charles C Thomas, Springfield, Ill., 1973.

Ansfield, F. J., Mackman, S., and Ramirez, G.: Newer concepts in chemotherapy of cancer. *Oncology* 26:114, 1972.

Averette, H. E., Weinstein, G. D., and Frost, P.: Autoradiographic analysis of cell proliferation kinetics in human genital tissues. *Am. J. Obstet. Gynecol.* 108:8, 1970.

Barlow, J. J., Piver, M. S., Chuang, J. T., Cortes, E. P., Ohnuma, T., and Holland, J. F.: Adriamycin and bleomycin alone and in combination, in gynecologic cancers. *Cancer* 32:735, 1973.

Baserga, R.: The relationship of the cell cycle to tumor growth and control of cell division: A review. *Cancer Res.* 25:581, 1965.

Bateman, J. R., Hazen, J. G., Stolinsky, D. C., and Steinfeld, J. L.: Advanced carcinoma of the cervix treated by intra-arterial methotrexate. *Am. J. Obstet. Gynecol.* 96:181, 1966.

Beck, R. E., and Boyes, D. A.: Treatment of 126 cases of advanced ovarian carcinoma with cyclophosphamide. *Can. Med. Assoc. J.* 98:539, 1968.

Bergsagel, D. E.: An assessment of massive-dose chemotherapy of malignant disease. *Can. Med. Assoc. J.* 104:31, 1971.

Berkson, B. M., Lome, L. G., and Shapiro, I.: Severe cystitis induced by cyclophosphamide: Role of surgical management. *J. Am. Med. Assoc.* 225:605, 1973.

Bloomfield, R. D.: Current cancer chemotherapy in obstetrics and gynecology. *Am. J. Obstet. Gynecol.* 109:487, 1971.

Blum, R. H., Carter, S. K., and Agre, K.: A clinical review of bleomycin—a new antineoplastic agent. *Cancer* 31:903, 1973.

Boesen, E., and Davis, W.: *Cytotoxic Drugs in the Treatment of Cancer*. Edward Arnold, London, 1969.

Boiman, R. E., Holzaepfel, J. H., and Barnes, A. C.: Intra-arterial nitrogen mustard in advanced pelvic malignancies. *Am. J. Obstet. Gynecol.* 72:1319, 1956.

Bruce, W. R.: The action of chemotherapeutic agents at the cellular level and the effect of these agents on hematopoietic and lymphomatous tissue. *Can. Cancer Conf.* 7:53, 1966.

Burchenal, J. H., and Carter, S. K.: New cancer chemotherapeutic agents. *Cancer* 30:1639, 1972.

Cavanagh, D., Hoyadhanakul, P., Comas, R., and Lindeman, J.: Regional chemotherapy: Pelvic scanning as an aid to catheter placement in intraarterial infusion. *Int. J. Gynaecol. Obstet.* 11:164, 1973.

Cavanagh, D., Martin, D. S., and Hernandez-Roman, P.: Closed pelvic perfusion: A new approach to the problem of advanced gynecologic malignancy. *Am. J. Obstet. Gynecol.* 92:996, 1965.

Chalmers, T. C., Block, J. B., and Lee, S.: Controlled studies in clinical cancer research. *N. Engl. J. Med.* 287:75, 1972.

Coggins, P.R., Eisman, S. H., Elkins, W. L., and Ravdin, R. G.: Cyclophosphamide therapy in carcinoma of the breast and ovary:A comparative study of intermittent massive vs. continuous maintenance dosage regimens. *Cancer Chemother. Rep.* 15:3, 1961.

Cohen, S. S., and Barner, H. D.: The death of bacteria as a function of unbalanced growth. *Pediatrics* 16:704, 1955.

Costanzi, J. J., and Coltman, C. A., Jr.,: Combination chemotherapy using cyclophosphamide, vincristine, methotrexate, and 5-fluorouracil in solid tumors. *Cancer* 23:589, 1969.

Cromer, J. K., Bateman, J. C., Berry, G. N., Kennelly, J. M., Klopp, C. T., and Platt, L. I.: Use of intra-arterial nitrogen mustard therapy in the treatment of cervical and vaginal cancer. *Am. J. Obstet. Gynecol.* 63:538, 1952.

DeVita, V. T.: Cell kinetics and the chemotherapy of cancer. *Cancer Chemother. Rep.* 2:23, 1971.

DeVita, V. T., and Schein, P. S.: The use of drugs in combination for the treatment of cancer: Rationale and results. *N. Engl. J. Med.* 288:998, 1973.

Duchatellier, M., and Israel, L.: A strategy of chemotherapeutic eradication based upon correlative variations in total cell population, growth fraction and resistance. *Europ. J. Cancer* **8**:263, 1972.

Exploitable Molecular Mechanisms and Neoplasia, a collection of papers presented at the Twenty-second Annual Symposium on Fundamental Cancer Research, 1968, at The University of Texas, M. D. Anderson Hospital and Tumor Institute at Houston. Williams and Wilkins, Baltimore, 1969.

Frei, E., III: Prospectus for cancer chemotherapy. *Cancer* **30**:1656, 1972.

Frei, E., III: Selected considerations regarding chemotherapy as adjuvant in cancer treatment. *Cancer Chemother. Rep.* **50**:1, 1966.

Frick, H. C., II: The efficacy of chemotherapeutic agents in the management of disseminated gynecologic cancer: Review of 206 cases. *Am. J. Obstet. Gynecol.* **93**:1112, 1965.

Frick, H. C.,II, Tretter, P., Tretter, W., and Hyman, G. A.: Disseminated carcinoma of the ovary treated by L-phenylalanine mustard. *Cancer* **21**:508, 1968.

Gerbie, A. B., Hathaway, H. H., and Brewer, J. I.: Autoradiographic analysis of normal trophoblastic proliferation. *Am. J. Obstet. Gynecol.* **100**:640, 1968.

Goolsby, C.D., Daly, J. W., Skinner, O. D., and Gibbs, C. E.: Combination of 5-fluorouracil and radiation as primary therapy of carcinoma of the cervix. *Obstet. Gynecol.* **32**:674, 1968.

Goss, R. J.: The strategy of growth. *In Control of Cellular Growth in Adult Organisms*, H. Teir and T. Rytomaa, Eds. Academic Press, London and New York, 1967.

Gottlieb, J. A., Baker, L. H., Quagliana, J. M., Luce, J. K, Whitecar, Jr., J. P., Sinkovics, J. G., Rivkin, S. E., Brownlee, R., and Frei, E., III: Chemotherapy of sarcomas with a combination of adriamycin and dimethyl triazeno imidazole carboxamide. *Cancer* **30**:1632, 1972.

Greenspan, E. M.: Thio-tepa and methotrexate chemotherapy of advanced ovarian carcinoma. *J. Mt. Sinai Hosp.* **32**:52, 1968.

Greenwald, E. S., Goldstein, M., and Barland, P.: *Cancer Chemotherapy*, 2nd Ed. Medical Examination Publishing Co., Flushing, N. Y., 1973.

Henderson, E. S., and Samaha, R. J.: Evidence that drugs in multiple combinations have materially advanced the treatment of human malignancies. *Cancer Res.* **29**:2272, 1969.

Howe, C. D., and Samuels, M. L.: Phase II studies of hydroxyurea (NSC-32065) in adults: Urologic and gynecologic neoplasms. *Cancer Chemother. Rep.* **40**:47, 1964.

Hreshchyshyn, M. M.: Vincristine treatment of patients with carcinoma of the uterine cervix. *Proc. Am. Assoc. Cancer Res.* **4**:29, 1963.

Hreshchyshyn, M. M.: Hydroxyurea (NSC-32065) with irradiation for cervical carcinoma: Preliminary report. *Cancer Chemother. Rep.* **52**:601, 1968.

Hreshchyshyn, M. M., and Graham, R. M.: 17—α-Hydroxyprogesterone caproate treatment of gynecologic cancer. *Am. J. Obstet. Gynecol.* **104**:916, 1969.

Hreshchyshyn, M. M., and Holland, J. F.: Chemotherapy in patients with gynecologic cancer. *Am. J. Obstet. Gynecol.* **83**:468, 1962.

Hryniuk, W., Foerster, J., Shojania, M., and Chow, A.: Cytarabine for herpes virus infections. *J. Am. Med. Assoc.* **219**:715, 1972.

Hulka, J. F., and Bisel, H. F.: Combined intra-arterial chemotherapy and radiation treatment for advanced cervical carcinoma: The McCall technique and results. *Am. J. Obstet. Gynecol.* **91**:486, 1965.

Hussey, D. H., and Samuels, M. L.: Combined therapy in advanced cancer: Hydroxyurea and radiotherapy. *Cancer Bull.* **23**:42, 1971.

Jacobs, E. M., Reeves, W. J., Jr., Wood, D. A., Pugh, R., Braunwald, J., and Bateman, J. R.: Treatment of cancer with weekly intravenous 5-fluorouracil: Study by the Western Cooperative Cancer Chemotherapy Group (WCCCG). *Cancer* **27**:1302, 1971.

James, Jr., D. H., and George, P.: Vincristine in children with malignant solid tumors. *J. Pediatr.* **64**:534, 1964.

Johnson, E. C., Ansfield, F. J., Ramirez, G., and Davis, H. L. Jr.: Further clinical studies of 5-fluorouracil (5-FU; NSC-19893) given by the multiple daily dose method in disseminated breast cancer. *Cancer Chemother. Rep.* **57**:59, 1973.

Julian, C. G., and Woodruff, J. D.: The role of chemotherapy in the treatment of primary ovarian malignancy. *Obstet. Gynecol. Surv.* **24**:1307, 1969.

Kaplan, S. R., and Calabresi, P.: Drug therapy: Immunosuppressive agents. *N. Engl. J. Med.* **289**:952, 1973.

Kelley, R. M., and Baker, W. H.: Progestational agents in the treatment of carcinoma of the endometrium. *N. Engl. J. Med.* **264**:216, 1961.

Kennedy, B. J.: Progestogens in the treatment of carcinoma of the endometrium. *Surg. Obstet. Gynecol.* **127**:103, 1968.

Kennedy, B. J.: Hormone therapy in cancer. *Geriatrics* **25**:106, 1970.

Knock, F. E.: Newer anticancer agents. *Med. Clin. North Am.* **48**:501, 1964.

Knock, F. E.: *Anticancer Agents.* Charles C Thomas, Springfield, Ill., 1967.

Krakoff, I. H., and Sullivan, R. D.: Intra-arterial nitrogen mustard in the treatment of pelvic cancer. *Ann. Int. Med.* **48**:839, 1958.

Krumbhaar, E. B., and Krumbhaar, H. D.: *J. Med. Res.* **40**:497, 1919.

Lee, Cheng-Chun, Castles, T. R., and Kintner, L. D.: Single-dose toxicity of cyclophosphamide (NSC-26271) in dogs and monkeys. *Cancer Chemother. Rep.* **4**:51, 1973.

Lefrak, E. A., Pitha, J., Rosenheim, S., and Gottlieb, J. A.: A clinicopathologic analysis of adriamycin cardiotoxicity. *Cancer* **32**:302, 1973.

Lokich, J. J., and Skarin, A. T.: Five-drug combination chemotherapy for disseminated adenocarcinoma. *Cancer Chemother. Rep.* **56**:761, 1972.

Lena, M. de, Guzzon, A., Monfardini, S., and Bonadonna, G.: Clinical, radiologic, and histopathologic studies on pulmonary toxicity induced by treatment with bleomycin (NSC-125066). *Cancer Chemother. Rep.* **56**:343, 1972.

Luce, J. K., Bodey, G. P., Sr., and Frei, E., III: The systemic approach to cancer therapy. *Hosp. Prac.* **2**:42, 1967.

Luna, M. A., Bedrossian, C. W. M., Lightiger, B., and Salem, P. A.: Interstitial pneumonitis associated with bleomycin therapy. *Am. J. Clin. Pathol.* **58**:501, 1972.

Malkasian, G. D., Jr., Decker, D. G., Mussey, E, and Johnson, C. E.: Preliminary observations on carcinoma of the cervix treated with 5-fluorouracil. *Am. J. Obstet. Gynecol.* **88**:82, 1964.

Malkasian, G. D., Jr., Decker, D. G., Mussey, E., and Johnson, C. E.: Chemotherapy of squamous cell carcinoma of the cervix, vagina, and vulva. *Clin. Obstet. Gynecol.* **11**:367, 1968a.

Malkasian, G. D., Jr., Decker, D. G., Mussey, E., and Johnson, C. E.: Observations on gynecologic malignancy treated with 5-fluourouracil. *Am. J. Obstet. Gynecol.* **100**:1012, 1968b.

Masterson, J. G., and Nelson, J. H., Jr.: The role of chemotherapy in the treatment of gynecologic malignancy. *Am. J. Obstet. Gynecol.* **93**:1102, 1965.

Mills, E. E. D.: Intermittent intravenous methotrexate in the treatment of advanced epidermoid carcinoma *S. Afr. Med. J.* **46**:398, 1972.

Moore, G. E., Bross, I. D. J., Ausman, R., Nadler, S., Jones, R., Jr., Slack, N., and Rimm, A. A.: Effects of chlorambucil (NSC-3088) in 374 patients with advanced cancer. *Cancer Chemother. Rep.* **52**:661, 1968.

Nathanson, L., Hall, T. C., Schilling, A., and Miller, S.: Concurrent combination chemotherapy of human solid tumors: Experience with a three-drug regimen and review of the literature. *Cancer Res.* **29**:419, 1969.

O'Bryan, R. M., Luce, J. K., Talley, R. W., Gottlieb, J. A., Baker, L. H., and Bonadonna, G.: Phase II evaluation of adriamycin in human neoplasia. *Cancer* **32**:1, 1973.

Omura, G. A.: Chemotherapy and hormone therapy in gynecologic cancer. *South Med. J.* **66**:689, 1973.

Omura, G. A., and Roberts, G. A.: Combination therapy of solid tumors using 1,3 bis (2-cholorethyl)-1-nitrosourea (BCNU), vincristine, methotrexate, and 5-fluorouracil. *Cancer* **31**:1374, 1973.

Patterson, W. B.: Contributions of surgeons to clinical cancer chemotherapy. *Oncology* **26**:277, 1972.

Perlia, C. P., Gubisch, N. J., Wolter, J., Edelberg, D., Dederick, M. M., and Taylor, S. G.: Mithramycin treatment of hypercalcemia. *Cancer* **25**:389, 1970.

Philips, F. S., Sternberg, S. S., Cronin, A. P., and Vidal, P. M.: Cyclophosphamide and urinary bladder toxicity. *Cancer Res.* **21**:1577, 1961.

Reitemeier, R. J., Moertel. C. G., and Blackburn, C. M.: Vincristine (NSC-67574) therapy of adult patients with solid tumors. *Cancer Chemother. Rep.* **34**:21, 1964.

Richardson, G. S., Hall, T. C., Green, T. H., and Ulfelder, H.: Chemotherapy of cervical carcinoma. *Ann. N.Y. Acad. Sci.* **97**:841, 1962.

Roy, D. K.: Treatment of advanced or recurrent carcinoma of the cervix by cytotoxic drugs. *Indian J. Cancer* **4**:32, 1967.

Scientific basis of cancer chemotherapy. In *Recent Results in Cancer Research*, G. Mathe, Ed., Springer-Verlag, New York, 1969.

Scott, R. B.: Cancer chemotherapy: The first twenty-five years. *Brit. Med. J.* **4**:259, 1970.

Sherman, A. I.: Progesterone caproate in the treatment of endometrial cancer. *Obstet. Gynecol.* **28**:309, 1966.

Shimkin, M. B., and Moore, G. E.: Adjuvant use of chemotherapy in the surgical treatment of cancer: Plan of cooperative study. *J. Am. Med. Assoc.* **167**:1710, 1958.

Shirakawa, S., Luce, J. K., Tannock, I., and Frei, E., III: Cell proliferation in human melanoma. *J. Clin. Invest.* **49**:1188, 1970.

Simister, J. M.: Alopecia and cytotoxic drugs. *Brit. Med. J.* **2**:1138, 1966.

Skipper, H. E., Schabel, F. M., and Wilcox, W. S.: On the criteria and kinetics associated with "curability" of experimental leukemia. *Cancer Chemother. Rep.* **35**:1, 1964.

Smith, J. P., and Rutledge, F. N., and Sutow, W. W.: Malignant gynecologic tumors in children: Current approaches to treatment. *Am. J. Obstet. Gynecol.* **116**:261, 1973.

Smith, J. P., Rutledge, F. N., Burns, B. C., Jr., and Soffar, S.: Systemic chemotherapy for carcinoma of the cervix. *Amer. J. Obstet. Gynecol.* **97**:800, 1967.

Smith, J. P., Rutledge, F. N., and Soffar, S. W.: Progestins in the treatment of patients with endometrial adenocarcinoma. *Am. J. Obstet. ynecol.* **94**:977, 1966.

Smith, J. P., Rutledge, F. N., and Wharton, J. T.: Chemotherapy of ovarian cancer: New approaches to treatment. *Cancer* **30**:1565, 1972.

Solidoro, A. S., Esteves, L., Castellano. C., Valdivia, E., and Barriga, O.: Chemotherapy of advanced cancer of the cervix: Experience in 55 cases treated with cyclophoshamide. *Am. J. Obstet. Gynecol.* **94**:208, 1966.

Stevens, D. A., Jordan, G. W., Waddell, T. F., and Merigan, T. C.: Adverse effect of cytosine arabinoside on disseminated zoster in a controlled trial. *N. Engl. J. Med.* **289**:873, 1973.

Sullivan, R. D., Miller, E., and Sikes, M. P.: Antimetabolite-metabolite combination cancer chemotherapy: Effects of intra-arterial methotrexate-intramuscular citrovorum factor therapy in human cancer. *Cancer* **12**:1248, 1959.

Sullivan, R. D., Wood, A. M., Clifford, P., Duff, J. K., Trussell, R., Nary, D.K., and Burchenal, J. H.: Continuous intra-arterial methotrexate with simultaneous, intermittent, intramuscular citrovorum factor therapy in carcinoma of the cervix. *Cancer Chemother. Rep.* **8**:1, 1960.

Symposium on vincristine, *Cancer Chemother. Rep.* **52**:453, 1968.

Takamizawa, H., and Wong, K.: Effect of anticancer drugs on uterine carcinogenesis. *Obstet. Gynecol.* **41**:701, 1973.

Tan, C., Etcubanas, E., Wollner, N., Rosen, G., Gilladoga, A., Showel, J., Murphy, M. L., and Krakoff, I. H.: Adriamycin—an antitumor antibiotic in the treatment of neoplastic diseases. *Cancer* **32**:9, 1973.

The Cell Cycle and Cancer, Vol. 1. In *Biochemistry of Disease*, A Series of Monographs, R. Baserga, Ed. Marcel Dekker, New York, 1971.

The Proliferation and Spread of Neoplastic Cells, a collection of papers presented at the Twenty-first Annual Symposium on Fundamental Cancer Research, 1967, at The University of Texas, M. D. Anderson Hospital and Tumor Institute at Houston. Williams and Wilkins, Baltimore, 1968.

Tisman, G., Herbert, V., and Edlis, H.: Determination of therapeutic index of drugs by *in vitro* sensitivity tests using human host and tumor cell suspensions. *Cancer Chemother. Rep.* **57**:11 1973.

Trussell, R. R., and Mitford-Barberton, G. de B.: Carcinoma of the cervix treated with continuous intra-arterial methotrexate and intermittent intramuscular leucovorin. *Lancet* I:971, 1961.

Wait, R. B.: Megestrol acetate in the management of advanced endometrial carcinoma. *Obstet. Gynecol.* 41:12, 1973.

Wallach, R. C., Kabakow, B., Blinick, G., and Antopol, W.: Thiotepa chemotherapy for ovarian carcinoma: Influence of remission and toxicity on survival. *Obstet. Gynecol.* 35:278, 1970.

Watson, J. D.: *Molecular Biology of the Gene.* W. A. Benjamin, New York, 1970.

Wolff, J. A., D'Angio, G., Hartmann, J., Krivit, W., and Newton, W.A., Jr.: Long-term evaluation of single versus multiple courses of actinomycin D therapy of Wilm's tumor. *N. Engl. J. Med.* 290:84, 1974.

Yarbro, J. W.: Molecular biology of anticancer agents. *Geriatrics* 25:135, 1970.

CHAPTER ELEVEN

Hyperalimentation

11-1 PURPOSE OF HYPERALIMENTATION

Hyperalimentation serves to provide adequate carbohydrate and positive nitrogen balance in patients who are undergoing catabolic processes (e.g., cancer or trauma) and/or patients who should not have oral intake. Use of hyperalimentation alone can provide absolute weight gain and is very effective in bowel rest, decreasing biliary, pancreatic, and intestinal secretions.

11-2 METHOD OF ADMINISTRATION

The parenteral solution is markedly hypertonic and therefore must be administered into a large central vein (subclavian or internal jugular entrance into superior vena cava). The catheter should be inserted under strict aseptic technique and maintained in sterile condition. The technique that we consider the safest is described below.

Preparation

There are four steps in preparation (procedure carried out in the operating room):

1. Place the patient in the Trendelenburg position, $\sim 15°$.
2. Shave the skin.
3. Prep with ether or acetone.
4. Prep with betadine.

Supraclavicular Approach (Fig. 11-1)

This approach is recommended because the vein is entered where it crosses the first rib and injury to the lung is avoided. With the patient in the Trendelenburg position, the external jugular veins usually become visible, indicating that positive venous pressure has been provided and air embolus will not occur at the time that the catheter is inserted through the needle. Engorgement of the external jugular veins indicates that the deep veins at the base of the neck are enlarged maximally; this facilitates the venipuncture. The neck is slightly flexed by placing a folded towel under the head; it is rotated 45° to the opposite side. This flexion of the neck relaxes the anterior scalenus muscle, and rotation contracts the sternocleidomastoid muscle; thus the two muscles can be easily differentiated. The hands are crossed on the abdomen, bringing the clavicle forward and increasing the costoclavicular space.

A local anesthetic is infiltrated into the skin at the lateral angle of the sternoclei-domastoid muscle and the clavicle. The anterior scalenus muscle is identified from the posterior border of the sternocleidomastoid muscle and traced down to the first rib. The subclavian vein crosses over the rib at the insertion of the anterior scalenus muscle. The index finger is held at this point to guide the needle anterior to the rib.

A 2-in. No. 14 needle is disconnected from a large intracatheter and attached to a small glass syringe. The tip is advanced through the anesthetized area and the needle inserted to a length of 1½-2 ins.; the finger is removed and the needle withdrawn with constant aspiration until a free flow of blood is obtained. During insertion, the needle transverses the vein, and it is then withdrawn until the tip is again within the vein. The trajectory of the needle for venipuncture is perpendicular to the axis of the vein (position I, Fig. 11-1). When the tip has been withdrawn to a point within the vein, it is necessary to change the

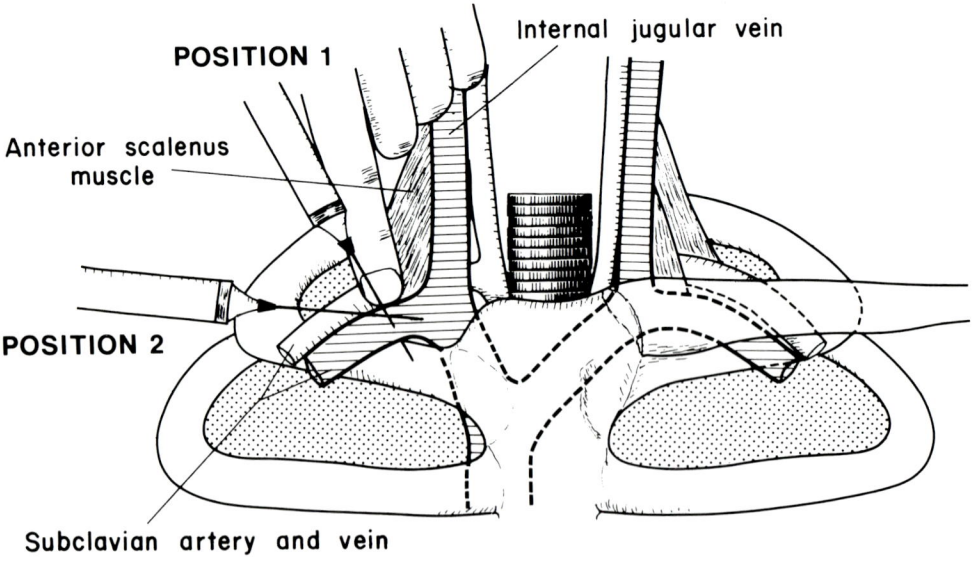

Fig. 11-1 Technique for placement of subclavian catheter: supraclavicular approach.

direction of the needle to facilitate passage of the catheter (position II, Fig. 11-1). The bevel of the needle at the time of insertion is cephalad; after venipuncture, rotation of the needle 180° in either direction brings the bevel caudad, thus preventing insertion of the catheter into the internal jugular vein. When the needle has been properly placed and free flow of blood can be obtained, the syringe is detached from the needle and the catheter is inserted.

Infraclavicular Approach

In this approach to the subclavian vein, the Trendelenburg position is established and a towel is placed beneath the dorsal vertebrae, hyperextending the shoulders. The head is averted and the field defatted with acetone or alcohol, surgically prepped, and draped. A local anesthetic is infiltrated into the skin and the subcutaneous tissue 1 cm inferior to the junction of the medial and middle thirds of the clavicle. A No. 14 needle with small syringe is advanced through the skin wheel with the syringe horizontal and the needle point directed medially and slightly cephalad (Fig. 11-2). A good point of reference can be established by firmly pressing the fingertip into the suprasternal notch to locate the deep side of the superior angle of the clavicle and directing the needle behind the fingertip. When free blood flow occurs, the syringe is raised toward the shoulder and the needle rotated, pointing the bevel to face the superior vena cava. Then, with the syringe removed and the patient performing a Valsava maneuver, the catheter is inserted to the predetermined depth. Fixation, dressing, and x-ray confirmation are performed after completing the described technique.

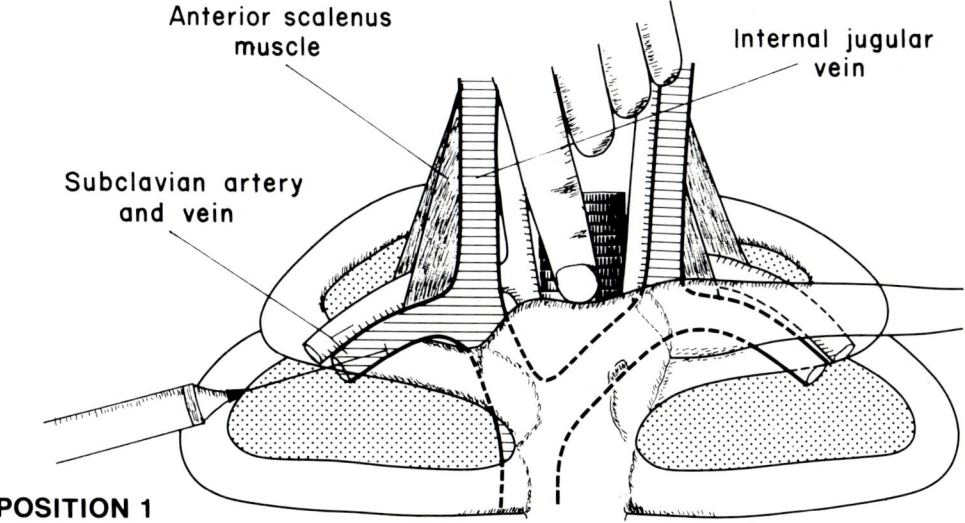

POSITION 1

Fig. 11-2   Technique for placement of subclavian catheter: infraclavicular approach.

Complications

Occasionally the subclavian artery will be entered alongside the subclavian vein. The color and ease of aspiration of the blood will signal this error. Simply withdrawing the needle and applying firm pressure suffice to control bleeding. This should not discourage further attempts to execute a subclavian vein puncture. On other occasions branches of the subclavian artery, such as the transverse cervicalis or suprascapularis, may be transected by the needle, causing local bleeding into tissues. Again, withdrawing the needle or catheter and applying firm pressure for several minutes usually suffice to control bleeding, although a small hematoma may result. Although A-V fistulae have been reported following inadvertent arterial puncture, these have undergone spontaneous occlusion within several weeks. Arterial puncture is more common in techniques that approach the internal jugular vein.

Pneumothorax usually occurs when the trajectory of the needle involves the apex of the lung. As the needle is advanced with a negative pressure in the syringe, the appearance of air in the syringe is indicative of puncture of the lung. At this point, the procedure should be abandoned and the patient observed closely. Approximately half of these patients will have a pneumothorax exceeding 50% and require chest tube decompression. Careful auscultation and serial chest x-rays are the best means of identifying patients in whom conservative therapy should be abandoned.

The parenteral solution administered is hypertonic and results in thrombosis if the catheter is threaded into any tributary of the vena cava. Proper placement of the catheter in a high flow vessel can be assured by the position of the radiopaque catheter on chest x-ray. Catheters that appear to be directed upward or laterally are in all probability positioned in a tributary, so that thrombosis is likely with administration of hypertonic alimentation fluids. Repositioning of the catheter is necessary.

One of the most serious complications of this technique is septicemia. True cannula sepsis is due to contamination from around the catheter or from the fluid bath. Before removing the catheter consideration should be given to other possible sources of sepsis. Cannula sepsis can be minimized by adhering to rigid sterile techniques in regard to both the insertion and the maintenance of catheters. Every 2-3 days the dressing and IV tubing should be replaced. The exit of the catheter and the surrounding skin should be prepped with betadine and a sterile occlusive dressing then applied. A catheter will last for several weeks if sterility is maintained.

11-3 BASIC NUTRITIONAL REQUIREMENTS

Calories. 2500-3500 daily.

Nitrogen. 8-16 g (75-150 g protein equivalent) daily; may increase to 30 g daily in severe trauma.

  1 g protein = 4 cal.

Carbohydrates. Necessary for protein utilization; usual requirement is 2000 calories, but for fever and severe trauma more are necessary.

  1 g of glucose = 4 cal.

Fats. In adults, not essential, especially for short-term management.

  1 g of fat = 9 cal.

Electrolytes. Very variable.

  Sodium. Depends on clinical situation. Weight changes and serum sodium must be monitored daily. Usually 125-150 meq/day needed for protein utilization.

Potassium. Minimum 40 meq/day, may be as high as 300 meq/day.

Magnesium. 10-20 meq/day.

Calcium. 10-20 meq/day.

Phosphorus. 25-50 meq/day.

Trace elements. Usually provided via plasma transfusions: zinc (needed for wound healing), iron, iodine, manganese.

Vitamins (daily requirement):

A-2500-4000 units.

C-250-500 mg.

D-400 Units.

E-10 units.

B_1-5-10 mg.

B_2-4-5 mg.

B_6-15 mg.

Niacin-50 mg.

Pantothenate-20 mg.

Folic acid-0.15-0.2 mg.

B_{12}-15-30 mg.

Biotin-150-300 mg.

K-10 mg every 3 days.

Water. Variable (2000-4000 cc daily).

1000 cc insensible loss; urine output and skin turgor must be monitored.

11-4 CONSTITUENTS OF HYPERALIMENTATION FLUIDS

1. 50% Dextrose: 50 g/100 cc H_2O.
2. 10% Hyprotigen (McGaw Laboratories):
    Protein-10 g/100 cc.
    Sodium-50 meq/1000 cc.
    Potassium-36 meq/1000 cc.
    Calcium-10 meq/1000 cc.
    Magnesium-4 meq/1000 cc.
    Chloride-36 meq/1000 cc.
    Phosphate-50 meq/1000 cc.
3. FreAmine (McGaw Laboratories):
    Amino acid mixture-8.5 g/100 cc.
    Sodium bisulfate->0.10 g/100 cc.
4. Vi-Syneral (Fisons):
    Vitamin A-50,000 units/10 cc.
        D-5000 units
        C-250 mg
        E-10 units
        B_1-50 mg
        B_2-5 mg.
        B_6-15 mg.
        Niacin-100 mg.
        Dexpanthenol-25 mg.

5. MVI concentrate (U.S.V. Pharmaceutical Co.):
   Vitamin A-10,000 units/10 cc.
              D-1000 units.
              C-500 mg.
              B_1-50 mg.
              B_2-10 mg.
              B_6-15 mg.
   Niacinamide-100 mg.
   Dexpanthenol-25 mg.
   Vitamin E-5 units.

11-5 SUGGESTED CONTENTS

Aggressive Approach

Starting with the highest concentration of dextrose, given slowly at first and gradually increased in rate to tolerance; for example:

500 cc	50% Dextrose
500 cc	10% Protigen
X meq	NaCl (or $NaHCO_3$)
X meq	KCl (*as needed*)
5 cc	MVI or other vitamin preparation
1000 units	Heparin (to prevent clotting at catheter tip)
1-5 mg	Folic acid/1000 cc bottle

The above is prepared in one bottle and started at 75 cc/hour; the volume can be increased every 1-2 days as needed.

Tolerance is determined by blood glucose levels (maintain between 100 and 200) and urine sugars. If urine sugars are constantly 4+, more dehydration in an already depleted patient may result. Ten units of regular insulin can be given by IV push every 1-2 hours as needed for 4+ sugars, but warily. A hypoglycemic syndrome can result, especially in patients who have a low renal threshold for glucose and in whom the *serum* glucose level is not appreciably elevated when insulin is administered.

When exogenous insulin has to be given frequently, it is added to the IV solution, starting with 50 units per bottle and increasing until the urine dextrose is 1+ to 2+. The infusion rate can also be adjusted to provide a serum dextrose of 150 mg %.

It is often necessary to begin another IV for H_2O infusion, since with severe glycosuria there is increased chance for hyperosmolar ketosis and coma. In some patients the pancreas has difficulty adjusting to the glucose load initially, and temporary glycosuria is common.

Conservative Approach

Use the following 10% dextrose solution, which can be given at a faster rate; the concentration of dextrose may be increased to 25% in 100 cc increments every 2-3 days.

With this regimen, there is a greater opportunity for the pancreas to react to the glucose load and hydration is usually adequate.

200 cc	50% Dextrose
500 cc	10% Protigen
200-300	H_2O
X meq	NaCl
X meq	KCl
5 cc	MVI/liter
1-5 mg	Folic acid/bottle
1000 units	Heparin

The following other orders are necessary:

Vitamin K-10 mg every 3 days.
Vitamin B_{12}-1000 meq every 2-4 weeks.
Iron-IM intermittently as determined by serum iron studies.
Magnesium, optional-may add 10 meq daily if desired.
Calcium, questionable whether it is needed-10 mg of calcium gluconate can be added every day.
Alcohol, good source of energy, provides 7 cal/g; 50-100 cc of 95% ethanol may be added daily in IV.
Occasional blood or plasma transfusion will provide adequate trace elements.

11-6 PRECAUTIONS

1. Test urine for sugar and acetone qid.
2. Take chest x-ray after insertion of catheter.
3. Maintain sterile dressing. Change every 3-4 days.
4. Use 100 cc Volutrol IV tubing to prevent inadvertent overload.
5. Take daily electrolytes to determine necessary NaCl and KCl to be added.
6. Use heparin in solution for the prevention of clotting within the catheter.
7. If an inadvertently rapid infusion occurs, coma and convulsions can result. To avoid this, follow these recommendations:

   5% D/W infusion.
   IV Valium to prevent seizures
   IV insulin (after checking dextrostix and blood sugars).
   Blood gases and HCO_3 as necessary.

8. Follow the request of most pharmacies that orders be written in exact concentrations *per liter* of solution; for example:

50 g	Protein
200 g	Dextrose
140 meq	Na
110 meq	Cl
65 meq	K
10 meq	Mg

    5 cc   MVI
    1 mg   Folic acid

This request obviates error in misjudging concentrations of various fluids, as well as errors caused by changing brands of protein hydrolysate in the pharmacy.

11-7 REPRESENTATIVE EXAMPLE

    (Patient: 50 kg female)
    Well hydrated; postoperative bowel resection
    Normal temperature; Cantor tube in place
    Electrolytes (serum)
        Na-136
        K-3.2
        CO_2-26
        BUN-10
        BS-130
        Cl-94
    Urine output, 1800 cc/24 hours
    Cantor tube, 800 cc/24 hours
Calculations:
    Fluid requirement
        1800 cc (urine)
         800 (cantor tube)
         800 (insensible)
        ─────
        3400 cc Total Output
        -400 (water of oxidation)
        ─────
        3000 cc intake/24 hours
    Nutrient requirement:
         50 g   Protein/liter-150 g total/24 hours ⎫
        200 g   Dextrose-600 g total/24 hours   ⎬ providing 3000 calories
                                                   ⎭
    Electrolyte requirement (per liter):
        140 meq   Sodium
         60 meq   Potassium
        160 meq   Chloride
         30 meq HCO_3
    Other:
          4 cc   MVI
        1000 units Heparin
          5 meq $MgSO_4$
          1 mg   Folic acid

For a change in constituents daily weights, urine output, N/G output, skin turgor, serum electrolytes, and CBC are evaluated.

Hyperglycemic Metabolic Acidosis

This serious complication occurs when inadequate amounts of endogenous insulin are secreted and insufficient amounts of exogenous insulin are given. This syndrome can develop rapidly in less than 6 hours or slowly over many hours. The persistence of 4+ glucosuria heralds the onset of this condition. Rapidly devloping hyperglycemic syndrome is due to an unrecognized rapid infusion rate. The clinical manifestations are usually abrupt: the patient complains of frontal headache, which is shortly followed by convulsions. Severe hyperglycemia that has developed over several hours and is not associated with severe acidosis does not produce convulsions. These syndromes can be avoided by prevention of hyperglycemia of more than 200 mg %.

Details of fluid preparation and administration can be found in the references. It is our opinion that amino acid mixtures such as FreAmine offer optimum sources of nitrogen and are to be preferred over protein hydrolysates.

REFERENCES

Allen, J. P.: Anabolism and growth in an infant receiving all nutrients intravenously. *Rocky Mt. Med. J.* **66**:34, 1969.

Dudrick, S. J.: Weight gain via vena cava. *Med. World News*, June 20, 1969.

Dudrick, S. J., Groff, D. B., and Wilmore, D. W.: Long term venous catheterization in infants. *Surg. Gynecol. Obstet.* **129**:805, 1969.

Dudrick, S. J., and Wilmore, D. W.: Long term parenteral feeding. *Hosp. Prac.* **10**:65, 1968.

Dudrick, S. J., Wilmore, D. W., Vars, H. M., and Rhoads, J. E.: Long term parenteral nutrition with growth, development and positive nitrogen balance. *Surg.* **64**:134, 1968.

Dudrick, S. J., Wilmore, D. W., Vars, H. M., and Rhoads, J. E.: Can intravenous feeding as the sole means of nutrition support growth in the child and restore weight loss in an adult? An affirmative answer. *Ann. Surg.* **169**:974, 1969.

Filler, R. M., Eraklis, A. J., Rubin, V. G., and Das, J. B.: Long term parenteral nutrition in infants. *N. Engl. J. Med.* **11**:594, 1969.

Groff, D.: Complications of intravenous hyperalimentation in newborns and infants. *J. Pediatr. Surg.* **4**:460, 1969.

Kaplan, M. S., Mares, A., Quintana, P., Strauss, J., Huxtable, R. F., Brennan, P., and Hays, D.M.: High caloric glucose nitrogen infusions. *Arch. Surg.* **99**:567, 1969.

MacPherson, B. H.: Intravenous nutritional support of the nonalimentating patient. *Am. Surg.* **35**:705, 1969.

Rea, W. J., Wyrick, W. J., McClelland, R. N., and Webb, W. R.: Intravenous hyperosmolar alimentation. *Arch. Surg.* **100**:393, 1970.

Scribner, B. J., Cole, J. J., Christopher, T. G., Vizzo, J. E.: Atkins, R. C., and Blagg, C. R.: Long term total parenteral nutrition, *J. Am. Med. Assoc.* **212**:457, 1970.

Wilmore, D. W., and Dudrick S. J.: Growth and development of an infant receiving all nutrients exclusively by vein. *J. Am. Med. Assoc.* **203**:140, 1968.

Wilmore, D. W., and Dudrick, S. J.: An in-line filter for intravenous solutions. *Arch. Surg.* **99**:462, 1969.

Wilmore, D. W., and Dudrick, S. J.: Safe long term venous catheterization. *Arch. Surg.* **98**:256, 1969.

Wilmore, D. W., Dudrick, S. J., Vars, H. M., and Rhoads, J. E.: Long term intravenous hyperalimentation. *Fed. Proc.* **27**:No. 2, 1968.

Wilmore, D. W., Groff, D. B., Bishop, H. A., and Dudrick, S. J.: Total parenteral nutrition in infants with catastrophic gastronintestinal anomalies. *J. Pediatr. Surg.* **4**:181, 1969.

CHAPTER TWELVE
Care and Management
of the Intestinal Stoma

12-1 COLOSTOMY

Planning and preparation materially aid the stoma patient to recover from the trauma of the operation and to return as quickly as possible to a normal life.

A good stoma is well constructed and is placed in an optimal position. It should be easily accessible to the patient and readily fit with an appropriate appliance. Whenever possible, the abdominal incision should be planned to accommodate the placement needs of the stoma. The most frequently made errors in stoma placement are: (1) too near a bony prominence, (2) on the belt line, (3) too close to the umbilicus, (4) too close to scars where valleys exist, and (5) on the undersurface of panniculus in obese patients. Another common error in the surgical procedure is to make the stoma flush to the skin, so that it is difficult for the patient to place the bag accurately. *Atlas of Intestinal Stomas* by Rupert B. Turnbull, Jr., M.D., and Frank L. Weakly, M. D. (C.V. Mosby Co., Publishers) describes the proper surgical technique.

The peristomal skin should be protected immediately after operation with a transparent adhesive bag, fitted so that *no skin is exposed.* This prevents the caustic intestinal fluid from irritating the skin and causing skin breakdown. The postoperative appliance should be open-ended so that fecal drainage may be emptied and the bag cleansed without removing it from the skin. The use of gauze dressings over the stoma in the immediate postoperative period is not recommended. A good postoperative appliance will have adequate adhesive qualities as well as a karaya ring for reinforcement and skin care. Tincture of benzoin may be applied around the stoma for extra adhesion. *Do not use benzoin compound* as it is extremely irritating to the skin.

The color of a stoma is the best indicator of its condition. A dusky stoma warns that the circulation may be impaired; a black stoma indicates that it is nonviable. Daily observations for color and warmth must be made. Also, the stoma must be dilated daily by the insertion of a gloved and lubricated little finger. The patient must learn to do this and must continue it after discharge.

310

Existing skin problems should be evaluated first as to their cause so that treatment can be selected accordingly. Common causes include tape burn, leakage, infection, allergic reactions, pressure sores, and ulcer or fistula formation. Good hygiene is the single most important tool with which to restore a healthy skin condition. Bathing the skin well and, if possible, allowing the air and mild warmth from a heat lamp or hair dryer to come into contact with the affected area will encourage healing without further treatment. Common skin problems are managed as follows.

A. Reddened or irritated skin.
    1. Wash with soap and water and dry area thoroughly.
    2. Apply thin layer of antacid to area (Maalox, Amphogel, Milk of Magnesia) with cotton swab and fan dry.
    3. Apply light coat of karaya powder, brushing off excess.
    4. Ensure proper fitting of appliance.
    5. Reinforce by making a picture frame of paper tape, half on adhesive edge and half on skin.
B. Excoriated skin, from *Monilia* or other infections.
    1. Wash with soap and water and dry area thoroughly.
    2. Apply Kenalog spray to all involved areas.
    3. Apply Mycostatin powder lightly, brushing off all excess.
    4. Ensure proper fitting of appliance.
C. Severe breakdown of skin.
    1. Expose to air for 30 minutes while preventing drainage.
    2. Apply aluminum hydroxide paste evenly with a tongue blade.
    3. Apply karaya powder until all moisture is absorbed.
    4. Ensure proper fitting of appliance.

Ascending and transverse colostomies have unpredictable flows, and the stool tends to be liquid or semiliquid. Irrigations have no real value under these conditions. Descending and sigmoid colostomies are more easily managed because of the firmer consistency of the stool, and hence irrigations can be utilized to establish control of fecal discharge. An irrigation is usually done daily but is adaptable to every other day or 3 times a week according to individual function. These irrigations should begin 5-7 days postoperatively and must be ordered by the physician. The medical and nursing staffs have a primary responsibility to teach the patient every aspect of this procedure to establish and maintain her confidence in the autonomous management of her bowel function (see Figs. 12-1 to 12-3).

Odor control is vital in colostomy care. Foods that are known to cause odor are asparagus, onions, fish, eggs, and cheese. Bismuth subgallate (200 mg, 2 tablets t.i.d) can be utilized for control of malodorous stool. (This substance also comes in powder form, in a 1 lb box, to be taken 2-3 tablespoons in water t.i.d.) This compound is especially beneficial with transverse and ascending stomas, and generally all of these patients should be discharged on it. There are many commercial products that can be placed directly in the bag to prevent odor. The placing of two aspirin tablets in the appliance is also effective.

Special diets are not recommended for colostomy patients; rather, each individual must establish her own optimum eating habits as she learns which foods are bothersome to her. Fried foods sometimes cause gas and diarrhea. Fibrous meat, oranges, coconut, and celery

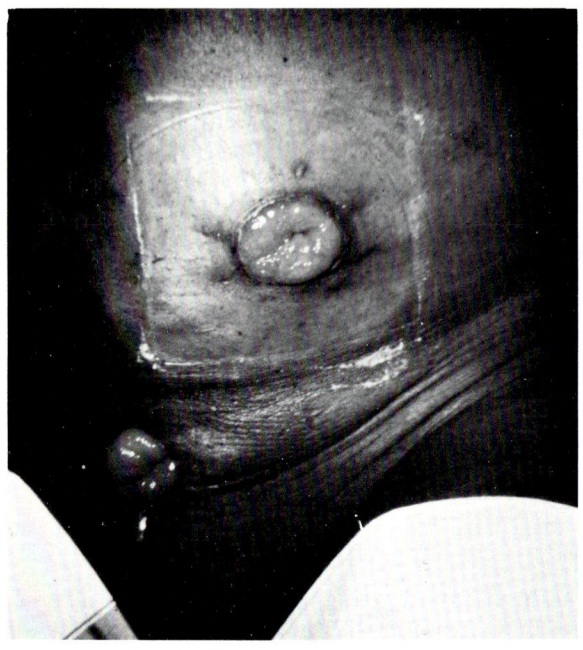

Fig. 12-1 Exposed stoma in preparation for dilation and irrigation.

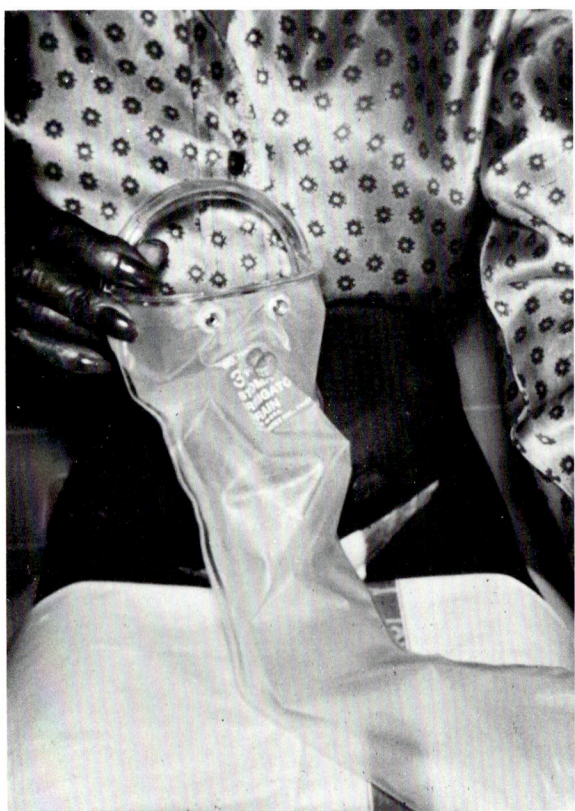

Fig. 12-2 Van Hove irrigation apparatus, held by patient who is about to place it over her stoma, belt it securely, and begin the irrigation procedure.

312

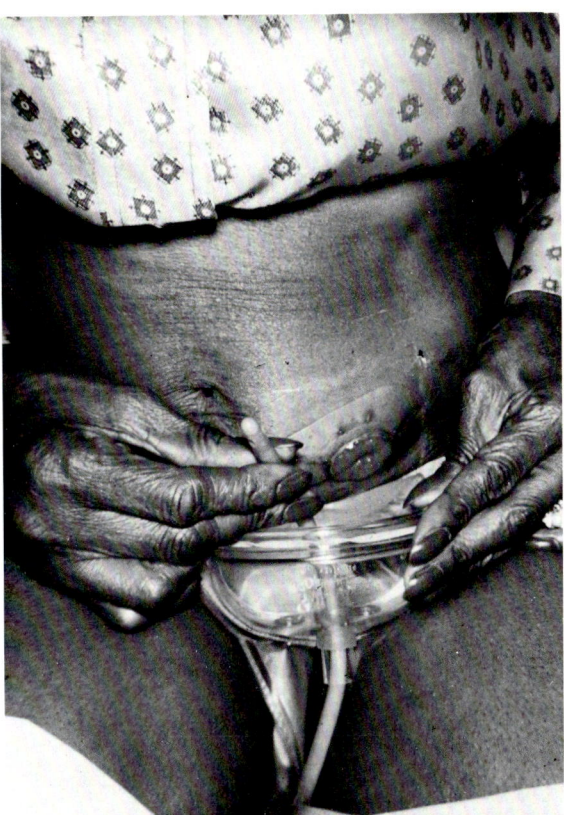

Fig. 12-3 A soft rubber tipped catheter is put into the Van Hove irrigation dome, lubricated, and then gently inserted into the stoma. Lukewarm water will flow from a receptacle placed at shoulder height through the catheter into the stoma and distal colon.

are difficult to digest thoroughly and should be avoided. Many patients think that skipping a meal before going out will ensure no accidents. On the contrary, this will cause much gas and can be more bothersome then a small amount of fecal drainage.

If diarrhea occurs, the patient should drink strong tea rather than coffee and eat bananas, applesauce, cheese, and peanut butter. Should the stool remain loose rather than having the consistency expected, Lomotil (1 tablet t.i.d.) may be taken daily to keep the patient mildly constipated. This will also help to prevent any bowel action other than the evacuation following an irrigation.

A wide range of colostomy equipment is available. Los Angeles County-University of Southern California Medical Center stocks Hollister colostomy bags and irrigating sets for general ward use. When a patient is discharged, a visiting nurse referral sheet is written so that an enterostomal therapist (ET) may begin visiting the patient at home the day after discharge. The ET will continue patient teaching and order the permanent equipment best suited for the patient for irrigation and for wearing. Before going home, the patient must learn *total self-care*. It is recommended that on discharge the patient be sent home with either (1) a bottle of antacid and karaya powder or (2) Kenalog spray and Mycostatin powder so that she and the ET will have something to work with should a skin problem develop.

Should the colostomy prolapse, the intestine should be ice packed to decrease any edema and then manually replaced (Figs. 12-4 and 12-5). If this is a common occurrence,

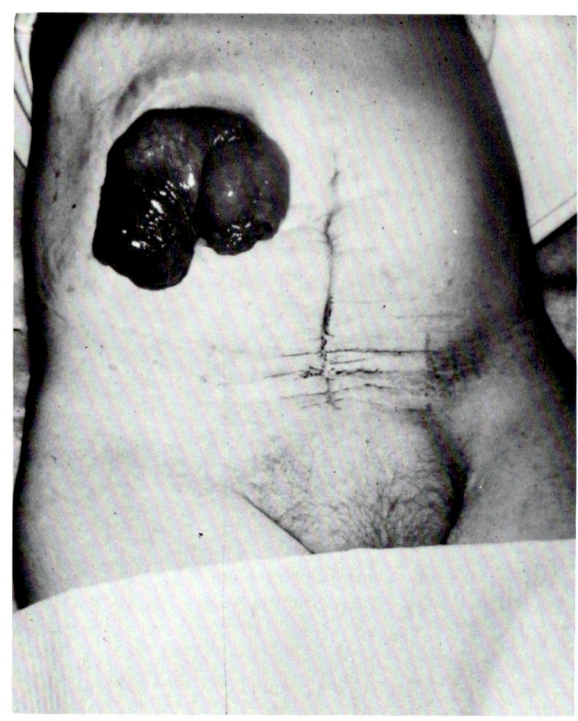

Fig. 12-4 Prolapsed double-barreled colostomy.

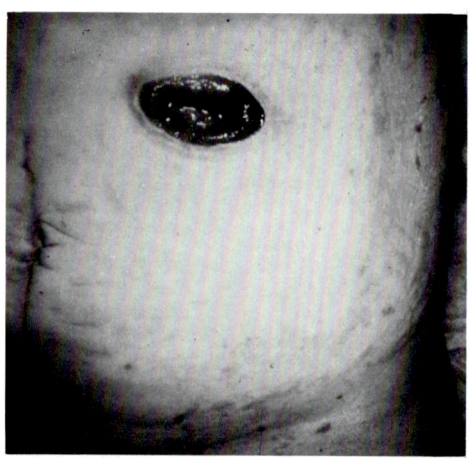

Fig. 12-5 Prolapsed colostomy after application of ice packs and manual replacement.

314

the patient should be instructed to wear a truss or an abdominal support of some kind, such as a mildly constricting panty girdle. Retraction of the colostomy stoma must be surgically revised.

12-2 ILEAL CONDUIT

The priniciples of stoma care as outlined above for colostomies are also applicable to ileal conduits. The surgical placement must be carefully considered, the peristomal skin protected (from leakage of urine) with proper appliance technique, and the stoma dilated with each appliance change (with ileal bladders the permanent appliance should remain on the skin for 5-7 days). Ileal conduit patients should take Mandelamine (I g PO q.i.d.) indefinitely to minimize recurrent urinary tract infections.

When a patient has more than one stoma, all personnel as well as the patient must be cognizant of which is the proper stoma for irrigation. Accidental irrigation of the ileal conduit can result in rupture of the intestine or reflux of contaminated urine into the renal pelvis.

Skin problems are treated similarly to those occurring with colostomies. Severe excoriation around an ileal bladder can be treated quite effectively by inserting a Foley catheter into the stoma and connecting it to straight drainage for 2-3 days. With the appliance remaining off for this period of time, mix karaya powder with a liquid antacid such as Maalox to form a smooth paste and put a heavy layer around the stoma. Do not remove the medication during this 3 day period; simply wipe off soilage and replenish the mixture when needed. If a *Monilia* infection is present, remove the appliance, insert a catheter, and place gauze soaked in Burrow's solution (diluted 1 oz in 1 qt of water) around the stoma. This should be done for 2-3 days or until the infection has cleared (Fig. 12-6).

Encrustations are caused by alkaline urine pooling in the bag. Under these circumstances the patient should change her bag more frequently and empty it often.

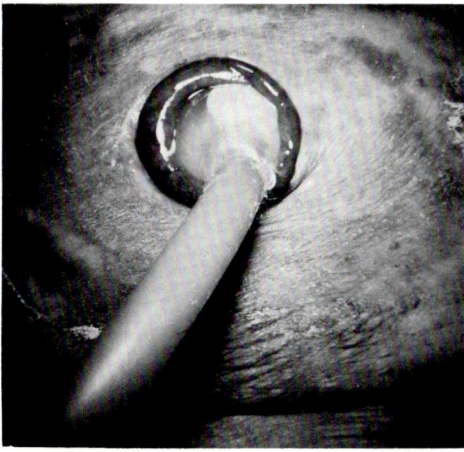

Fig. 12-6 Insertion of a Foley catheter into an ileal conduit stoma to divert the urine away from the skin, making it possible to expose the *Monilia* infected skin to air, and/or to apply medication as described in text.

Deposited crystals in the appliance can be dissolved with full strength vinegar. To rinse the appliance, close the bottom valve, pour in 1 cup of white vinegar (yellow will discolor), stopper the disk opening, and soak the bag for 20 minutes. Then discard the vinegar, wash the bag with soap and water, and allow it to air dry. Foul odor from ileal bladders is caused by a large amount of mucus and alkaline urine. This can be decreased if the patient drinks cranberry juice daily and ingests greater volumes of liquids. Ascorbic acid can also be taken to acidify the urine.

Pseudoepitheliomatous hyperplasia, a "wart-like" skin condition growing up around the stoma, is caused by the constant urine bath and usually suggests too large an opening in the faceplate of the appliance. The opening in the appliance should measure exactly to the size of the stoma plus 1/8 in. The patient should bathe the skin with full strength vinegar and also put 2-3 tablespoons of vinegar into the empty bag before going to bed. The faceplate of a properly fitting bag will eventually push the skin flat again.

These appliances are usually provided through the hospital facility or procured through a local manufacturer. It is suggested that a visiting nurse referral be written on discharge, so that an ET can make a home visit soon after discharge to reassure the patient regarding self-care at home.

The American Cancer Society offers an inexhaustible supply of resources to benefit the ostomy patient. Their services include the counseling of stoma candidates preoperatively by people who have stomas themselves; the organizing of ostomy clubs where stoma patients can meet together and assist each other; and the free distribution of books, pamphlets, and visual aids to patients and for use in inservice education programs.

A very appropriate adage when caring for the stoma patient is "An ounce of prevention is worth a pound of cure."

REFERENCES

Fowler, I. J. and Benfield, J. R.: Care and management of the intestinal stoma: Viewpoint of the enterostomal therapist. *SCANcer* (American Cancer Society): **5**, No. 3, 1973.

Hollister, Inc., *Managing Your Colostomy*. Chicago, Ill. 1971, 20 pp.

Katona, E. A.: Learning colostomy control. *Am. J. Nursing* **67**: No. 3, 1967.

Rowbotham, J. L.: Current concepts of stomal care. *N. Engl. J. Med.* **279**:90, 1968.

Turnbull, R. B., Weakly, F. L.: *Atlas of Intestinal Stomas.* C. V. Mosby Co., Publ., 1967.

CHAPTER THIRTEEN

General Aspects
of Tumor Immunology

13-1 GENERAL CONSIDERATIONS

In the early part of this century Paul Ehrlich hypothesized that malignant neoplasms were antigenic and as such they could be recognized by the hosts' immunologic mechanisms as foreign protein. This attractive hypothesis, if valid, has considerable significance for clinical medicine. First, the concept of an immunologic response to a tumor antigen suggests that there may be antibodies or cell mediated effectors to these antigens in the peripheral circulation of a patient bearing a malignancy. If either of these components exist, the possibility of assaying the blood for their presence would lead to a diagnostic tool for the detection of malignancy. This possibility has been realized in the recent past by the identification and determination of plasma carcinoembryonic antigen (CEA) in patients with cancer. The second profound implication of Ehrlich's hypothesis involves possible methods of cancer immunotherapy. If, indeed, the human organism musters an immunologic response to cancer similar to that seen in infectious diseases, it is conceivable that this response may be augmented to result in a new therapeutic modality.

Unfortunately, the era immediately surrounding Ehrlich's influence became preoccupied with carcinogens and genetics as the bases of malignant transformation, and very little experimentation was done to substantiate or refute his hypothesis. In the 1930s and 1940s some transplantation experiments were done in animals, but these lay victim to the valid criticism that transplanted neoplasms were recognized by the host as nonself because of differences in histocompatability antigens (HLA) and not because these tissues indeed had acquired neoantigens. Beginning with the work of Phren and Main in the mid-1950s, tumor transplantation experiments were performed on inbred animals that were genetically identical, i.e. syngeneic (Table 13-1). These experiments substantiated

A portion of this chapter was previously published in
Contemporary Obstetrics and Gynecology McGraw-Hill, New York, November, 1974.

TABLE 13-1 TRANSPLANTATION IMMUNOLOGY

Genetic Relationship	Antibody	Transplantation Antigens	
		Old Term	New Term
Identical, same individual	Auto	Auto	Syngeneic (autochthonous)
Identical twin	Iso	Iso	Syngeneic
Different individual, same species	Iso	Homo	Allogeneic
Different species	Hetero	Hetero	Xenogeneic

Ehrlich's hypothesis in that malignant tissue was rejected when transplanted from a donor to a genetically identical recipient, whereas normal tissue was not. Thus an immunologic response was clearly demonstrated in the animal system, and subsequent experimentation showed this immunologic response to be capable of preventing and destroying tumor growth.

In recent years, considerable evidence has been accumulated which confirms the existence of such a host defense mechansim in the human organism. This was suggested strongly by several indirect proofs. Some of these proofs lay in the observation that patients with immunologic deficiency disease (e.g., hereditary telangiectasia ataxia and Wiscott-Aldrich syndrome) and those on chronic immunosuppressives (e.g., renal transplant patients) have much greater incidences of malignant disease than matched controls. The correlation between increasing frequency of malignant disease in the aged and decreasing immunocompetence has also been defined. Hundreds of reports of spontaneous regression of well documented malignancies, especially hypernephroma, malignant melanoma, neuroblastoma, and gestational choriocarcinoma, were compiled to substantiate the role of the host defense mechanism.

13-2 MECHANISMS OF IMMUNITY

Over the past two decades a core of experimental endeavors has succeeded in demonstrating the mechanisms of tumor immunity (Fig. 13-1) in both the animal and human systems. *In vitro* work with human malignant tumors suggests very strongly that most malignant cells possess tumor antigens which represent new molecular sites or neoantigens when compared to corresponding normal tissue cells. These neoantigens are apparently located on the cell surface and in most instances are capable of evoking a weak immunologic response in a manner similar to transplantation antigens. As with most antigens, the immunologic system reacts by producing both antibodies and cell mediated (lymphocyte) effector arms. (Fig. 13-2) It would appear that the antigen or an antigenic message diffuses from the malignancy through regional lymphatics to neighboring lymph nodes. In the lymph system the antigenic message is processed by a macrophage, (Fig. 13-3) and the macrophage in turn emits a message (probably in the form of RNA) that is capable of transforming uncommitted lymphoid stem cells into lymphoblasts; these then proliferate into many "attack" lymphocytes capable of a cytotoxic effect on the malignant cells. These committed "attack" lymphocytes are of the "T" cell variety and

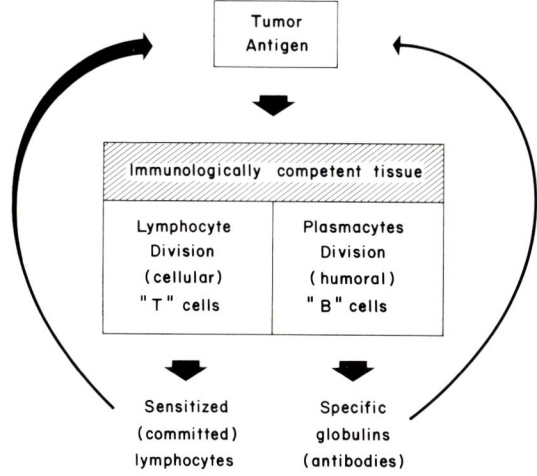

Fig. 13-1 Mechanisms of immunity.

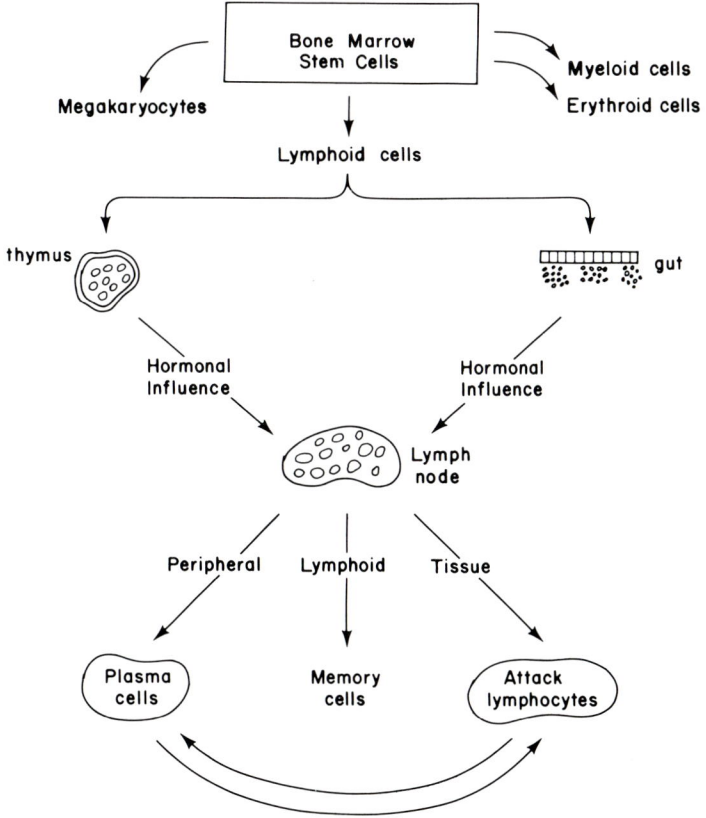

Fig. 13-2 Development of immune system.

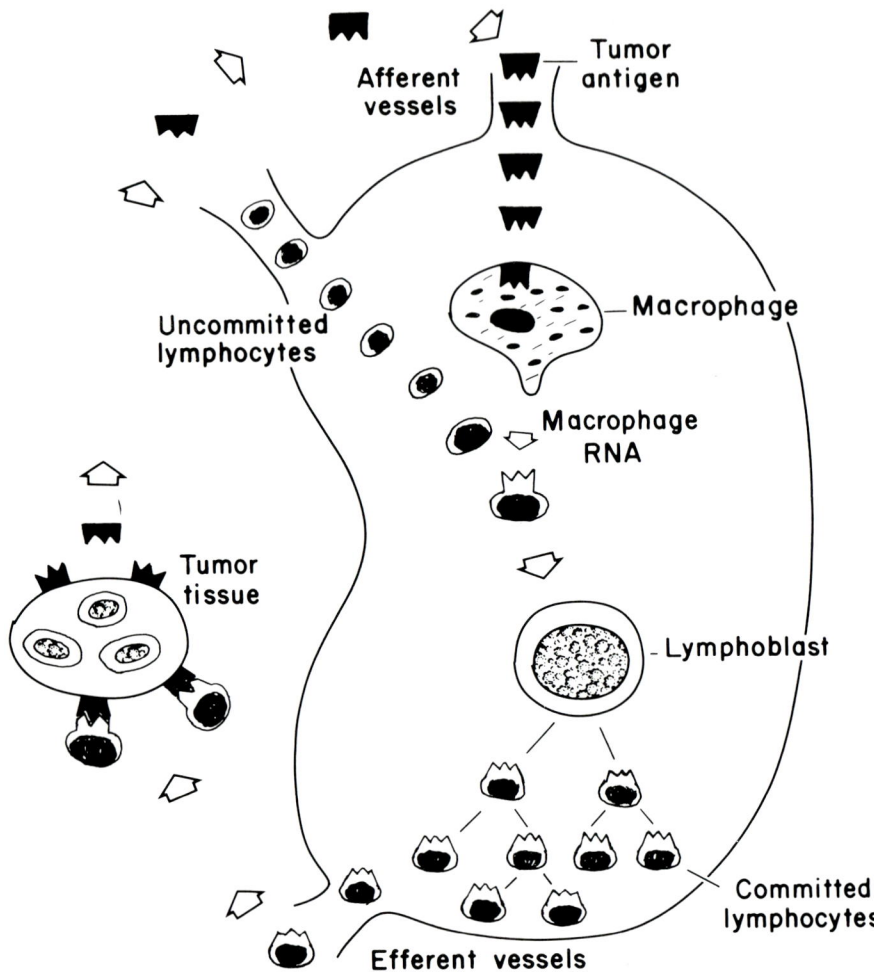

Fig. 13-3 Mechanisms of sensitization of small lymphocytes.

are thymus dependent. The exact mechanism of the thymic influence is ill understood in the human organism but is suspected of being hormonal. The T cell lymphocytes now committed to the "tumor associated antigens" (TAA) flow out into the peripheral circulation via efferent lymphatics and are capable of depositing themselves in and around the malignant tumor, causing a cytotoxic effect under prescribed circumstances.

The other arm ("B" cell) of the immunological response is also excited by most tumor associated antigens. Here, too, an interpretation of the antigenic message probably takes place in regional lymph nodes, where lymphoid stem cells of the B variety are influenced by a macrophage processed message in the direction of the production of plasma cells. Stimulated plasma cells are capable of producing large amounts of immunoglobulin, some of which is converted into tumor antibodies. These are, however, considered to be much less effective in delivering an injurious effect to the malignancy. If clearly identified in future investigations, antibodies to malignant neoplasms would have their greatest promise in affording a more dexterous method for immunodiagnosis. This stimulation along the plasma cell line is also thought to be under a hormonal influence of extrathymic lymphoid tissue (probably intestinal). This is unclear in the human being but has been thoroughly worked out in the chicken, where the lymphoid tissue of the bursa of Fabricius has been identified as the central control center for the production of antibody. Our best indirect evidence to date suggests that the analogous tissue in the human organism lies in the neighborhood of Peyer's patches within the intestine.

The spectrum of immunoglobulins produced against tumor associated antigens in the human organism is a subject of intense investigation but is confused at this time. Varying studies utilizing cytotoxicity assays as well as immunoflourescence have demonstrated the presence of antibodies directed against tumor associated antigens. As stated above, the "killer effect" of these antibodies appears to be quite small in comparison to the cell mediated component of the immune mechanism.

13-3 "T" CELL LYMPHOCYTES

Whatever the mode of action of thymic influence on precursor cells, the resulting immunocompetent T lymphocyte is most responsible for cell mediated reactions and is involved in a cooperative effort with bursa dependent (B) lymphocytes. T cells occur in the peripheral blood as well as in the thoracic duct lymph. They have also been found deep in the cortical areas of the follicular structure of the lymph node and in the periarteriolar areas of the spleen. T cells proliferate during the primary response to the processed antigen, and the cellular products of this proliferation may either participate in the immune expression or survive as memory cells. Lymphocyte kinetic studies show a mixture of "long lived" and "short lived" populations in the blood and thoracic duct. The difference between these two kinetic populations may be largely a matter of degree of immunologic commitment, for both appear to be capable of exerting an injurious effect on tumor cells. Because of its long life span and the ability to recirculate, it is the small lymphocyte that is the logical candidate for initial antigenic recognition and memory retention. It has been shown both *in vitro* and *in vivo* that after appropriate stimulation small T cell lymphocytes undergo blastic transformation. The deficit of blastic transformation *in vitro* in response to antigenic agents in thymectomized rodents and chickens as well as athymic infants indicates that thymic integrity is a prerequisite for response by the small lymphocyte. Experiments by many investigators have demonstrated that T lymphocytes are capable of exerting an injurious effect on malignant cells *in vitro*. The lymphocyte attaches to the cell membrane of the malignant cell, and in 48-72 hours there appears to be a vacuolization which progresses to cytolysis in most cases. Although the nature of this injurious process is ill understood, some evidence suggests that it is RNA dependent. Study of the cells *in vitro* suggests that cytoplasmic bridges between the attack lymphocytes and the malignant cell are established.

Undoubtedly the lymphocyte has been the most ignored cell in the human organism. It becomes more apparent each day that the sophistication of this cell is far beyond our previous conceptions. Recently elucidation of the role of soluble factors from antigen stimulated lymphocytes, including transfer factor (TF), lymphocyte transformation activity (LTA), lymphotoxin (LT), and migratory inhibition factor (MIF), has resulted in a clearer understanding of the diverse means available to lymphoid tissue to act both as a cytotoxic effector and as the initiator of an augmented response to immune reactions. (Fig. 13-4).

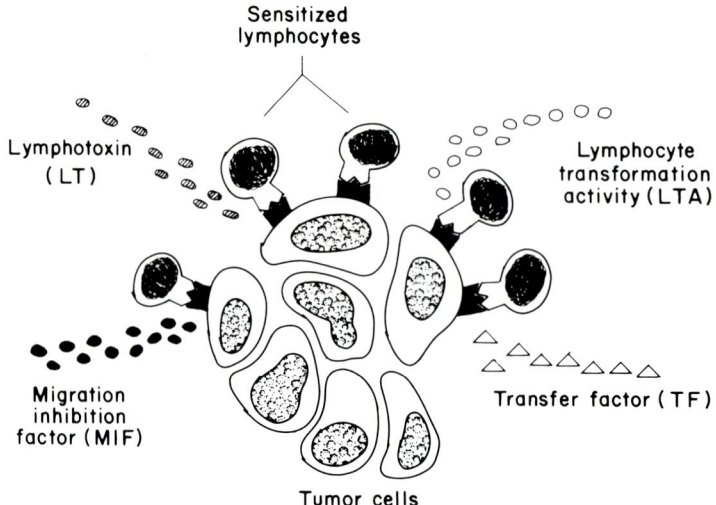

Fig. 13-4 Lyphokinin production.

Transfer factor is a heat stable, low molecular weight substance capable of initiating transformation and clonal proliferation of the recipient lymphocytes in the presence of sensitizing agents. A nonsensitized recipient, when exposed to transfer factor, will exhibit a prompt onset of delayed hypersensitivity. In fact, this may be passed from human donor to recipient by antigen sensitized cells, by cell lyophilisates, or by dialyzable material of these lyophilisates. This factor is undoubtedly released *in vitro* from intact cells in the presence of a specific antigen and can be recovered in dialysates of the medium. Augmentation of the patient's immune response by the infusion of transfer factor holds one of the greatest hopes for immunotherapy.

Lymphocyte transformation activity can be obtained from the supernatant of antigen sensitive lymphocytes in the presence of the antigen and shares with TF the ability to confer on previously unchallenged recipients a state of delayed hypersensitivity specific for stimulating agent. The exact interplay of LTA and TF has yet to be clarified.

Another heat stable substance, with a molecular weight of approximately 90,000, which is capable of destroying a wide variety of target cells in culture, results from the exposure of reacting lymphocytes to either nonspecific stimulants (such as PHA) or specific antigens. This substance, called lymphotoxin, has been isolated from several systems *in vitro*. Indeed, the effect of this cytotoxic material on target cells is apparently irreversible after incubation for 24 hours or more. Experimental evidence suggests that LT depresses RNA and protein synthesis in the target cells and thereby leads to their demise.

The interaction of antigen-sensitive lymphocytes with the corresponding specific antigen is also responsible for the production in the lymphocyte and the subsequent release of a protein substance that is capable of creating an interference of macrophages, diverting their migration from antigen containing areas. This substance, migratory inhibition factor, has proved to be a sensitive indicator of delayed hypersensitivity. In our experiments many patients demonstrating anergy by skin test methods have lymphocytes that fail to inhibit macrophage migration. Like cytotoxicity assays, MIF has been used *in vitro* to demonstrate the presence of tumor associated antigens in both ovarian and cervical malignancies.

13-4 "B" CELL LYMPHOCYTES

The B cell lmphocyte has a life span in the neighborhood of days to weeks, as compared with months to years for the T cell lymphocyte. Like the T cells, many B cells originate in the bone marrow. They can be localized in the lymph nodes, spleen, and Peyer's patches and tend to be identified in areas apart from the T cells (Table 13-2). In the lymph node they are usually found in the subcapsular or medullary portion of the node, whereas in the spleen they occur in the peripheral white pulp and red pulp. Their location in Peyer's patches is usually in the central follicle, unlike the T cells, which are usually found in the perifollicular structure. The B cells appear to have little role in cell mediated immunity and are involved primarily in the induction of humoral immunity and antibody synthesis. It is unknown whether or not a memory, which is one of the hallmarks of the T cell, exists among B cells. The production of antibodies in response to tumor associated antigens appears to be less consistent than sensitized lymphocyte production. The possibility exists that the degree of cellular cooperation leading to antibody formation depends on special properties of the stimulating antigen, such as the physical and chemical nature of the carrier and the antigen, the site and mode of antigen entry into the body, localization, and concentration.

13-5 ANTIBODY

Antibodies (immunoglobulins) are specific serum proteins that are synthesized in response to an antigenic stimulus by the cells of the gut-dependent lymphoid sytem (B cells). Five distinct classes of immunoglobulins with characteristically different chemical structures and biologic functions have been discovered. All are similar in basic molecular structure (Fig. 13-5), having two light chains, which may be either of two types, and two heavy chains, which are specific for the class of immunglobulin. In both the heavy chains and the light chains, there are constant and variable regions of amino acid sequence. The constant region is determined by the genetic inheritance, whereas the variable region differs with the specificity of the antibody for its corresponding antigen. The binding sites of the antibody are found in this latter region of the molecule. Both the heavy chain and the light chain may contribute to the specificty of the antibody, but, of the two, the heavy chain contributes more to the reaction with the antigen. Isolated heavy chains

TABLE 13-2 COMPARISON OF "T" CELL AND "B" CELL

	"T" Cell	"B" Cell
Origin	Bone marrow	Bone marrow
Location		
Lymph node	Deep cortical	Subcapsular
	Perifollicular	Germinal centers
Spleen	Periarteriolar	Red pulp
Peyer's patch	Perifollicular	Central Follicle
Function		
Cell mediated immunity	Yes	No
Humoral immunity		
Induction	Yes	Yes
Antibody synthesis	No	Yes
Life span	Months to years	Days to weeks

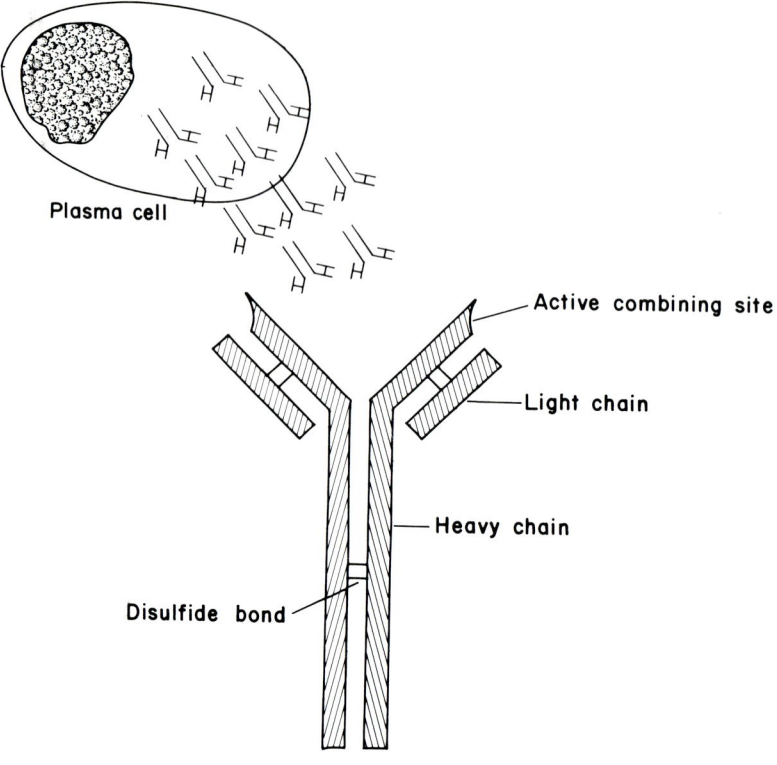

Plasma cell

Active combining site

Light chain

Heavy chain

Disulfide bond

Fig. 13-5 Basic structure of immunoglobulins.

usually bind to specific antigen, whereas light chains as a rule do not; but a combination of light and heavy chains from specific immunoglobulins is much more effective than heavy chains alone.

The term complement refers to a complex effector system of eleven distinct serum proteins that serve primarily to amplify the effects of the interaction between specific antibody and antigen. Of these, IgM and three of the four classes of IgG are known to activate the complement system, but IgA does not. Definite information is not available for IgE and IgD, but in the currently available data IgE antibodies do not seem to activate the complement system. This activation of the complement system can lead to several important biologic effects, including immune adherence, phagocytosis, chemotaxis, and facilitation of intracellular killing.

The most plentiful and probably the most important immunoglobulin in man is IgG. Antibodies to most of the bacteria, virus neutralizing antibodies, precipitating antibodies, hemagglutins, and incomplete hemolysins are among the types of antibody found in the IgG peak. The active synthesis of IgG occurs predominantly in the plasma cells from the medullary portion of the lymph nodes and in the red pulp of the spleen. Whereas IgG is produced as a late response to antigens, IgM is the first antibody to appear after a primary antigenic stimulus, the first to appear in phylogeny and ontogeny, and the last to leave in senescence. A powerful activator of the complement system, IgM is the predominant antibody formed as a response to gram negative bacteria. Plasma cells that synthesize IgM are also found in the red pulp of the spleen and in the medullary cords of the lymph nodes. The biologic functions of IgA, IgE, and IgD are not well understood at this time.

Weak cytotoxic antibodies have been demonstrated in some tumor systems such as human malignant melanoma and adenocarcinoma of the ovary. The cytotoxic effect is often limited to changes in membrane permeability and does not exhibit the devastating quality seen with lymphocytes. The class of immunoglobulins to which these cytotoxic antibodies belong is probably IgM, but further investigation is necessary to clarify this matter. Tumor specific circulating antibodies have been demonstrated by immunoflourescence, hemagglutination, complement fixation, and various other immunochemical tests.

13-6 BLOCKING ANTIBODY

The question that naturally arises in the reader's mind is why so many patients succumb to their malignancies in spite of the host's defenses. If, indeed, the human host has the capability of mustering a dual-armed immunologic defense, then why do people die of malignant tumors? One answer to this query has been elucidated by the work of the Hellströms and others in demonstrating a blocking serum factor that is probably a circulating antigen-antibody complex. These investigators have demonstrated in both the animal and human systems that patients with progressive disease have a circulating serum factor which can "coat" the malignant cells and thereby abrogate the effect of the cell mediated attack on the tumor. This phenomenon may indeed explain the immunologic tumor enhancement (Fig. 13-6) of transplanted cells (which possess tumor associated antigens), as occasionally observed *in vivo* using the animal system. Also, it may explain the mechanism of tumor enhancement in the development of human autochthonous neoplasms. It offers a solution for the seemingly paradoxical situation in which tumors grow progressively *in vivo* despite the fact that their cells are inhibited by autochthonous

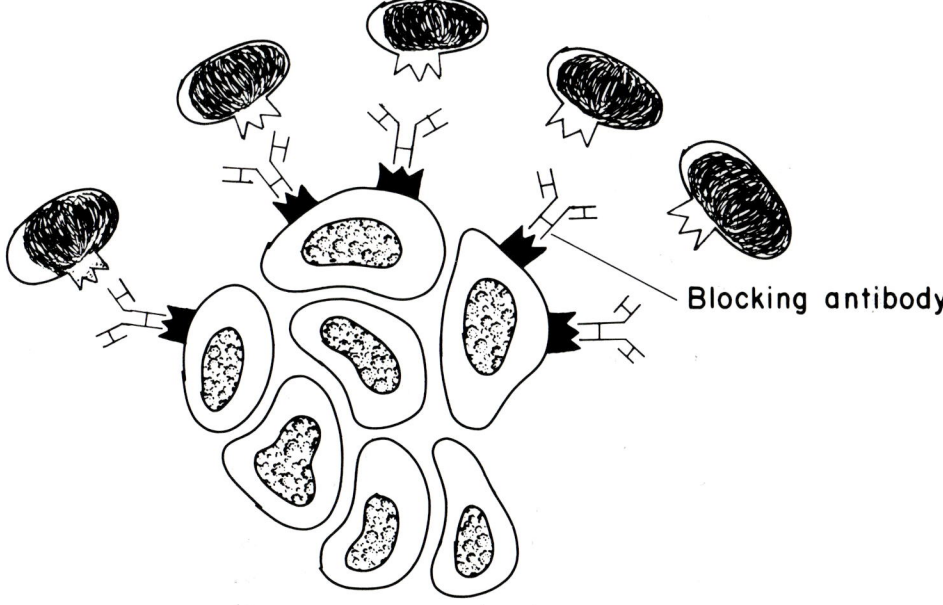

Fig. 13-6 Tumor enhancement.

lymphocytes *in vitro*; presumably the neoplastic cells are protected from destruction by serum factors (blocking antibody). This, in addition, suggests a pathway for therapy; suppression of blocking antibody production may lead to an augmentation of the host defense mechanisms and thereby act as a counterplay to tumor enhancement.

Recently it has been reported that sera from patients with regressing disease are capable of counteracting the blocking activity of progressive sera. This suggests very strongly that regressive sera contain a factor that can combine with the target cells and cancel the effect of the blocking molecules. It is not known whether the blocking and nonblocking molecules differ with regard to immunoglobulin class, complement binding ability, or specificity for tumor antigens. Indeed, it has been suggested by some that the "deblocking factor" is not antibody but antigen which ties up the blocking antibody and thus exposes the tumor associated antigens to the cell mediated attack.

13-7 SUMMARY

Several theoretical concepts have been substantiated during the last two decades. It has been demonstrated unequivocally that most human malignancies possess tumor associated antigens or molecules which can be recognized by the patient's host defense mechanism as nonself and to which the patient can muster an immunologic response. This response takes the form of both thymus dependent and extra-thymic-dependent lymphocytes that are capable of either direct or indirect effect on malignant cells. The small T cell lymphocytes appear to be the primary "killer cells." At least four types of lymphokines have been identified as originating from T lymphocytes, and these substances are capable of implementing and augmenting the host's reaction to its malignancy. In general it can be stated that the effect of the T lymphocyte is beneficial, as *in vitro* studies consistently demonstrate the T cell lymphocyte to be capable of producing an injurious effect on the malignant cell. B cell lymphocytes are primarily concerned with immunoglobulin production, and their proliferation is apparently under the influence of extrathymic lymphoid tissue thought to be centered in the intestinal tract. Undoubtedly a spectrum of immunoglobulins is produced in response to tumor associated antigens, but very few are consistently capable of an injurious effect on the malignant cell.

Antibodies directed toward tumor associated antigens have been demonstrated, especially with techniques such as immunoflourescence, complement fixation, and hemagglutination, but their role remains unclear. This is especially evident when one considers the presence of serum blocking factors, which have been tentatively labeled as blocking antibody. Unfortunately, there appears to be "antibody" that is capable of abrogating the cytotoxic effect of T cell lymphocytes on malignant cells. This blocking concept is particularly satisfying to the oncologist because it conveniently explains the ability of a malignant tumor to flourish at the 5 or 10 cell stage in spite of an immunocompetent host.

Certainly the future will demand investigation along many directions in the field of tumor immunology. First and foremost, the tumor associated antigens must be identified, (Fig. 13-7) isolated, purified, and, hopefully, used as a basis for sensitive assays such as the radioimmunoassay. This would presumably lead to early diagnosis and maximum curability. Immunization or augmentation of the immune response may be possible in the form of antigen vaccines. Clearer understanding of the mechanisms of action of T cell lymphocytes would lead to an ability to augment their processes and create more effective immunotherapeutic techniques.

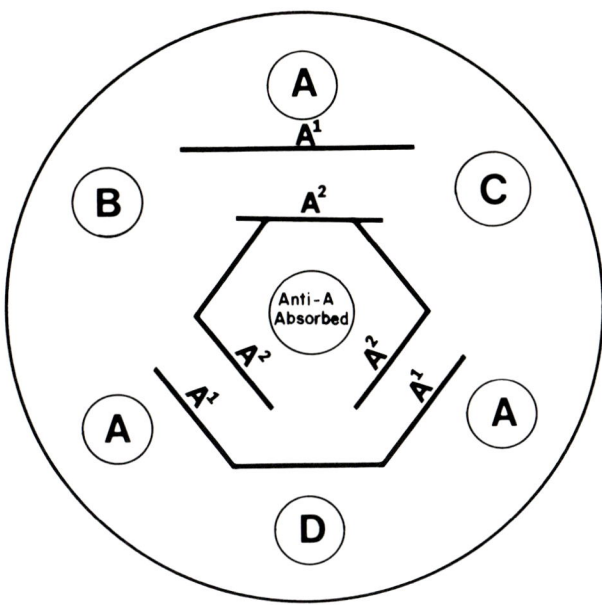

Fig. 13-7 Ouchterlony double diffusion.

The progress of immunotherapy can take three approaches. The first is nonspecific immunotherapy, which is an attempt to increase the patient's immune response with substances known to stimulate the immune system, such as mixed bacterial toxins or fractions of the tuberculous bacillus (BCG). The second is active immunization of a patient's malignancy with vaccines prepared from her own tumor or from one of similar histologic type. The rationale for this, of course, is based on animal studies demonstrating that a growing tumor does not induce a maximun immune response in the host. Efforts are thus made to increase the patient's tumor immunity by altering the tumor specific antigens in such a way that they become more antigenic, or by simultaneouly stimulating the patient's lymphoreticular system with agents (immunologic adjuvants) that enhance the immune response to tumor antigens. Agents such as BCG or crude pertussis vaccine can act as potent stimulants when combined with active vaccines. Third, passive immunotherapy of human cancer is possible with antisera produced in foreign species or in volunteer human donors. Indeed, sera from patients cured of a similar malignancy may contain high titers of cytotoxic or unblocking factors and improve the results of any type of cancer therapy. Another attempt at passive immunotherapy utilizing specifically sensitized lymphocytes is actively under way.

It should be stated at this point that all of these approaches to immunotherapy are indeed quite investigational. Pilot studies are under way in all of these areas, and these should be carefully evaluated before widespread use of these techniques. A great deal of conflicting evidence has resulted from the use of BCG, with both dramatic responses and severe complications being reported simultaneously. The practicing physician should be patient and await long-term follow-up of these pilot studies. There have been many empirical attempts at immunotherapy of human cancer in the past, and there is no doubt that occasional patients have benefited, and some impressive regressions have been induced. However, at the present time, the future of immunotherapy in human cancer, although bright, is unclear, and we must await further knowledge.

13-8 IMMUNOLOGY GLOSSARY

Adjuvant. A substance that when mixed with an antigen enhances its antigenicity.

Agglutinin. An antibody that produces aggregation or agglutination of a particulate or insoluble antigen.

Allele. An alternative gene acting at the same locus on the chromosome.

Allergen. A substance (antigen or hapten) that incites allergy.

Allergic death. Death of an antibody producing or antibody carrying cell presumed to result from overstimulation by antigen. It can be active or passive.

Allergy. A state of specific increased reactivity to an antigen or hapten such as occurs in hay fever. The term is most commonly used to designate states of delayed sensitivity due to contact allergens and immediate sensitivities due to Prausnitz-Küstner antibodies.

Alloantibody (isoantibody). An antibody produced by one individual that reacts specifically with an antigen present in another individual of the same species. The term "isoantibody" is commonly used in blood work and "alloantibody" in tissue transplantation work.

Alloantigen (isoantigen). An antigen that incites the formation of antibodies in genetically dissimilar members of the same species.

Allogeneic. Pertaining to genetically dissimilar individuals of the same species.

Allogeneic disease. A systemic illness resulting from a graft-versus-host response when the graft contains immunologically competent cells and the host is immunologically incompetent (e.g. runt disease).

Allograft (homograft). A graft derived from an allogeneic donor.

Alloimmune. Specifically immune to an allogeneic antigen.

Anamnestic response (recall phenomenon, memory phenomenon). Accelerated response of antibody production to an antigen which occurs in an animal that has previously responded to the antigen.

Anaphylactic antibodies (anaphylactogenic antibodies; see Prausnitz-Küstner antibodies). Antibodies that produce "true anaphylaxis."

Anaphylaxis, acute. Systemic shock (often fatal) that develops in a matter of minutes after reexposure to a specific foreign antigen.

Anergy. Absence of a hypersensitivity reaction such as would be expected in other similarly sensitized individuals.

Anti-antibodies. Autoantibodies against hidden antigen determinants formed in antibodies (gamma globulin molecules) which are presumed to become exposed during distortion of the antibody molecule on complexing with antigen. The term is also used in a less restrictive sense to designate antibodies against uncomplexed antibody molecules incited in allogeneic or xenogeneic animals.

Antibody (Ab). A substance (commonly, if not always, a gamma globulin) that can be incited in an animal by an antigen or by hapten combined with a carrier and that reacts specifically with the antigen or hapten. Some antibodies occur naturally without known antigen stimulation.

Antibody reaction site (antigen binding site, antibody combining site). The local inverted surface site on antibody which reacts with the antigen determinant site on antigen.

Antibody response. The production of antibody in response to stimulation by antigen (see also **Immune response**).

Antigen (Ag). A substance that can react specifically with antibodies and under appropriate conditions can incite an animal to form specific antibodies. *Extrinsic:* An antigen that is not a constituent of the cell. *Instrinsic:* An antigen that is a constituent of the cell. *Occult:* A self-antigen that does not reach antibody forming tissues.

Antigen determinant. A small, three-dimensional everted surface configuration on the antigen molecule that reacts with the antibody reaction site on the antibody molecule.

Antigenic paralysis. See **Immunologic tolerance.**

Antigen tolerance. See **Immunologic tolerance.**

Auto. Self or same.

Autoantibodies. Antibodies produced by an animal that react with the animal's own antigens. The stimulus is usually not known but could be the animal's own antigens or cross-reacting foreign antigens.

Autoantigen. A "self-antigen" that incites the formation of autoantibodies.

Autochthonous (indigenous). Found in the part of the body in which it originates, as in the case of a disease; **autochthonous tumor**—tumor borne by the host of origin.

Autograft. A graft derived from the same animal to which it is transplanted.

Autologous. Derived from the subject itself.

Bursa of Fabricius. A cloacal structure in aves containing lymphoid elements (B-cells) presumed to govern the production of humoral antibodies.

Cell associated antibodies (cell bound antibodies). Antibodies in or on cells. The constitute both antibodies of antibody forming cells and cytophilic antibodies.

Chimera. An individual composed of genetically dissimilar tissues.

Clone. A population of cells derived from a single cell by asexual division.

Committed cell. A cell committed to the production of antibodies specific for a given antigen determinant. Committed cells include primed cells, memory cells, and antibody producing cells.

Complement (C′). A multifactorial system of one or more normal serum components characterized by their capacity to participate in certain antigen-antibody reactions.

Complement activation. Promotion of the killing or lytic actions of complement.

Complement fixation. The fixation of C′ to an antigen-antibody complex.

Cryoglobulin. Globulin that precipitates from serum at 0-4°C.

Cutaneous anaphylaxis. An immediate type of skin sensitivity reaction to specific antigen mediated by anaphylactic antibodies.

Cytophilic antibodies (cytotropic antibodies). Antibodies with affinity for cells that depend on bonding forces independent of those which bind antigen to antibody.

Delayed sensitivity. A specific sensitive state characterized by a delay of many hours in onset time and course of reaction. It is transferable with cells but not with serum.

Desensitization. The procedure of rendering a sensitive individual insensitive to an antigen or hapten by treatment with the agent.

Determinant group. That part of the structure of an antigen molecule that is responsible for specific interaction with antibody molecules evoked by the same or a similar antigen. When antibody is formed in response to a protein to which distinctive chemical groups (hapten) have been conjugated artificially, the structure of the determinant groups is very often identical or closely similar to that of the hapten.

Fab (fragment antigen binding). A segment of the IgG antibody molecule, derived by papain treatment and reduction, containing one antibody reaction site. Under oxidizing conditions Fab fragments recombine to form the divalent molecule $F(ab)_2$ devoid of the Fc segment of the original molecule.

FC (fragment crystallizable.) A segment of the IgG antibody molecule derived by treatment with reducing agents in the presence of urea.

Freund's adjuvant. *Complete:* Freund's water-in-oil emulsion of mineral oil, plant waxes, and killed tubercle bacilli used to incorporate with antigen to stimulate antibody production. *Incomplete:* Freund's mixture without tubercle bacilli.

Gamma globulin. A fraction of serum, based on electrophoretic mobility, composed of a number of molecular classes and subclasses of immunoglobulins and other nonantibody globulins.

Germinal centre (synonyms: **lymphocytopoietic nodules, secondary nodules of Ehrlich**). A reactive change in the cortex of a lymph node, thymus, Malpighian body of the spleen, or any accumulated mass of lymphocytes consisting of a loosely packed, roughly spherical collection of cells that are larger and have paler, more open nuclei than the surrounding cortex of closely packed small lymphocytes. They usually include many cells with mitotic figures.

Graft versus host reaction (GVH). Immune response of grafted cells against the host.

Half-life. Time taken to decrease to half. When the rate of decrease is exponential (i.e., the rate of disappearance at any given time is proportional to the amount present at that time), the half-life is a constant quantity.

Hapten. A substance that combines specifically with antibody but does not incite the formation of antibody unless attached to a high molecular weight carrier. Some antigen determinants, such as simple chemicals, represent the entire hapten.

Hemagglutinin. An antibody that reacts with a surface antigen determinant(s) on red cells to cause agglutination of the red cells.

Hemolysin (amboceptor). An anti-red cell antibody that can specifically activate C' to cause lysis of red cells.

Hetero-. Other or different; often used to mean "of a different species."

Heterophile antigens. Antigens common to more than one species.

Histocompatibility antigens (transplantation or HLA antigens). Antigens coded for by "histocompatibility genes" that determine the compatibility of grafted tissues and organs.

Homologous. See **Allogeneic.**

Homologous disease. See **Allogeneic disease.**

Humoral antibodies. Antibodies present in body fluids (humors).

Immune. The state of being secure against harmful agents or influences.

Immune clearance. Clearance of antigen from the circulation due to complexing with antibodies.

Immune response. A specific response which results in immunity. The total response includes an afferent phase during which responsive cells are "primed" by antigen, a central response during which antibodies are formed, and an efferent or effector response in which immunity is effected by antibodies or immune cells.

Immunity. The state of being able to resist and/or overcome harmful agents or influences. *Active:* Immunity acquired as the result of experience with an organism (usually specific and due to antibodies); also innate. *Passive:* Immunity due to acquisition of maternal antibody or injection of antibody. *Adoptive:* Immunity produced by the acquisition of immune lymphoid cells.

Immunize. The act or process of rendering an individual resistant or immune to a harmful agent.

Immunocompetent cell (antigen-sensitive cell). Any cell that can be stimulated by antigen to either form antibodies or give rise to cells which form antibodies, including inducible cells, primed cells, and memory cells.

Immunogen. An antigen that incites specific immunity.

Immunoglobulins (Ig). Classes of globulins to which antibodies belong.

Immunologically competent cells. Term introduced by P. B. Medawar to indicate cells are able to respond to contact with any particular immunogen by manifesting or developing a specific immunologic capacity. Such responsiveness would include the formation of specific antibody, or the ability to react in delayed-type hypersensitivity reactions or in homograft rejection.

Immunologic enhancement. Enhanced survival of incompatible tissue grafts (tumor or normal tissue) due to specific humoral blocking factors.

Immunologic paralysis. Absence of normal specific immunologic response to an antigen, resulting from previous contact with the same antigen, administered in a quantity greatly exceeding that required to elicit an immunologic response. The normal capacity to respond to other unrelated antigens is retained. The term "immunologic paralysis" is usually employed when specific unresponsiveness is induced in adult life, while "tolerance" has been used when unresponsiveness is induced before the immunologic apparatus is fully developed. It is not clear that there is any essential distinction between the mechanisms involved in each case.

Immunologic tolerance (antigenic paralysis, immunologic suppression, immunologic unresponsiveness, antigen tolerance). Failure of the antibody response to a potential antigen after exposure to antigen. Tolerance commonly results from prior exposure to antigens. *Feeding tolerance:* Tolerance to foreign antigens acquired by their ingestion. *Fetal tolerance:* Tolerance acquired by exposure to antigens during fetal life. *Genetic tolerance:* Tolerance that results from genetic identity; example: identical twins, inbred animals, and tolerance of the F_1 hybrid to parental tissue. *Parity tolerance:* Tolerance to self-antigens, thought to be acquired during embryonic and fetal life. *Split tolerance:* Failure to develop one but not the other of the following: the delayed sensitivity or the humoral antibody response.

Iso—. Identical (from Gk. *isos* = equal).

Isoantibody. See **Alloantibody.** Term used in blood grouping studies to designate an antibody formed by one individual that reacts with antigens of another individual of the same species.

Isoantigen. See **Alloantigen.** "Isoantigen" is commonly used in blood work.

Isogeneic. See **Syngeneic.**

Isograft. See **Syngraft.**

Isoimmune. See **Alloimmune.**

Isologous. See **Syngeneic.**

Lymphocyte. Round cell with scanty cytoplasm, diameter 7-12 μ. In stained preparations cytoplasm is transparent, lacking basophilia but at times containing azurophilic granules. The nucleus is round, sometimes indented, with chromatin arranged in coarse masses and without visible nucleoli. Lymphocytes may be actively motile.

Lymphoid cell(s). Any or all cells of the lymphocytic and plasmacytic series.

Lymphoid follicle (germinal center, lymphocytopoietic nodule, secondary lymphoid follicle). A collection of proliferating pale-staining cells in lymphoid tissue such as the cortex of lymph nodes.

Lysosome. Membrane bound structure in the cytoplasm of cells that commonly contains large amounts of hydrolytic enzymes. Lysosomes often fuse with phagocytic or pinocytic vesicles to form phagolysosomes.

Mast cells (tissue mast cells, blood basophils). Two types of cells of different origin and morphology, but similar structural and functional chararcteristics, namely, large basophilic granules, cytophilia for P-K antibodies, and the capacity to store and release heparin and to act as mediators of inflammation on contact with antigen.

Memory cells. Cells that can mount an accelerated antibody response to antigen. They may consist of short-memory and long-memory types.

Natural antibodies. Antibodies that occur naturally without deliberate antigen stimulation. Some are known to arise as a result of natural exposure to antigen.

Oncogenic. Capable of causing normal cells to acquire neoplastic characteristics. The term is usually applied to viruses, such as adenoviruses.

Prausnitz-Küstner antibodies. Homocytotropic antibodies of the immunoglobulin class IgE that are responsible for cutaneous anaphylaxis. (Abbreviated P-K antibodies.)

Precipitin. An antibody that reacts specifically with soluble antigen to form a precipitate.

Ribosome. Cytoplasmic particles (usually about 150 Å in diameter) composed of ribonucleic acid and protein, which are considered to be the sites at which protein synthesis takes place. In fully differentiated cells of the pancreas or liver most of these particles are attached to membrane surfaces within the cytoplasm, but in embryonic tissues and many tumor cells the particles appear free in the cytoplasm.

Runt disease. Condition of dwarfing that follows the injection of mature allogeneic immunologically competent cells into immunologically immature recipients. Characterized by failure to thrive, lymph node atrophy, hepato- and splenomegaly, anemia, and diarrhea.

Second-set graft rejection. Accelerated rejection of a second graft due to immunity developed to a primary graft.

Sensitive. A state of increased capacity to respond specifically to an antigen or hapten.

Sensitize. The process of increasing the specific reactivity of a subject or cell to an agent. Commonly used to designate the process of increasing reactivity due to specific antibodies or "immune cells."

Sessile antibody. Antibody that is attached to tissues sufficiently firmly to resist removal by, for example, washing or perfusion.

Shwartzman reaction. A local nonimmunologic inflammatory reaction with hemorrhage and necrosis produced by the injection of bacterial endotoxin.

Syngeneic (isogeneic). Pertaining to genetically identical or nearly identical animals such as identical twins or highly inbred animals.

Syngraft (isograft). A graft derived from a syngeneic donor.

Univalent antibodies (functionally univalent antibodies, nonprecipitation antibodies, incomplete antibodies, blocking antibodies). Antibodies that behave as though they are functionally univalent and hence do not cause precipitation and agglutination in saline.

Vaccination. Injection or ingestion of an immunogenic antigen(s) for the purpose of producing active immunity.

Vaccine. A suspension of dead or living microorganisms that is injected or ingested for the purpose of producing active immunity. Solutions of antigens such as toxoids and pollen extracts are sometimes referred to as "vaccines."

Wheal-flare rection. A skin sensitivity reaction of the P-K type due to histamine, characterized by an edematous elevation and erythematous flare.

Xenocytophilic antibody (heterocytotropic antibody). An antibody produced by an individual of one species that possesses cytophilic properties for cells of another species. It may not be cytophilic for cells of the species of origin.

Xenogeneic (heterologous). Pertaining to individuals of different species.

Xenograft (heterograft). A graft derived from an animal of a different species than that of the one receiving the graft.

RECOMMENDED READING

Alexander, J. W., and Good, Robert A: *Immunobiology for Surgeons.* W. B. Saunders, Philadelphia, 1970.

Good, Robert A., and Fisher, David W.: *Immunobiology.* Sinauer Associates, Stanford, 1971.

Gordon, Benjamin Lee, II, and Ford, Denys K.: *Essentials of Immunology.* F. A. Davis, Philadelphia, 1971.

Halborrow, E. J.: *An ABC of Modern Immunology.* Little, Brown, Boston, 1973.

Harris, Jules E., and Sinkovics, J. G.: *The Immunology of Malignant Diseases.* C. V. Mosby, St. Louis, 1970.

Humphrey, John H., and White, R. G.: *Immunology for Students of Medicine,* 3rd Ed. F. A. Davis, Philadelphia, 1970.

Turk, J. L.: *Immunology in Clinical Medicine.* Appleton-Century-Crofts, New York, 1969.

Weir, D. M.: *Immunology for Undergraduates.* Williams and Wilkins, Baltimore, 1971.

Index

335